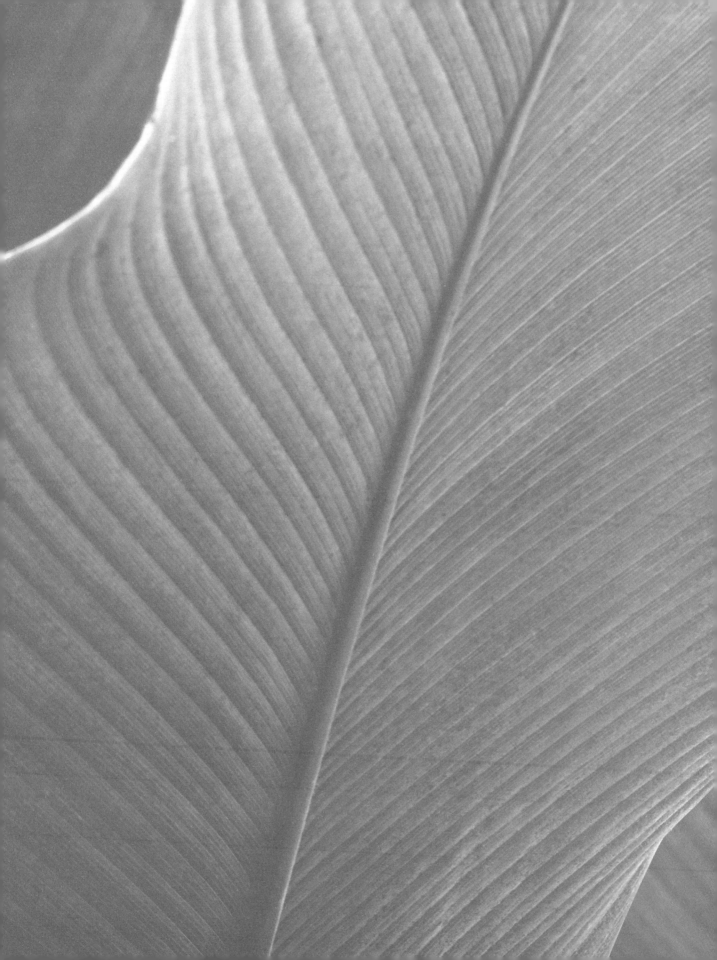

Nourish

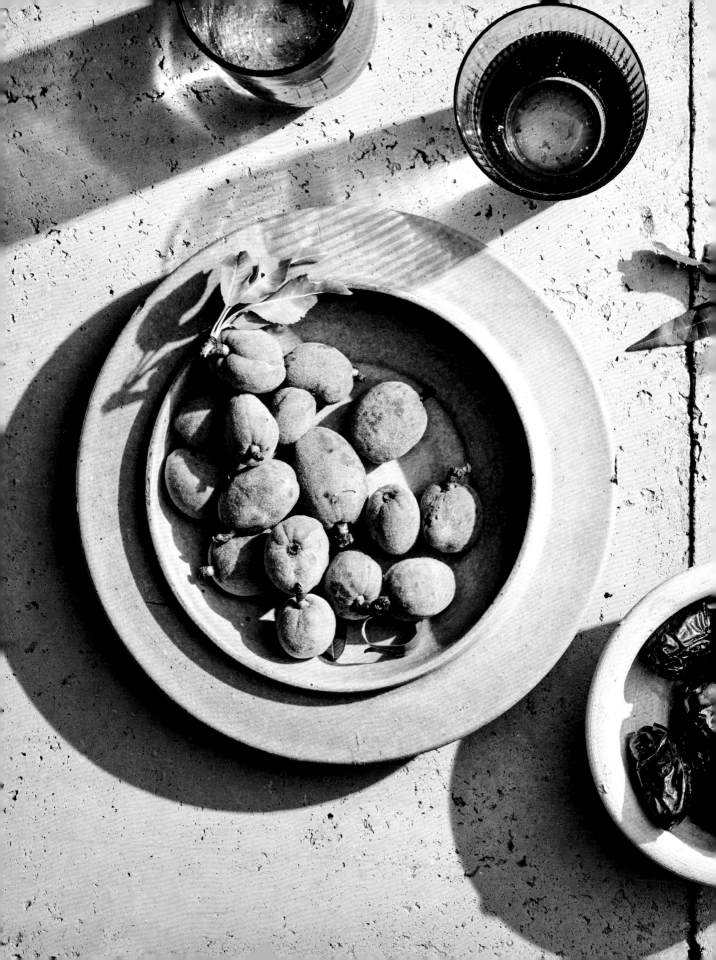

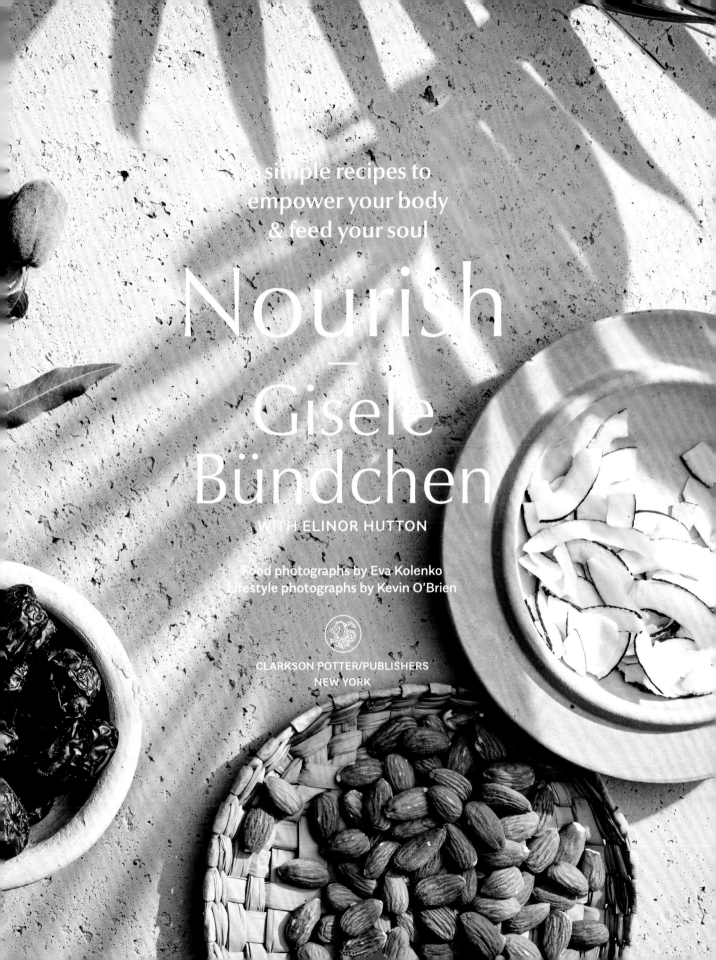

simple recipes to
empower your body
& feed your soul

Nourish

—

Gisele
Bündchen

WITH ELINOR HUTTON

Food photographs by Eva Kolenko
Lifestyle photographs by Kevin O'Brien

CLARKSON POTTER/PUBLISHERS
NEW YORK

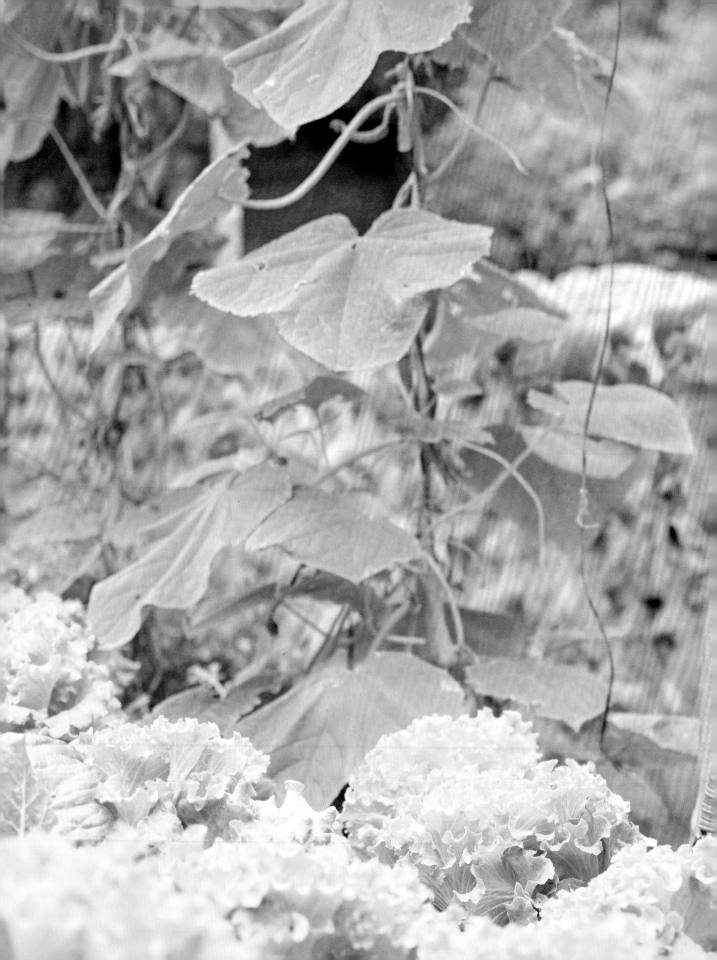

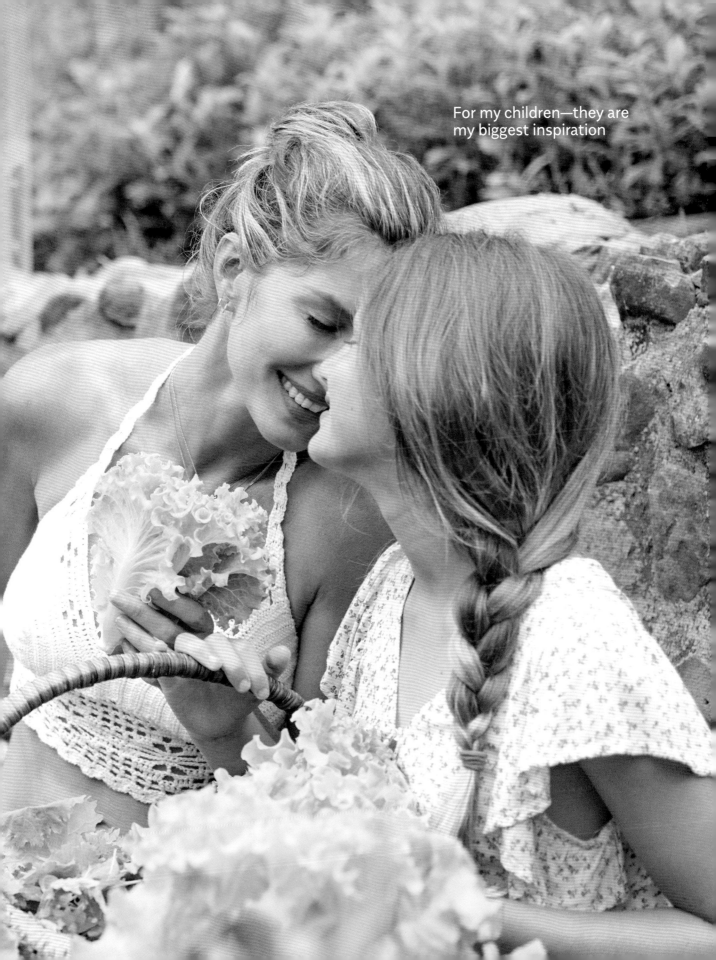

For my children—they are
my biggest inspiration

Contents

Everyday Vegetables

Favorite Proteins

Crunchies & Condiments

Sweets

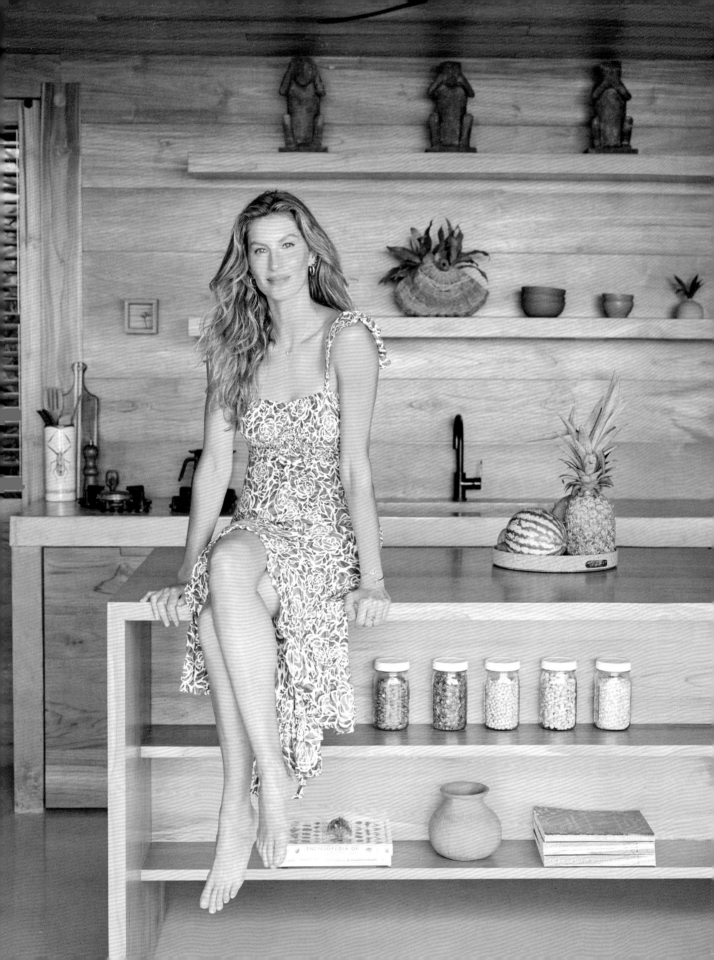

Introduction

Health is true wealth.
I have learned this the hard way.

My experiences have taught me that feeling good both mentally and physically is my greatest asset, because when life is difficult, it's my health that holds me up. Being strong is something I am proud of and work hard at, and what I eat and how I eat affects my quality of life and my health more than almost anything else I do. I find happiness, contentment, and wellness through food, and I take so much satisfaction and joy in treating my body kindly. Eating nutritious food nourishes my body and feeds my soul.

When it comes to the food I love most, I turn to simplicity. I want all the benefits of real, nutritious food with no fillers or fake stuff. I also don't want restrictions or complications from diets. Luckily, simple food—like fruits, vegetables, smoothies, occasional meat and fish—usually tastes best and is the easiest to prepare, too. Not to mention, it gives me joy. I don't just eat to satisfy my hunger or for instant gratification—though of course both are happy by-products. Most important, I've found that eating simply provides me with happiness, health, energy, and well-being. This plus good sleep and a daily exercise routine improves my bodily functions, from easy digestion to physical strength to a clear mind. Food is the fuel that drives us. Eating delicious, organic, natural foods and sharing meals with my family where we all feel fully nourished and cared for are deeply meaningful to me. It makes me feel whole.

In life, you reap what you sow. If you give love, you will receive love. And if you eat well and take control of what you choose to put in your body, you will feel strong, mentally resilient, and comfortable in your own skin. But it's a choice. It's up to you. The consequences are yours alone, good or bad. Taking responsibility for my health changed my life, and I'm grateful for the courage and discipline it took to get to this point. Today I feel stronger than I ever did before. It was a long road to get here, but I'm so happy that here is where I am. I surround myself with positive energy. I am loving to myself. I really believe that we become what we think and what we eat.

Here is my story,

Healing

Breaking a Cycle

To understand why I am how I am and why I eat what I eat, I need to explain how I got here. Realize that I had never expected or even dreamed of becoming a household name. I grew up in a small town in rural Brazil, a middle child in a family of six girls. My sisters and I were inseparable. Our family life was simple and loving. Our day-to-day meals were modest—tons of rice and beans and fresh produce—whereas our celebrations were always feasts centered on meat (which is the custom in the south of Brazil—and in Germany, where both sides of my family emigrated from in the late 1800s). My mother always had us helping her in the kitchen and with household chores every day; only after we finished those tasks were we allowed to go outside to play with friends until sundown. I felt so free! I have the best memories of my childhood.

By the time I was 13, I was very tall—taller than everyone else in my grade—and as a result I was incredibly self-conscious. I had terrible posture, always stooping to seem shorter than I was in an effort to fit in. To cure me of my constant stooping, my mom enrolled me and my sisters in a modeling course. While I was with that class, on a field trip to the mall, a scout spotted me and encouraged me to enter a modeling competition. That encounter changed the course of my life.

I came in second place in the modeling contest and went to Ibiza, Spain, for the world final. There I was signed by the Elite Modeling Agency. They told me that as soon as I finished the school year, I should move to São Paulo, Brazil, to share an apartment with some other girls (all models) and try to get cast in modeling jobs. So I did. I wasn't driven to become a model; I just did what was suggested—an opportunity presented itself, and I took it.

My parents helped me pack a suitcase—we filled it with my older sisters' hand-me-downs—and they dropped me off at the bus station in our town. Since I had never been to São Paulo by myself, my father gave me money to take a cab from the bus terminal to the apartment. But on the 24-hour bus ride to the city, I came up with a new plan: use that money to buy some better-fitting clothes so I could be better dressed for castings (all my pants were too short for me). The tradeoff was that I'd have to make my way to the apartment on my own. With the address written on a scrap of paper in my pocket, I dragged my suitcase onto one subway and then another. When I got to the right neighborhood, only then would I take a much cheaper cab to the apartment, and would end the day still having most of the money my parents gave me.

This would have been a great plan, except that I was a kid traveling alone for the first time, and without any big-city experience. I was naïve and had no idea that someone would steal my wallet out of my backpack. Without any money, ID, or any idea what to do next (this was before cellphones!), I sat down on my suitcase and cried. A woman walking by gave me a couple of coins, which I used to call the apartment, where the chaperone gave me directions for walking the remaining mile to the place. Sweaty, exhausted, and devastated, I finally arrived.

From that next day on, I went to castings all day, all around the city, sometimes ten in a row. Models were needed for television commercials, bridal magazines, catalogs, fashion shows—everything. I learned quickly how to deal with rejection. After all, I might stand in various lines for the entire day, going from one place to another with my book (a portfolio of my photos), and not get a single job. When I did get a booking, most paid the equivalent of $50, so I had to book a lot of jobs just to pay my part of the apartment rent to the agency.

Then a few months later, I was sent to Japan to do catalog work, which paid better. Most

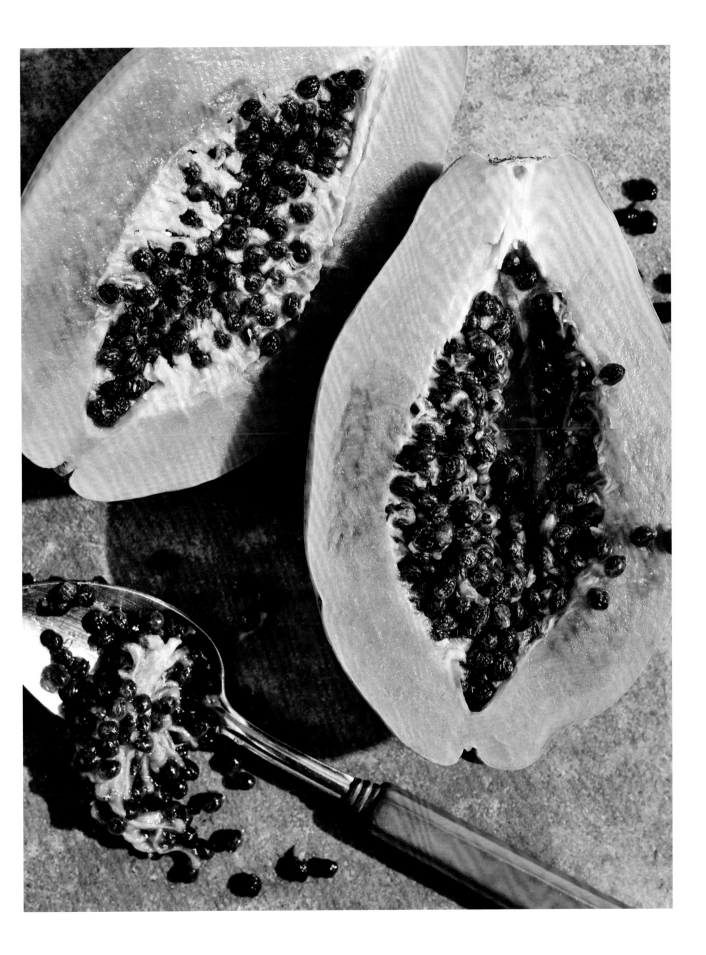

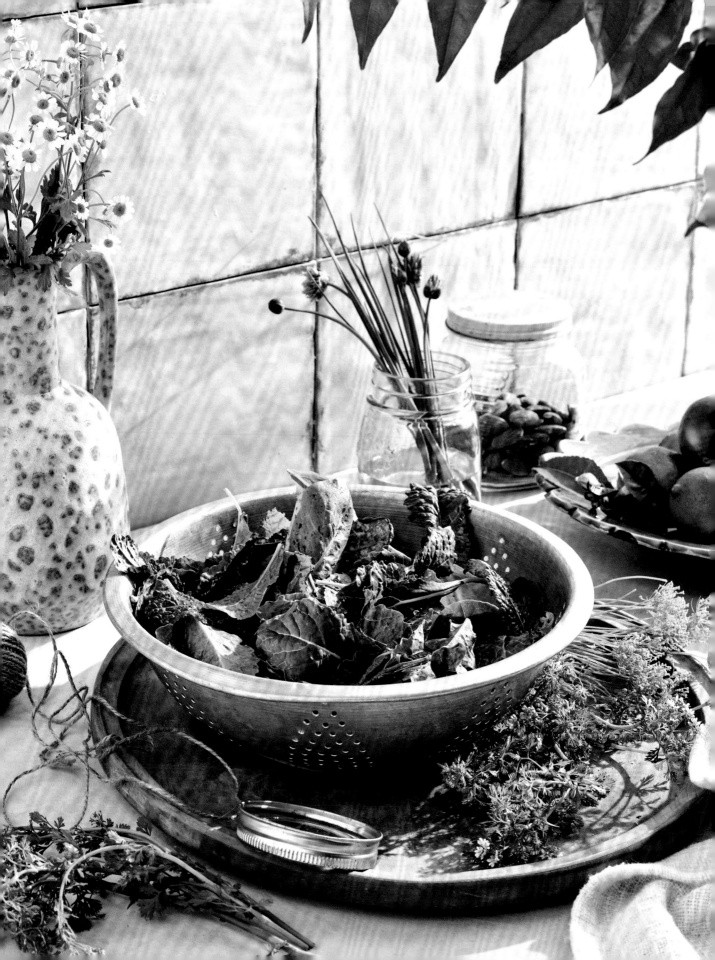

models I knew were cycled through Japan for a period of time, just to help pay their expenses. It was easier to find work there, as a driver from the agency would take everyone to the castings, which were all grouped in a particular part of town. I often booked two shoots a day, one from 6 a.m. to 1 p.m., and another from 2 p.m. to 7 p.m. While I never again lived in a place with a chaperone after the São Paulo stay, I was lucky in Japan to have been assigned a 16-year-old Brazilian roommate, as I couldn't speak any language other than Portuguese at that time. After three months there, I made enough money to pay back my living expenses to the agency and to send some money home to help my parents. It was then that I realized this modeling career might really be worth pursuing, and that I might be able to make something of it. It was hard work, and uncomfortable most of the time. But I could tell, even at that young age, that this was a once in-a-lifetime chance. The money was helping my family, and I had nothing to lose. I never lived at home with my sisters and parents again.

After the Japan trip, I moved back to São Paulo briefly, and then on to New York City. There, life was even more competitive. The fashion look in the '90s was "heroin chic," and I did not fit that picture. Life was a struggle; I could barely pay my rent and buy food. I was fully responsible for taking care of myself—doing my own cooking and laundry (all those chores my mom had us do paid off, big time), taking the subway, and through it all, attempting to communicate, almost always in places where I didn't speak the language. But somehow I got by. I worked a lot of showrooms, wearing clothes for designers before the show models arrived. But by the time I was 16, I started going to castings for fashion shows. Then in 1998, I walked in the Alexander McQueen show. That was a big shift in my career. I started doing multiple fashion shows in multiple countries each season. I walked the runways for all the big names: Chanel, Dior, Versace. I flew in hundreds of planes, zigzagging from Paris to London, to Milan, to New York City, and on and on. I felt I could never turn down a job, as money at home was still tight.

Then, in 1999, on my nineteenth birthday, *Vogue* declared the "The Return of the *Sexy* Model," with me on the cover. That same year, VH1 awarded me Model of the Year.

Despite all the work experience and street smarts I had acquired, I was still a girl: a bit socially naive and very trusting. My life was far from that of a regular teenage girl. For example, I never got to go to high school; instead, my education came from the school of life. I learned English by repeatedly listening to music on cassette tapes. I still struggled to understand what people were saying, but I'd never admit it. (This is when I started to learn about the language of energy; it's amazing how much can be said in this way.) Though I was doing well professionally, my self-esteem was low. I needed constant validation and approval. Perhaps this need came from not having my parents in my everyday life. Because it was so expensive and time-consuming to fly home from wherever I was living, I saw my family only once a year. I was lucky to have developed a few friends along the way, but everything I did revolved around work. Thinking about who I was becoming and what I wanted from life were never top of mind. Instead, I worried that one day my whole career would just disappear, as the industry was so fickle. I worked continuously and constantly. I was so happy to have been given a chance, but I was truly exhausted.

Plus, I was a people pleaser, and I was conditioned to never say no. After all, how could I do that when I had worked so hard to get here and was being given this big chance? I thought I was worthy of love only if I made everyone happy and comfortable, so I always put others' needs ahead of my own. I was scared to see some of my roommates doing drugs, but I didn't want to feel like an outsider, so that's when I started smoking cigarettes. On shoots, I would do anything—physically contorting myself, jumping and running in 6-inch heels all day, hoping that would result in better shots and make the photographers happy. Modeling is all about being in a silent movie, playing a role, facing outward. I was so caught up in this strange world that I nearly lost myself.

Of course, I didn't eat well. During show season, I barely slept, since the call times were so early (4 or 5 a.m.) and travel was so disruptive. A typical day: Breakfast was often my beloved mocha frappuccino and a cigarette. To get through the day (which could last upwards of 14 hours), I would drink more caffeine and eat whatever was on set—candy, pastries, you name it. When I needed a break from everyone's fussing with me (fixing my clothes and hair, touching up my makeup), I'd have a cigarette. (Ironically, cigarette breaks gave me a moment of peace, during which I had some space to breathe.) A real meal might come late at night, but it consisted of whatever was easy, like junk food or pizza, or my favorite, french fries. To wind down, I would drink red wine. Then the next day, the whole thing started again.

to take over my life, and soon I was unable to be in a closed space anywhere. My hands would get sweaty, and I would feel like I was going to faint. I was the picture of good health on the outside, but on the inside I felt like I was dying. Anxiety bloomed in all sorts of situations that I couldn't avoid, like simply being in a room where the windows couldn't be opened, or being in a tunnel or on an airplane. After a few months of trying to hide this anxiety from others, and especially from myself, I found myself one night on my apartment balcony in New York City. I was having trouble breathing, and I felt so desperate that I actually thought about jumping.

Everything stopped.

This feeling was something new, and totally surprising. I had never even thought of myself as in any danger from my feelings, despite the panic

Don't be afraid to be yourself

I told myself that my vices were a function of my lifestyle. Smoking helped me fit in and feel calm during high-intensity work and in social settings. Caffeine gave me energy, then alcohol soothed me and helped me relax at the end of the day. Food was comfort. I justified this lifestyle by seeing all around me how those vices could actually be much worse. I told myself that this pattern "worked" for me. Here I was, successful, at the top of my game. Like the headlines seemed to be saying at the time, I had it all. Right? *I have it all*, I told myself.

By now, I was 22. And one day, while I was in the elevator of my apartment building, I had a panic attack. I felt like the walls were closing in on me and my heart started racing. I got through the attack, but it started happening more and more often, and eventually I had panic attacks most days. I couldn't slow down my life, so I just worked around my issues. Avoiding elevators, I walked up and down the stairs everywhere I went. Then I had a panic attack on a plane. My anxiety began

attacks that left me feeling helpless. But here I was, contemplating ending everything. The anxiety and depression had wound their way so deep inside of me that I didn't realize how bad it had become. The weight of my deteriorating mental health, which I had been carrying around so "well," suddenly became very heavy.

Then one thought pushed through from deep inside of me, from a part of my subconscious that I had been ignoring: *I want to live*. That jolt of insight broke the moment. I didn't want to die, but I was not happy, and I was not at all okay. These realizations hit me, one after another; it was a flood of emotions and awareness. I had been holding so much in, in pursuit of this career and this life, and of making everyone happy, of having it "all" that I wasn't even aware of my own feelings. But there was that thought again, now stronger: *I want to live*.

I had repressed all the things I didn't know how to cope with. I was always very busy, and believed I should just be happy for my successes. I

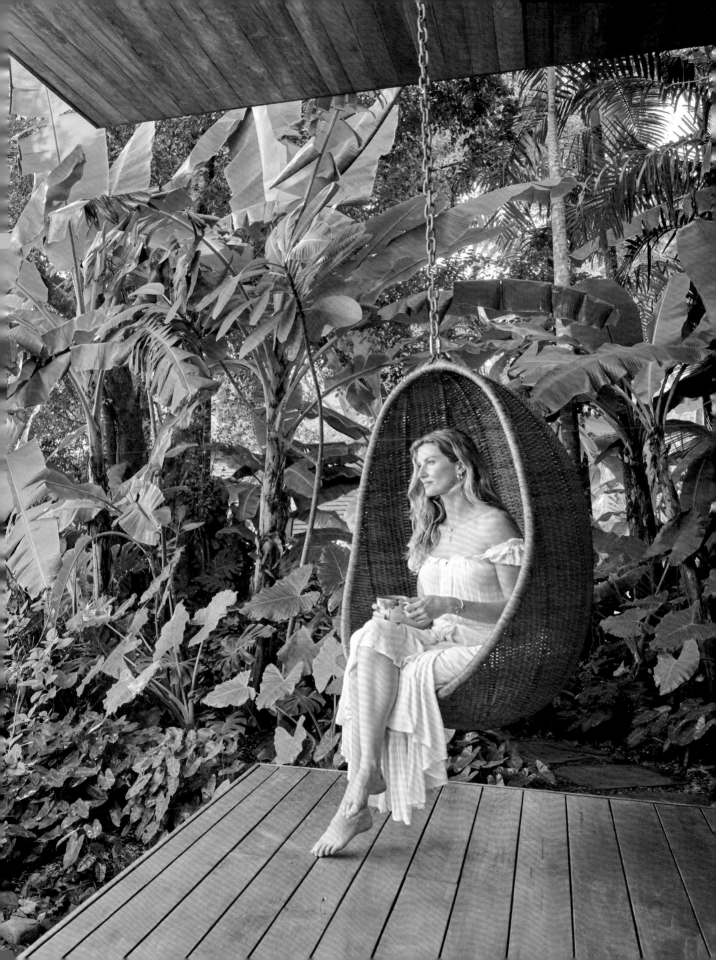

I am very grateful for all of the opportunities in my life. I have a great career and have been compensated well for working the last almost thirty years of my 43-year-old life! I travel a ton for jobs, and even when I am at home, my schedule is bananas. So, my family has had the benefit of working with various chefs over the years, who provided some consistency in the kitchen when I was unavailable. I am aware that this is not an option many people have—and I am so thankful for the help. Together, we have experimented with many different ways of eating and nourishing our bodies. I have brought my culture and ideas to these chefs, and they have showed me delicious recipes, surprising ingredients, and new techniques. They have been amazing teachers, and I am so grateful for all the nourishment they have given me and my family. Our health is also a testament to them!

could eat pizza and fries, and I could chain-smoke, and I could have minimal sleep, but still my career was going great, so why change things? Why stop? Those unconscious choices created the condition I found myself in.

There's a metaphor for my anxiety that really captures how I felt: an angry dog in the basement. Everyone has an angry dog—a hurt or vulnerability or unresolved trauma—and sometimes, instead of dealing with it, you put it in the basement. I didn't want to address those issues with anxiety and my fears; maybe I didn't even realize they were there. But the problem with putting an angry dog in the basement is that eventually it will come out biting. And that was how I felt that night on the balcony. That night, I opened the basement door and looked down at that very angry dog and I had to deal with it. It was scary and intimidating and overwhelming.

I felt like all of a sudden I didn't know myself. That all these years, while I had been trying to please everyone around me, I had been ignoring myself. I had allowed anxiety and depression to consume me, and I wasn't even aware of it.

I met with many doctors, who ran all sorts of tests. In the end, they all offered depression and anxiety medication, but, for me, taking those pills didn't feel right. Back in Brazil, when I was a child, my grandmother had a garden and she used to mix up all sorts of teas and natural remedies for everyone who needed them. People would come from all over the neighborhood, seeking her help. She always had something that would make them feel better. So, I've always preferred natural solutions whenever possible. I hoped there was an alternative to those prescriptions.

I eventually met with an osteopath, Dr. Dominique. He wasted no time; my anxiety and depression were crippling me. I was burnt out. My adrenal glands—which control the production and distribution of various hormones—were fatigued to the point that he called me "Adrenalina." He said he had never seen a person so young with such burned-out adrenal glands as mine. Critically, he had ideas that did not require medication but that could make a big difference: radically changing my diet, adding certain supplements and vitamins, and altering my lifestyle. His first suggestion was an extreme one: cut out caffeine, nicotine, all sugars, alcohol, and gluten. Essentially, I needed to reboot my body.

I balked. Giving up these items sounded impossible, not to mention unpleasant! While I never thought of myself as addicted to these things, my cigarettes and coffees and late-night pizzas and wine gave me comfort, as well as all sorts of other benefits. I wasn't sure I could do what he asked of me and still lead my life. He said a diet and lifestyle change would strip away all these crutches and give my body a chance to reset and heal. He explained that it takes three months to establish a new habit, so that was how long I would need to be on this path to wellness. Only then could we re-evaluate my health. I pushed back, thinking that there must be another way to solve this problem—one that was less extreme.

But then he asked me simply: "Do you want to live?"

And I said, "Yes, I want to live."

Resetting

I'm not going to lie. This new regime was difficult. Not only was I giving up refined sugar, but also any food that turns into sugar or creates inflammation in the body, like carbs, desserts, and alcohol.

Going cold turkey on caffeine and nicotine was also challenging. In the first couple of weeks I had crushing migraines. In fact, this reset was the hardest thing I had ever done in my life. The process made me question my choices and my concessions. *Why was I not taking better care of myself? Why was I not happy anymore? What has gone wrong?* I felt like I had to knock my life down to the studs and build myself back up again. I was unsure of what the results would be, and I wondered if I would have the discipline and strength to follow through. Nevertheless, I threw myself into it completely because, ultimately, I wanted my life back! I wanted to feel happy again.

But to my surprise, I did not get my old life back. I got a whole new life instead. A better one. A healthier one.

Three months later, my doctor said I could move on. I had successfully established new habits and, truthfully, gained a new lifestyle. My anxiety quieted down. My depression lifted. I felt more in control, more present. I felt as if the cells in my body had shifted, too. I noticed an increase in energy and a greater ease in how my body moved and functioned. Our mind can play tricks on us, ignoring some things and overemphasizing others, but the body doesn't lie. My body was so much happier. And my mind followed suit.

After all the turmoil and soul searching, and all the restrictions, I had changed. I felt like a new person. Before I began this experience, I hadn't felt connected to my inner thoughts and feelings; I had manipulated my body and my mind to fit others' expectations. I had conditioned myself to put others' needs before my own. Now, I saw I could break those patterns. Now, I treasured self-reflection and self-love. I started to identify those times when I didn't want to do something, and little by little it became easier to say no. I strived to put my needs and my feelings first. I pursued

RESET REGIME

When my anxiety and depression had reached a breaking point, my osteopath prescribed a diet that I was to follow for three months. It was designed to be anti-inflammatory and easy to digest—but that didn't make it any easier to follow. It was very restrictive! But I do credit that diet with changing my lifestyle for the better. Even today, about twenty years later, I still feel its effects. I am so grateful for the health and clarity that this reset gave me, and the path it set me upon. If you have similar issues, talk to your doctor or nutritionist before starting any new regime.

Approved Foods

High-quality fats, like extra-virgin olive oil and ghee

Nuts (all except peanuts, which are inflammatory) • I was instructed to soak almonds and walnuts for easier digestion (and remove the skins of almonds), which I still do today.

Green vegetables • Leafy, soft, hard, raw, and cooked—I ate them all. Vegetables of other colors were not allowed.

One daily portion of lean animal protein • my favorites were chicken, beef, duck, fish, and eggs.

Broth • I sipped broth often as a beverage and used it to make simple soups, adding some shredded vegetables or chicken depending on what was in my fridge.

Herbal teas

Popcorn • I think my doctor let me have popcorn just to be nice!

Restricted foods

Carbohydrates/grains	**Sugar** • processed sugar as well as natural sugars
Beans/legumes	
Dairy products	**Caffeine**
Fruits	
Non-green vegetables	**Alcohol**

health as my priority, determined to find calmness and clarity, above all.

My experience in addressing my anxiety proved how important those everyday decisions about what to eat and drink were to my physical and mental health. That gave me new insight into the true value of food. I now understood the meaning of "Let thy food be thy medicine."

I am forever grateful for this experience, which opened my eyes to a new way of eating and, ultimately, of living. Instead of running endlessly on the hamster wheel, I realized that being conscious and deliberate about the choices in my life had a long-term effect.

But I felt I couldn't—and didn't want—to sustain a restrictive diet forever. I love food. I love sharing a meal with friends and family. So, I had to find a middle ground—one where I would have my mental health, but also be able to eat more than green veggies, nuts, and the occasional animal protein. For example, I knew it was both unrealistic and unappealing to never eat any kind of sugar, including the natural sugars resulting from the digestion of whole grains, fruits, and more colorful vegetables. So, I started to reintroduce certain foods back into my diet. For instance, after three months going without any, nothing tasted as good as fruit. The first mango I ate—wow! It was pure joy, so sweet and simple. Dates were caramelly, sticky. An avocado tasted creamier than ever before. Most of all, I enjoyed eating a wider variety of foods again. I carefully monitored my reactions, and became fascinated with the whats, hows, and whys of nutrition, as well as my body's reactions.

It was during this slow reintroduction of certain foods that my birthday arrived; I hadn't had any sweets yet! Friends had gotten me a cake on set—I didn't want to be rude and refuse it. Plus, I was feeling confident; I felt so good! But the effect of that sugar on my newly reset body was profound. The cake was so sweet that it gave me a terrible migraine. Rather than a disappointment, though, this was a revelation. And instead of being sad that I couldn't eat something I used to love so

much, I was amazed that my body had sent out a message so clearly. Refined sugar (like white sugar, not the natural sugar found in fruit) does not agree with me, and this was the proof. If I wanted to feel good, I needed to be conscientious about what I ate. My body was just reminding me of this, but now I was listening.

Not only did I want to be mindful of what I added back into my diet, and how those foods affected my health and well being, but I also started to pay attention to how my body processed food. I knew that fruits and other carbs eventually are turned into sugar, so I learned how best to consume them so my body can get the most from them. For instance, eating fruit by itself was one such solution. Fruit is digested differently if it is consumed alone, rather than when mixed with other foods, like veggies or animal proteins. If a mango is in your stomach with some harder-to-digest foods—say, meat or vegetables—it will not pass through your system and digest as fast, and then it will start to ferment, making you feel bloated. But a mango eaten on its own is digested in much less time, and with much less work for your body. These were the sort of insights I loved discovering. Finding ways to eat consciously and deliberately made everything feel more nourishing. Streamlining my digestion also gave me more energy and clarity.

Bringing Mind and Body Together

I started asking bigger questions of myself. Like a frog in the well who sees only the life right above his head, I now felt like I had climbed out of the well and realized my little patch of sky was just a tiny piece of the whole.

Striving toward greater consciousness became my constant desire. I made the effort to listen to myself. My intention was to always be unpeeling the layers, liberating my true self. I constantly asked, *What really is my truth? What am I living for?*

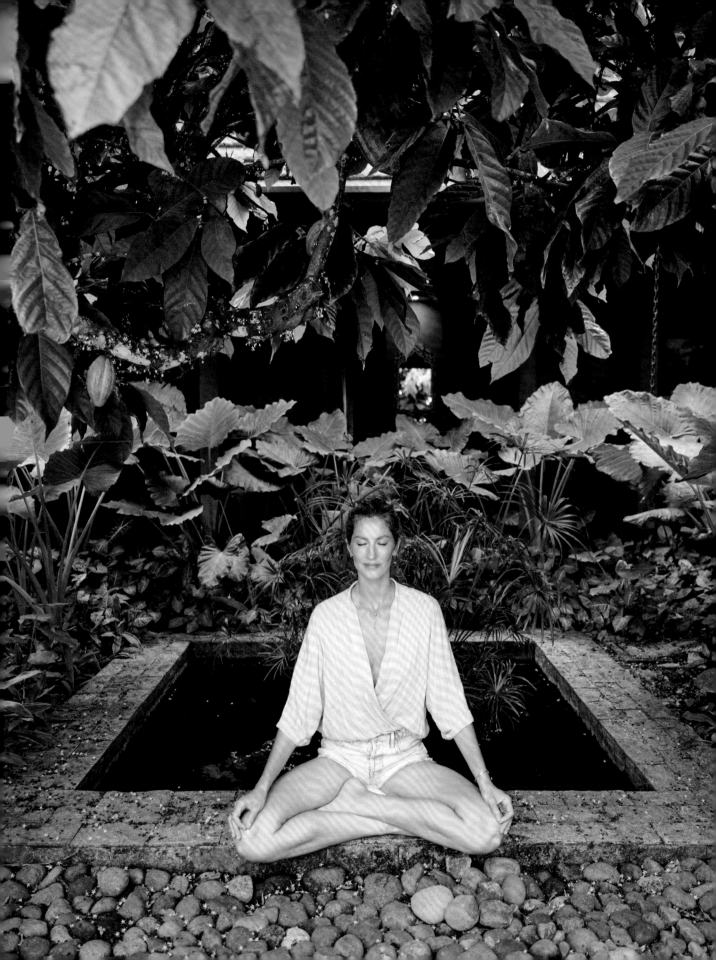

Ultimately, I wanted to be happy. And how could I be happy if I wasn't myself? Diving deeper within and getting to know myself became my priority.

I began praying every night, just like my grandmother had taught me. In my early modeling days, I was often not able to converse with anyone because of the language barrier so praying and writing in a diary before bed was my way to reflect. But I had fallen out of that habit. I started again and it gave me strength and clarity.

One night, I prayed for a long time. A message—that's the only way I can describe it—came to me to start doing yoga. So strange! I was barely familiar with yoga, and I had never practiced it. Yoga wasn't as popular then, in the early 2000s in the United States. I met with a yoga teacher, and after talking with her about my need to lessen my anxiety, calm my mind, and

work, and meditation all helped me create a new structure for my day. And after a few months, I was able to relax faster and felt more in touch with my body—and more connected to myself.

Blessing my food became a part of my new life, too. When I sat down, I would float my hands above the plate. I'd take three deep breaths, connecting and feeling gratitude for what I was about to eat. It reminded me of Reiki, a Japanese form of energy healing in which energy flows between a practitioner's hands and your body. I could feel that kind of energy exchange with my food. Giving this blessing at each meal also felt intentional. I used to eat on the go, consuming food without thinking, distracted by other things. Pausing right before I begin to eat gives me a moment of deep gratitude and quiet. I feel more connected and more conscientious about what

The strength that you build within will last forever

breathe calmly again, she suggested Hatha yoga. She also came up with a routine for me: 15 minutes of breath work, 15 minutes of meditation, then 30 minutes of asanas (moving yoga). I tried it—and it helped me so much! So I committed to it every day. Like prayer, yoga gave me peace and a way to connect with myself. Though my exact sequence has changed some in the last twenty years (now I do asanas first, as I find the movement helps my body and mind to relax so I can settle into meditation easier), I still do a variation on what she taught me to do almost every morning.

This yoga practice also provided a new routine for me. Instead of having that morning cigarette and coffee, I now woke up early to go on a walk or run, then do my yoga routine. Instead of winding down with a glass (or bottle) of wine at the end of a long day, I took a walk or meditated. I was removing habits from my life that weren't serving me and replacing them with habits that supported my feeling my best. Yoga, breath

I've chosen to put in my body. It makes me more aware of the nutrients I am about to consume, which will fuel me and keep me nourished and healthy. Food is a gift I give myself, to help me function at my best. So, blessing my meals helps me reinforce that gift.

All these new experiences, new lessons, and positive changes made me feel I was now on a new wavelength. When you're constantly being stimulated—whether by people, work, or just rushing about—it is hard to find stillness and silence. But with a new ability to create silence in my mind, I found joy again. I was calmer and life was slower, there wasn't as much pressure, not as much rushing. Doing things mindfully makes them feel more special. It makes the ordinary feel extraordinary. In short, bringing my full attention to eating, breathing, and moving my body made it all meaningful, as well as joyful. It made me realize how life is sacred.

Finding My Food Path

In the years following these experiences, I continued to adjust my eating habits in an ongoing quest to optimize my health, while balancing my desire to eat delicious food and enjoy life. I'm a curious person, and I love going deep with whatever I am thinking about. I am grateful to have worked with various chefs, who have exposed me to new practices and ideas about food. How I eat and what I eat are the result of constant experimenting and learning what feels best to me—a path I will always be on. Not every new eating plan that I tried worked well for my body, but I learned a lot from all of my experiences.

I was vegan and/or vegetarian for a couple of years. Animals have always been a huge part of my life. My dogs, cats, horses, and chickens are my family. Before modeling, I even considered becoming a veterinarian. I loved the idea of aligning this passion with what I ate (or didn't eat).

Being vegan and vegetarian closely aligned with the food I now love best: vegetables and fruits. But no matter how many lentils, dark leafy greens, nuts, and seeds I ate, I became anemic. Iron supplements didn't help. I was tired and had no energy. All this was alleviated easily if I ate a little red meat, even just a couple times a month. Also, relying on legumes almost exclusively for protein meant I ate so many beans that it affected my digestion. Being gassy and bloated is not fun, of course, and it's not ideal for a job where I often wear bikinis or lingerie! What I learned from this experience is that while I couldn't commit to being a vegan or vegetarian, I could apply what I learned in a piecemeal way. For example, I was introduced to, and now crave, plant-based milks like coconut and almond milk (see recipes for these and others on pages 68–72); I digest them much easier than conventional dairy milk. I also conceptualize meals differently now. Instead of the conventional meat-starch-vegetable combination that dominates many Western meals, I started thinking about a meal based on the produce, not the protein.

The lesson here—of wanting to be vegan or vegetarian, but not physically able to—was humbling. It taught me to be flexible, listen to my body, and do what felt best for it, even if that wasn't what I wanted at first. This approach might have felt half-assed to me at another time, when I was less mature, but now I knew the benefits of paying attention to one's body. In that way, not being vegan or vegetarian felt like being attuned

CAFFEINE

My relationship with caffeine has taken many twists and turns. I gave it up cold turkey for three months, after my anxiety had peaked and I began my doctor-ordered reset. But I came back to it gradually. Caffeine tends to make me agitated, but I have often relied on it to help me wake up, especially when I had to travel so much and work in different time zones.

When I was training for a half-Ironman race, waking up at 4:30 a.m. to bike for two hours, I returned to drinking coffee. I made myself just one coffee with fresh hemp milk and foam—very moderate, and so delicious. But it was a Band-Aid. While I was able to get through the workout, I just didn't feel right. I was a bit shaky (not just from the physical exercise) and not feeling grounded.

Because I have struggled with anxiety in the past, feeling jittery can be a trigger, sending me in an uneasy direction that could stay with me all day. So, my friend who was training with me had a great idea to skip the coffee and replace it with one of my favorite foods, dates. I stuffed a few dates with almonds and kept them in my pocket while I biked, nibbling on one every few miles. While of course the dates didn't wake me up like coffee does, they did provide boosts of energy, and I preferred that. It wasn't the same, but it was good enough. Similarly, if I want to feel calm, I try to point my actions toward achieving that calmness. I have to allow myself to feel what I am feeling and evaluate what works best for me at the time. The path or result isn't always consistent, but my listening to the effect is.

These days, I don't drink any coffee. I found a dandelion tea that is caffeine free, which serves as a great replacement (see page 48). It tastes delicious and it doesn't leave me feeling jittery. I love it!

to my needs. And I found enjoyment in forging my own path.

At least 80 percent of my diet is still plant based. Eating a small amount of animal protein gave me the energy and nutrients my body required and was a much easier and more efficient way to ingest the iron I needed than from exclusively vegetarian whole-food alternatives. I now eat meat usually only once or twice a week. I am also committed to being as responsible a meat eater as I can be, so I always try to buy from small producers who treat their animals ethically.

For a while, I tried a raw-food diet. There was something appealing about how clean eating raw feels, similar to how it feels to do a juice cleanse. I started to see my body as an engine, and eating raw felt like feeding my body the best, purest fuel. When I was eating raw, I focused on the source of my vegetables and fruits in a way I had never done before. Eating organic and non-GMO produce became a focus, and I really felt and tasted the difference, as if the fruits and veggies were more alive. The producers at the farmer's market make tremendous efforts to use natural fertilizers to grow their crops and compost their scraps, creating soil that is incredibly fertile. That super soil then feeds more nutrients into the plants, producing fruits and vegetables that are more delicious and nutritious.

Giving my body this density of nutrients not only felt great physically but also appealed to me from an environmental point of view. I could support my local farmers and avoid food that had been shipped from all ends of the earth. It was so inspiring that I started a little garden of my own to supplement my shopping. I still have a garden today, and my kids and I love picking the veggies and eating some of them on the spot. Growing our own food also encourages my kids to try a wider variety of produce.

Through my experience with raw diets, I also grew to like the taste and texture of uncooked vegetables. Now, I keep a ton of prepped raw carrots, cucumbers, celery, radishes, and more in my fridge. My kids will plow through a whole plate of these in the minutes before dinner. And

ALCOHOL

While my drinking patterns were never dangerous or abusive, I wasn't always at peace about alcohol. Before my healing journey began, I was drinking most nights. After taking three months off to heal, I drank much more moderately and mostly in social settings. If I went to a party, I'd have a drink to be a part of things and to loosen up. But the next day I would inevitably feel foggy and get a headache. This made it hard to wake up early and be able to go through my morning routine of breath work, yoga, and exercise.

In thinking about why I was doing that to myself, I realized that my drinking was a crutch; it served to make awkward situations bearable. Often I was in a place I didn't want to be in, or I was otherwise uncomfortable, but the alcohol helped to numb my feelings. Finally becoming honest with myself made it easier to let it go. I needed healthy boundaries regarding the people I spent time with, as well as the things I did with my time. And I wanted to keep my promises to myself to start each day strong.

I still am learning to say no and to prioritize my needs and comfort. Once I analyzed why I was drinking and the physical results and lack of motivation that came of that, I found I didn't really need or want the drinks anymore. I stopped completely over two years ago; it feels great.

blending raw cashews, a pillar of raw dieting, yields one of my favorite sauces (see Ginger-Cashew Sauce, page 223), a Creamy Cauliflower Soup (page 131), and a frozen Banana Dream Pie (page 247).

However, the raw diet didn't work for me in its entirety, because I was freezing cold all the time. No matter how much I exercised, how much tea I drank, or what clothes I wore, I could not stay warm. It was as if processing all those raw vegetables left my body with no energy remaining to heat myself. But I will forever grow produce and buy the highest-quality vegetables and fruits. I cook my vegetables less too, thereby retaining more nutrients; besides, I now prefer a little crunch (but no more raw broccoli, please!). Everything is an opportunity for learning and growth.

I discovered juicing and having juice fasts during this time, as well. Detoxing with fruit and vegetable juices a few times a year was good for my body, as well as my mind. Before I had children, I would do juice cleanses for up to five days, sometimes in silence. After the kids came, I juiced whenever my body needed a reset, like after traveling or as a happy ritual on the equinox or solstice. Juice detoxes always left me feeling rejuvenated, especially when combined with meditation, dry-brushing my skin, and breath work. While temporarily challenging, the positive effects on my bodily functions and the clarity of mind were real. But doing a cleanse requires attention and commitment, neither of which I always feel able or willing to undertake, so I have had to adapt.

In the last year or two, I've done fewer juice cleanses, and for now (at least) it's not a part of my life. Instead, I have been experimenting with replacing a single meal with a smoothie (see page 39), a practice I learned from my friends the Valente brothers, while keeping the rest of my normal diet. As a mother, I found it hard to put aside a few days for a juice fast. And as someone who works a lot, I found it difficult to fit the fast into my schedule, as much as I wanted to prioritize my health. Instead of the rigidity of needing to pause for a few days, I prefer the ease of simply making a smoothie for myself for breakfast, lunch, or dinner. Plus, today, smoothies feel more gentle, mentally and physically, than a juice cleanse. I know the only constant in my life is change, so I won't make any promises about the future. But I feel great now, drinking these smoothies.

Experimenting with all these different ways of eating helped me find *my* way. A good meal is one of the pleasures of life, something I really, really

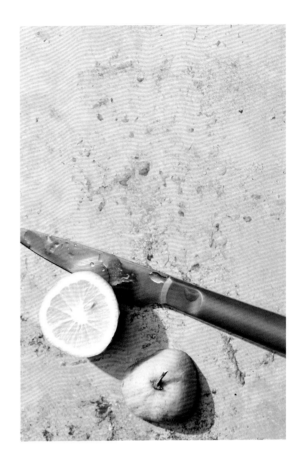

enjoy. It didn't feel like me to reject foods just because they weren't "allowed." I needed to find balance and my own flow. My path was not always straight, but the zigging and zagging were part of the process and gave me valuable insight.

The most important thing I learned from this time is that I still have so much to learn! We are all so different from each other, and our own bodies age and evolve, too. What makes me feel good today might be different from what makes me feel good tomorrow. Change is constant: life changes, circumstances change, physical needs change, emotional needs change. But what is unchanged are curiosity and the desire to feel good—they both drive me. I now try to always be listening, learning, and adjusting. Healing is a process.

With discipline comes freedom

How I Eat Today

A Balanced Lifestyle, Not a Diet

To arrive at how I eat today, I had to reconfigure my outlook on instant gratification. I had to start listening to what my body needed, not just what it wanted because of what it was used to. I used to be on a roller-coaster, living with the daily effects of the foods and drinks I consumed. If I wanted a frappuccino, I had one and dealt with the repercussions later—a sugar and caffeine high, then a crash, a headache soothed by a cigarette. And it would progress from there. As I've described, the effects eventually got more serious, affecting my physical and mental health. It was a cycle, and I was conditioned by social pressure, by media, and by society to think it was normal. Everyone I knew ate this food, drank these drinks, did this to their bodies, so it had to be okay, right? I didn't see the pattern of my everyday choices or its repercussions. I saw only my immediate wants and how to satisfy them.

In the process of learning about nutrition and making changes for my health, I tried many diets. But diets were rigid, and I wanted choice and flexibility—something that would work for my lifestyle, tastes, and body. To find a solution that was sustainable, I realized that I needed something bigger than a simple fix: an attitude change. Instead of thinking about what food I needed to stop eating, I started to reframe eating three times a day as an opportunity to choose wholesome, healthy foods that made my body feel as good as possible.

Adding intention here really changed how it felt to pursue my health. Instead of following a diet or list of rules, I listened to my body with health as my priority—and found joy in giving myself this care and attention. The way I eat now is a lifestyle. I think about why I'm eating, as well as what I'm eating, making sure it is what is truly best for me. Only then could I tune into my body

and respond accordingly. For the last twenty years, I have stuck with this goal—health above all—even as the details changed and life evolved. This long view helped me reframe the way I think about and consume food. I continue to define and redefine what makes me feel at my best.

Now, when I eat a perfectly ripe peach or a pile of blanched green beans, I appreciate them for both their taste and their impact on my health. Since the food I eat affects my bodily systems, my energy, and my mental health, it also determines how I feel and what I am capable of achieving. Rather than giving in to impulse and to riding the highs and lows, I appreciate how my body feels when I eat well, and I make choices to achieve that as often as possible.

I've been experimenting with the effects of different foods on my physical and mental health for more than twenty years. I want to feel the pleasure of eating great food *and* I want my body to feel at its best. For me, peace and contentment come when I am aligned physically and mentally.

I love to eat nutritionally dense foods. This ends up being mostly plants, and specifically lots of the best-quality vegetables and fruits. People make a distinction between food that is "good for you," meaning nutritious, and food that is "good," meaning delicious. As if you cannot have both! I don't want to choose between nutritious and delicious. Something that tastes good but makes my body react badly doesn't work for me. It is so empowering to eat food that makes my body feel so good. It's a loving act to myself. Each time I eat, I have the opportunity to add a constructive thing to my life, to feel good. I am so grateful that I can give that to myself every day.

But let's be real here—what about truffle fries? Baguettes with French butter? Gelato? Or any other foods I crave while eating out, while on vacation, and on special occasions? Don't get me wrong; these exceptions still happen occasionally, especially when I am traveling or am with family

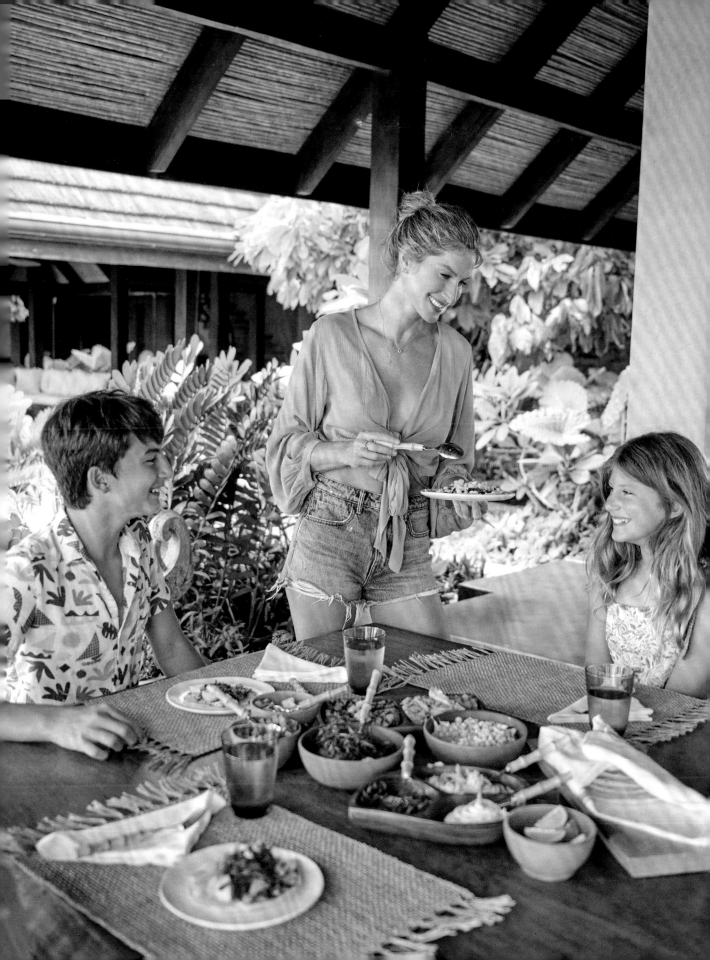

and friends. While these foods don't all nourish me in the same way as fruits and vegetables do, they do provide joy or inclusion, and that is important, too. So, I still have them when I feel like it. But listening to and knowing my body is key! I now know ahead of time what effect I may feel and I can take that into consideration. For example, while I know that refined sugar will make me feel awful the next day, I still sometimes have it. I'm human! But I take steps to minimize the effects. First, I eat it separately from other meals, which will ease digestion (I find afternoons the best time, not directly following a meal or at night). Second, the rest of the day I am sure to eat other nutrient-dense foods that fully support my health goals. And third, I actively try to find satisfying treats that are made of more gut-friendly ingredients. As I mentioned before, flexibility is key. Never say never—life is too short. I've found that when I eat mostly nutritious food, then eating something like a dessert or gluten once in a while doesn't have a negative impact on my overall long-term health—as long as I continue to listen to my body and achieve balance accordingly.

That said, I refuse to eat junk food. Period. No McDonald's or shelf-stable cupcakes or candy for me. My body is my temple, and my temple is sacred. Eating that sort of processed food is not being loving to myself. Better options exist when I want a treat: a Baru Nut Bar (page 233), Buttered Popcorn (page 217), or a Pecan Bar (page 234). These are made from real ingredients; they are not only better for me but taste better too.

To me, this means I'm not giving up anything; instead, I'm making a choice to feel good. After what I have been through healthwise, rejecting junk food is no longer difficult. But it is a choice. It's a priority you have to set and a commitment you have to stick with, numerous times a day.

EVERYDAY CHOICES, EVERYDAY IMPACT

Embrace flexibility · I love having a smoothie every day, but when I am traveling, I eat plain fruit instead—plus, I can try local varieties.

Consider your options · Change your mindset from focusing on avoiding processed foods and instead explore all the delicious healthful food that exists. To start, there's a whole rainbow of produce in the world; try something new and have fun!

Listen to your body · Sometimes a craving is a need in disguise. When my body tells me to eat red meat, it's often because I need more iron.

Opt for nutritionally dense foods · Simple foods—roasted veggies, soups, salads—are widely available and contain tons of nutrition. Even sweets can be nutritious (see pages 55–57).

Exceptions still happen · I can't resist a carrot cake—what can I say? Make your choices easier on your body by considering when you eat; the afternoon is best for sweets, so you're not processing them with another meal in your system.

Listening to your body is important, but your body does send all sorts of messages, including cravings, moments of nostalgia, and impulses. It's up to you to strive to make positive decisions. Remember: this way of eating is not a diet, it is a lifestyle; and it's up to you.

While at home, it's easier to eat organic, nourishing food, so that is what I do: fruits, salads and soups, vegetables of all kinds, the occasional meat or fish. If I want something sweet, I usually choose a more nutrient-dense version, like a homemade fruit ice pop (see page 62) or my

Find the things that are best for you and stay true to them

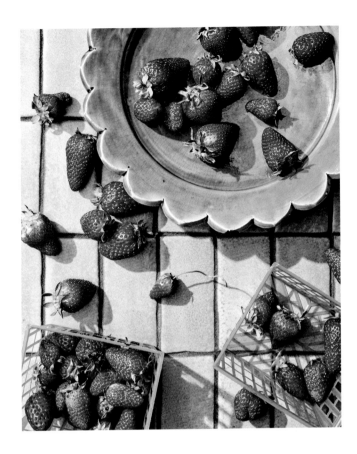

well-being without making it the subject of every meal or feeling like I am missing out. I enjoy food too much to stress about it!

My goal is to find balance, *always*. Food is the fuel that gives me energy and health, and my choices prioritize that. I want goals that I can manage, that make me feel capable and accomplished, not goals that are so difficult they place me in a position to not meet them. I love knowing what to do to encourage my well-being, and then doing it! You get only one body in this life. I want to surf and ride horses with my kids; I want to live without pain and anxiety. I want to be strong in mind and body and make choices that help me feel my best for as long as I live.

Getting into Specifics:
Organic, non-GMO, Local, Seasonal, Ethical

This is likely clear by now: I care a lot about what food I eat. And it's so important to me that the food I eat and serve my family has the highest value. Meaning it offers the most antioxidants, healthy fats, vitamins, and minerals, and that it will be digested easily so our bodies can unlock and access these nutrients.

The reason I insist on organic food is simple: it's better. Why? Because it's usually the freshest you can find. Since it hasn't been sprayed with toxic pesticides and other chemicals, the produce doesn't last as long in a box, on a truck, or on a shelf. Additionally, those toxic chemicals used to ward off pests and extend shelf life can be ingested and have negative effects on your health. Plus, the toxic pesticides deplete the soil that plants grow in, as well as the wider environment and ecosystem. If the soil is depleted, it can't grow nutrient-rich foods.

If I'm eating an arugula salad with roasted vegetables, I want the nutritional benefits of an arugula salad and vegetables—that's the whole idea. Those vegetables and fruits need to be organic so they can be brimming with all their natural benefits. All of that said, eating a wide

favorite dates. In addition to being delicious, these sweets are whole foods, so they satisfy my body more than white flour and refined sugar—plus I don't feel sluggish afterwards.

When traveling, I have less control over my food options. I always do my best to choose the most nourishing foods available—often the simplest dishes have the best ingredients. I bring my own food when possible and convenient, especially when I know I won't have many options, like on an airplane. At a friend's house, my desire to be polite and respectful is my priority. I try everything and am grateful that someone has cooked for me. Sometimes eating smaller portions lets me be involved without going overboard. Going out to eat with friends is similar—I always like to relax and enjoy the experience. Even when the meals are not my ideal, I am thankful for the food and care that I am receiving. One off-track meal is not going to destroy my progress, and I can make a special effort to eat especially nutritious food for the next few meals. I can still focus on my

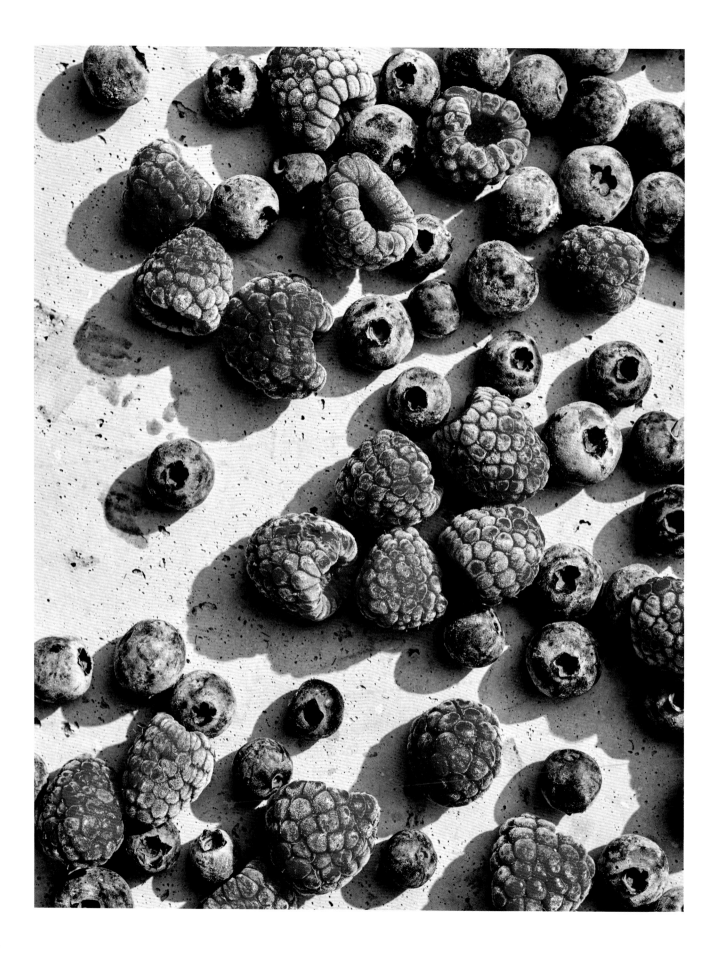

variety of produce is the most important thing; plus, organic certification can be expensive, so some small farms may choose to bypass the stamp, yet still opt out of using sprays and chemicals on their farms. Go to your local farmer's market and ask questions—or try growing your own veggies (many urban centers have plot-share community gardens, too). When we lived in Tampa, the kids and I loved going to Meacham Urban Farm—we used to get most of our organic produce from them. It's so special when you know who is growing your food.

I have similar reasons for choosing non-GMO food (GMO means "genetically modified organism"). Genetically modified foods are altered at the cellular level to make them hardier or more attractive—essentially to defend against pests and disease and to grow and ripen in artificial ways. These alterations are made to benefit food businesses (among other reasons) and not necessarily the people who will ultimately consume the food. In general, I avoid foods that have been genetically modified, like most soy, canola, and corn products and many processed foods. I don't want or need anyone changing my food to look a certain way or to be a certain shape or size. As I tell my kids all the time, when choosing something to eat, look to nature.

The expense involved in making these choices is worth mentioning. I am fortunate enough to be choosy. But not everyone can cover the extra costs of buying organic, sustainable, grass-fed, free-range, and GMO-free foods. But sometimes it's important to consider the long view; disease can be traced to what we put in our bodies. I am betting on the fact that organic and non-GMO foods are at least partially responsible for my long-term health! To me, paying a surcharge at the farmer's market every week is less expensive in the long term than having health problems later in life. A CSA (community-supported agriculture) organization that sells weekly boxes of organic produce is a great option, too, as the food is often less expensive than shopping for it piecemeal. Frozen organic produce is another option, as it's almost always less expensive than fresh—and is

usually picked at peak ripeness and flash-frozen to preserve all the nutrients and natural flavor.

Eating locally is as much a social issue as an environmental one. Supporting your local farmers and food producers is good for the local economy, and I like being a part of the community I am living in. It's also nice to know that the produce I buy from a local farm was not picked green and has not traveled for days on a ship or in a refrigerated plane or truck. Local eating also has some specific health benefits, like consuming regionally produced raw honey to help alleviate allergies.

Seasonality is important for a couple of reasons. First, seasonal food tastes the best because it's usually coming from local growers and traveling the least distance from farm to kitchen. Shopping seasonally also has the benefit that you're buying food when it's at its most plentiful, meaning prices are usually their most affordable. Plus, you're helping local farmers make a living. (I think of organic farmers as magicians, and if you ever tried to grow something you will see that growing food is truly an art!) Ripe, seasonal organic produce doesn't last as long as conventional, so if you can't eat it all within a few days, buy less at a time or cook or freeze the excess to enjoy later.

Eating ethically is complicated for me, as it likely is for many people. I love animals. If I could live my best life without eating animals or animal products, I would (see page 21 for my experience as a vegan). But my body just functions better if I eat a bit of meat and fish—plus, a little cheese here and there is something I enjoy. I buy meat and fish from ranchers, fisheries, and producers who treat their animals humanely—as far as possible from factory farming. "Humanely" is defined in all sorts of ways, including the animals having access to high-quality food and water, having space to grow and have a good quality of life, and not being fed GMO products or excessive antibiotics, among many, many other considerations.

If we all make the effort to eat intentionally, especially in regard to these factors, the impact could be huge.

CREATING A VALUE SYSTEM
WITH YOUR KIDS

As anyone with children knows, sometimes you need a dinner-table strategy to get the conversation rolling beyond the "nothing" they did at school that day. We used to go around the table and do "roses and thorns"—each of us talking about one good thing and one bad thing that happened that day. But since meeting the Valente Brothers (see page 58), we have another conversation starter: the 753 Code. This code, and their book of the same name (learn more at 753code.com), introduces the jiujitsu philosophy through a set of fifteen values outlining a moral code that I have come to appreciate tremendously—for myself and my children. The values are separated into three categories: spirit, body, and mind.

Spirit • rectitude, courage, benevolence, respect, honesty, honor, loyalty.

Body • exercise, nutrition, rest, hygiene, positivity.

Mind • awareness, balance, flow.

While I obviously talk a lot about nutrition in this book, I know the health of one's body is very much connected to one's mind and spirit. Remember, my struggles with anxiety and depression were greatly affected by both my diet and my lifestyle. Investing in the mind, body, and spirit is so important to me; I'm constantly trying to be a better person, for myself, my family, and others. I want to instill a positive foundation and moral compass in my children as well.

So, we started using these fifteen elements from the 753 Code framework to discuss our own successes and areas of improvement over dinner. And let me tell you, it's been amazing. We have really deep conversations, and I can see how my kids have developed critical thinking skills and accountability. They love it. Benny actually said to me, "If everyone followed the 753 Code, the world would be a better place." I agree! It gives my kids a clear idea of what our values are, and we get to discuss the nuances of difficult situations together. I feel like it's my role as their guardian to help them find tools to best navigate their lives. We all need to take responsibility for how we want to grow

and live in the world. It is my responsibility as their mom to help them develop strong moral roots and the ability to self-reflect. It's also so meaningful to share my experiences with them—things I am working on or am proud of, and things I could have done better. We don't always go through all fifteen of these elements; usually we talk about the ones we struggled with or felt good about that day. This framework helps me, and it helps them; we are on this journey together. Mealtimes have become sacred for us. Not just for nourishing our bodies, but also to feed our minds and spirits, as well as our relationships with each other.

SOME TOOLS TO HELP
REGULATE EMOTIONS

When things are difficult, these are some tools my kids and I use to help us turn around:

Three deep breaths • This is something I taught my kids when they were very little. Taking three deep breaths can help calm and stabilize you at a time when you feel out of control. It's so simple, but it works.

Exercise • Whether it's running in the yard with the dogs for a few minutes, going on the trampoline, or just doing a few stretches between meetings, doing something physical is so helpful to body, mind, and spirit. It can clear your mind and help put things in perspective.

Fresh air • A little sunshine and change of scenery can alter a mood very quickly. Taking a walk, even a quick one, gives you an opportunity to think and process.

Taking a quiet moment • Lying down, taking a few concious breaths, and allowing your thoughts and emotions to flow gives you a chance to recenter and reflect. We are conditioned to always be producing or doing something, and that can create guilt when we aren't—but sometimes there is nothing more nourishing than just being.

My Daily Routine

I feel better and healthier now in my forties than I did in my twenties! After burning out my adrenal grands when I was younger, I had to find a new routine. My old way of living—not sleeping enough, eating nothing of value, drinking loads of sugary coffee drinks and wine every night before bed—made my digestion a mess and provoked anxiety attacks and depression.

The goal of my new routine was to help me live the longest while having the best quality of life. Changing my lifestyle has proved to be vital to improving my health and well-being. When I am traveling, it can be difficult to keep consistent, but at home—whether in Florida or in Costa Rica—I relish my daily routines and spending time with my family. Every day is a gift, so I try to make each one count and stay in the present, while also practicing flexibility—rigidity can create stress. I'm always adjusting and optimizing, but I here are the things I aim to do on an ideal day:

- **Wake up early:** That's usually before sunrise and before my kids.

- **Scrape my tongue:** I use a copper tongue scraper, which is meant to be beneficial for bone health.

- **Start hydrating:** Right when I wake up, I drink a glass of lukewarm water with a lemon squeezed in it and a pinch of high-mineral salt (I like Celtic salt). Putting a gentle, alkaline thing in your stomach wakes up your system.

- **Moving meditation/meditation (see page 20):** This sets my mood and intentions for the day. If I'm proactive about having this time, I always have a better, more productive day.

- **Dog walking:** I walk the dogs for at least 30 minutes. Sometimes I'll make calls if I need to catch up with work, but I really love to go without my phone and just enjoy the quiet time.

- **Oil pulling:** I do it with ayurveda oil (or unrefined virgin coconut oil) for about 10 minutes, as it's good for the gums! For efficiency, I usually feed the dogs while I do it.

- **Exercise:** These days, I usually do a combination of weight training and cardio.

- **Breakfast:** The type of breakfast I crave depends on my workout. If I've lifted weights, I like some protein, like boiled eggs or a smoothie (see pages 55–57) with a scoop of unflavored protein powder.

- **Morning work time:** When I am not on set, I do Zoom calls and meetings at home. I usually have a dandelion tea with honey at some point. I have an alarm set on my phone every hour to remind me to get up from my computer between meetings to do some lunges or stretches for 5 minutes so I don't feel stiff from sitting.

- **Lunch:** Ideally this is at least four to five hours after breakfast: Unless I'm having a big meal at dinner (like going out with friends or having people over), this is usually my main meal of the day. This is also when I usually take my supplements (see page 45).

- **Afternoon work time:** I usually have another herbal tea.

- **Dinner:** Ideally this is at least four hours after lunch, and a couple of hours prior to bedtime. I usually have a light dinner (unless I'm entertaining or being entertained) so I don't go to bed with a full stomach and can sleep more comfortably.

- **Dog walking:** It's important to move after eating and before going to sleep.

- **Bedtime:** Before bed, I drink some chamomile tea and sometimes take some magnesium (see page 45). If I'm at home, I usually go to sleep early, between 9 and 10, so I can get at least seven hours of sleep and still wake up early. Rest is absolutely vital—don't underestimate its power!

Cleanses, Past and Present

I still travel quite a lot for work. With so much travel, it's easy to feel unsettled. This can affect my sleep, my digestion, my mental health, and more. I used to do a cleanse a few times a year to reset my body, feel my best, function on high-intensity jobs, and be the rock for my family. But I've recently stopped doing cleanses, as they have started to feel too extreme at this moment in my life.

Instead I've been experimenting with drinking particular smoothies (see pages 55–57) as a replacement for a meal, often having one for breakfast or for dinner. A three- or four-ingredient smoothie is easier for my body to digest than one with a multitude of ingredients. Plus, they are pure nutrition, combining sweet fruit and almond meal (the residue of making almond milk, not the storebought flour made from grinding almonds), which adds some protein and reduces the glycemic effect of the fruit. Drinking these smoothies is much easier for me to accomplish than a full day (or days) of juicing, as I used to do with my equinox or solstice cleanse. I've found smoothies to be gentler on my system, and I wake up feeling light and energized.

If I am feeling sluggish or have been traveling a lot, getting back to the simple routine of a smoothie (or two, on occasion) a day can turn me around. Further, prioritizing my health every day, instead of just those special two times a year, is a reminder that I must put on my oxygen mask first. It is a way to say yes to myself, to my health, and to a happier and more fulfilling life.

MANAGING STRESS

Yoga, meditation, exercise, sleep, and a great diet are all ways that help me stay balanced, healthy, and feeling good. But of course I cannot control outside forces, some of which create stress. So, I have a few things I do when something has happened or I become overwhelmed with what's ahead.

Just breathe
At any point during the day, I take a moment to close my eyes and do a few breathing exercises. It helps me to calm myself and bring me back to the present moment.

Stretch
Stretching or doing a yoga pose or two can have a similarly grounding effect as deep breath work.

Visualize
Imagine a connection to something bigger than yourself. If I'm feeling very stressed, I do a quick visualization to reset: I imagine a cord from my belly going down my pelvic floor and connecting to the center of the earth; I visualize anything that isn't serving me to be released into the earth so it can be transformed. I feel any worry leave my body, and then a cord of bright golden light comes from the center of the Earth and goes up through my pelvis, traveling up my spine, filling me up with good energy.

These techniques help de-escalate my feelings about what has happened or what I anticipate will happen, and anchors me to the present, where I focus on just one thing. I have been meditating so long that I can usually calm myself and feel grounded fairly quickly by just breathing. If you're new to meditation, know that repetition helps build the practice. Breathing exercises are so powerful—and we all have access to them anytime.

Connect with your breath and listen to your body

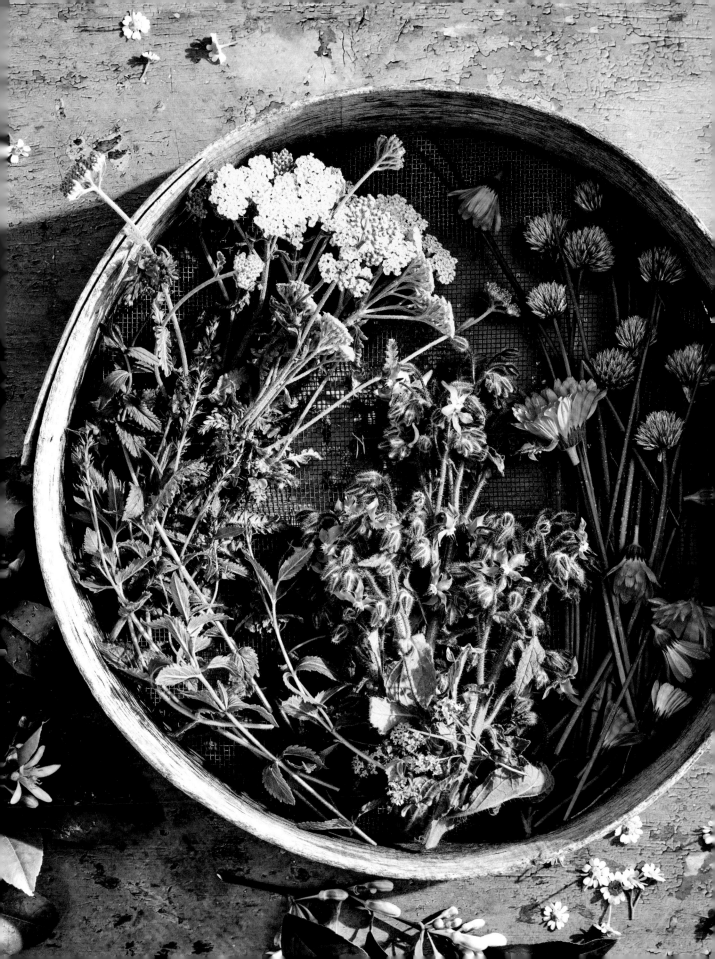

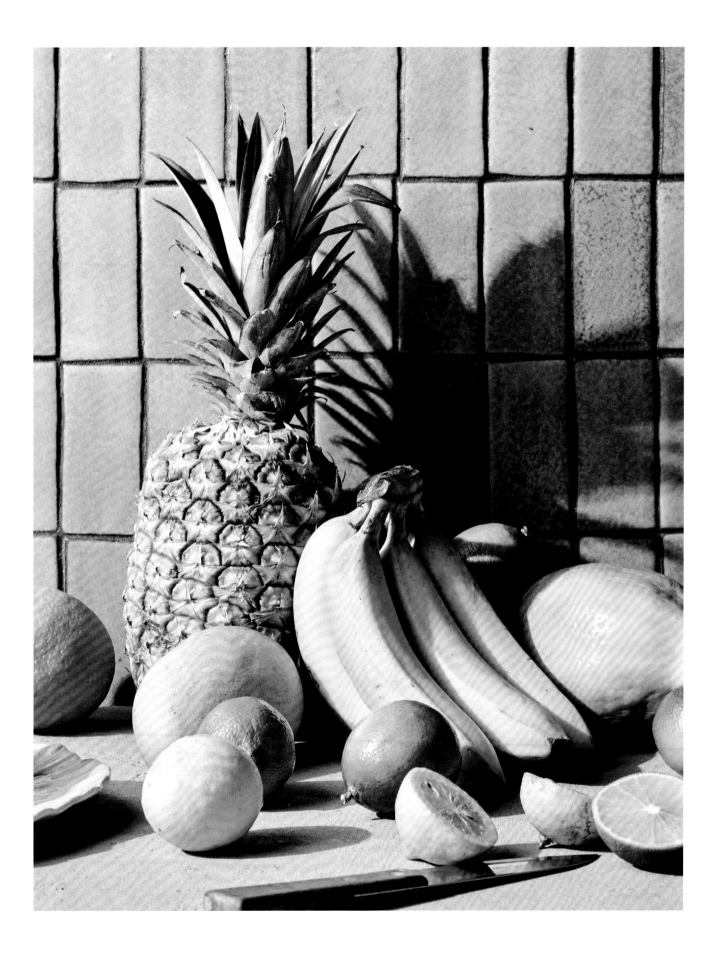

With Purpose and Intention

This book is a reflection of how I eat. I have included all the details of my pantry and my recipes, as well as tips for the kitchen—it's all helpful for learning *how* to care best for your body. But that's meaningful only if you understand the big picture: the *why*.

What I really want readers to take away from this book is that your health is your wealth and your body is your temple, so take good care of it.

You can go through life doing things like you have always done them, staying in your comfort zone and finding reasons why it is too hard to change or make choices that will best support your health. Or you can make conscious choices and make your health and well-being a priority, knowing that in the end you will be the biggest beneficiary of this effort.

I don't have all the answers, nor does anyone else in your life. No one knows you like you. Be the director of your own movie. Find what makes you feel your best. Don't take your blessings for granted; instead, build on them! Having purpose and intention in everything you do will impact your relationships, your happiness, and your success, as well as your health. The power in where I chose to put my attention is one of the most important things I've learned. Compassion that doesn't start with the self is not compassion.

Plus, I'm a Cancer, with a moon in Scorpio. This means I feel things very intensely. Anything superficial is meaningless to me. For me, if I'm not fully present in whatever it is I'm doing, I feel I'm cheating myself out of life. Every day, every opportunity, comes only once, and I want to make the most out of every experience. I always want to be doing my best and improving.

I pride myself on growing every day of my life, even when things are hard. And especially then. I know by now—in my forties—that the one thing I can rely on is change. Instead of fighting it, I've learned to lean into it. When something really difficult happens, there are different ways to look at it. The first way is to wonder when it will end, when there will be a break—all you can see is the difficulty of it. The second way is to accept what it is and see it as an opportunity to learn, gaining strength from going through hard things, and growing in the process. I try to take that second route every time. No matter what the results are, I want to know at the end of the day that I was fully present and engaged and that I learned from it. After all, nothing is more meaningful than our experiences. For me, that's what life is all about.

Never stop evolving and growing

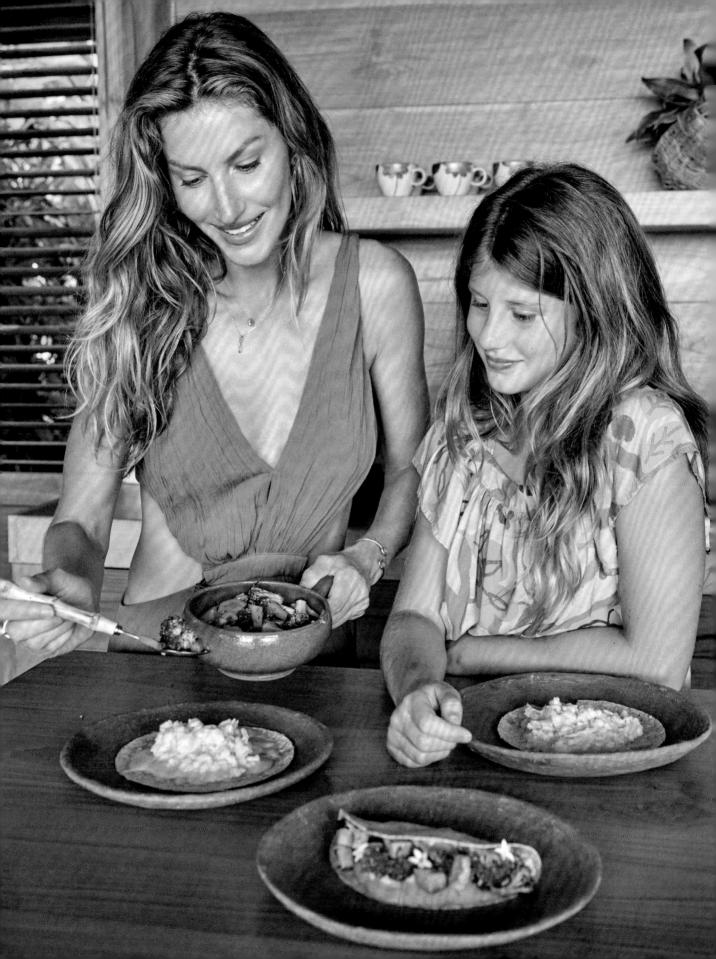

Using This Book

Simplicity Is Key

Yes, I do cook, way more often than I used to. I am lucky to have learned from incredible chefs who helped us at home for many years—they can make anything taste amazing! They have inspired me and taught me so much. But I am not a chef, not at all. I just love food! So, in this book I share some of the things I love to eat and how I like to cook. They are not complicated recipes; you won't find aspirational meals not centered in the real world. Given our society's obsession with appearance and other superficial things, it is important that I describe how I really eat, and how my eating habits have changed my outlook on life and my health.

Above all, I describe the way I eat as *simple*. My diet is mostly plants, and the way I prepare them is usually straightforward. Yes, I have a few more complex special-occasion meals, like a variety of tacos on taco night (page 202) and a handful of sweets I make for special occasions (see pages 233–49), and these do require a longer list of ingredients. But in general I share the idea that food doesn't need to be fussed over to be delicious. Many of the dishes I prepare have barely five ingredients. I joke that I could live the rest of my life seasoning everything with just olive oil and salt. (Okay, maybe garlic, too!) If you have excellent produce (and good olive oil and salt), that is all you need. The main ingredient is the star. As I've said earlier, when the produce is organic and it is grown from high-quality seed and in high-quality soil, it doesn't need much else—it's delicious as is. Why make things more complicated?

Also, I believe that simpler combinations of foods are easier on our bodies to digest. When you eat a piece of fruit without anything accompanying it, that fruit goes through your system much faster and easier than if you had combined it with other foods. This is not to say I wouldn't eat a whole breakfast bowl, but often I go for the simpler version, just to help my gut (which many people consider our second brain). I find this to be especially true when you combine fruit with animal protein, as animal protein needs extra time to be digested; with that additional time, the fruit remains longer in your system and can ferment, causing discomfort or bloating. Just splitting enjoyment of these two ingredients by a few hours can make for easier digestion.

Note that *simple* is not the same as *easy*. I love food to be as simple and the preparation as streamlined as possible—both for fewer food combinations but also for my personal taste. Most of the recipes here are made with whole foods, some of which need prepping. I recognize there is work and time involved in baking a loaf of bread (see page 92), making homemade Almond Milk (page 69), or blending a batch of Hummus (page 180)—and time can be hard to find, especially if it's already difficult finding work-social-family-life balance. So, I include some strategies and tips for planning and organizing your meals so you're set for success—see pages 38–42. Also, there's no need to jump right into the deep end; you can ease yourself into this way of eating and living by making just one or two of these recipes a week. Like anything else in life, the more you do it, the easier it becomes. Be kind to yourself and set attainable goals for yourself, working toward them incrementally.

Also, every meal need not have multiple components. When you are cooking meals from scratch, it's easier to have fewer things to execute, obviously. That said, if you want to customize the recipes a bit, making them more substantial, or for your kids, or just mixing things up a little, check the "Make It Yours" section included with many recipes. I most often pair these recipes with more veggies, adding a side of roasted vegetables or a salad, but this feature gives more ideas and variations. (See page 44 for more details.)

Eating with Intention

The serving sizes for these recipes are moderate. Brazilian culture does not encourage overeating, especially when compared to the supersizing of nearly everything served in the United States. After eating, I don't want to feel overly full, lethargic, or bloated. I have had to learn how to gauge my fullness and satisfaction. Just because I like the taste of something, that doesn't mean I should eat it without limit or without concern for my body's wants or needs. Smaller portions and prioritizing the most nutrient-dense options give me the taste of everything I love but don't result in overindulging.

My plate is mostly filled with vegetables, and occasionally with a small portion of meat or fish. This strategy keeps me focused on the most important part of my diet: plants. It is difficult to eat too much salad, raw or cooked vegetables, soup, or fresh fruit. Replacing a meal once a day with a smoothie (see pages 55–57) also makes me feel amazing, while ensuring that at least one meal of the day is very healthy.

In addition to blessing my food (see page 20), I try to eat mindfully, meaning I do so slowly, so that my stomach has a chance to catch up with my mouth. I don't watch television or look at my phone while I'm eating (unless it's popcorn, which I do love to eat while watching movies!). Being distracted by these things means I can miss the cues my body is giving when it has had enough. I like to say food is my fuel. So, I like the most efficient, effective fuel for my body; I try to eat no more and no less than I want and need.

Lastly, since eating is one of the best pleasures of life, why not celebrate it? Make it special! Why not use a nice napkin or bowl or eat outside if it's nice? Or put some fresh flowers on the table or light a candle at dinnertime. If you are in a pleasant place with people you love, eating will be a much more enjoyable experience, beyond just the food. Celebrating a meal in these additional ways adds to the satisfaction of the experience.

Planning Ahead

In the best of circumstances, eating healthy is simple: focus on eating real food and what is in season; eliminate processed foods; and include small amounts of high-quality dairy, meat, and fish, if you like. Let's be real, though—that can be time-consuming and expensive, too. And most of us don't have help in the kitchen! In this book, I have tried to make these recipes as easy and flexible as possible. They are simple, fresh, and delicious. I hope you enjoy!

Meal Planning and Prepping

When I was growing up, food and cooking were central to our family and social life. My mom worked full time as a bank teller, and my dad was an entrepreneur; he also taught negotiation courses, wrote some books, and later became a sociologist—so he was on the road a lot. With six hungry girls at home, there was a lot of food preparation to be done every day. My mother was in charge of this, and she did a great job. She was very organized—she had to be. You can't make any meal for eight people in half an hour without having planned ahead. She always created a list on the weekend for all the meals we would eat during the week ahead. She would use this list to shop, of course, and also to prep ahead.

5 QUICK TIPS TO GET ORGANIZED

Have a menu for the week.

Make a shopping list.

Buy the best-quality produce.

Know where and when to spend your money.

Prepare items ahead of time, so your refrigerator and pantry have delicious things ready to go.

I learned from my mother how to plan meals and prep ahead. Not only does it make eating well an easier reality (who wants to scramble at the end of the day to shop and cook?), but having a plan ensures you will use all the food you purchase for the week. This limits waste—of your money and of food! The goal is to walk into the kitchen and know what you will cook, or at least have the key ingredients you need. All this takes is a few hours a week to set up: making a shopping list and then prepping some basics to have on hand ahead of time that will make weekday cooking more efficient.

These are some of the items I like to make ahead. Try a few—your future self will thank you.

- **Smoothies** (pages 55–57): Since I usually have at least one smoothie a day, I juice the fruit the night before and place it in the blender jar, then into the fridge. (I use fruit juice in my smoothies rather than water and ice, which keeps them nutritionally dense.) Then, in the morning, I add my frozen fruit, then just blend and drink. An extra bonus is that the smoothie is super-cold.

- **Alternative milks** (pages 68–72): I make a couple milks at the same time, as everyone in my family has a personal favorite. For instance, if you're blending almonds for almond milk, it's just as easy to next blend cashews or coconut for those milks. After straining, remember to save any residual almond meal to add to your smoothies.

- **Broths** (pages 122–24): While broth takes a few hours to cook, the process is almost entirely hands off, whether you do it in a pot or a slow cooker. The end result lasts a long time in the freezer and can be the foundation for a delicious last-minute soup. Broth makes everything taste good and it adds so much nutrition—I add it to almost everything! (Which is why I usually make a double batch.)

- **Roasted nuts and chickpeas** (see pages 116 and 213): I always like to have something crunchy in the pantry to add protein and texture to soups and salads.

THE IMPORTANCE OF WATER

We all know how important it is to drink water, and lots of it. Water is life! I aim for ten glasses (or three of my large water bottles) of plain, lukewarm water every day. (My mom always said to drink water close to your own body temperature, so it doesn't give your system a shock.) I start the day with a big glass of warm water into which I have squeezed half a lemon and dropped in a pinch of Celtic salt. This helps wake up my body and gets some minerals into it right away.

In addition, I drink a ton of hot tea. Some of my favorites are chamomile, fennel, and fresh mint, as well as dandelion (which I drink instead of coffee, with a little honey; see page 48). I also have a collection of specialty teas and a recipe for a Ginger-Lemon Healing Tea (page 75) if anyone in the family has a sore throat. See my pantry list on page 48, as well as the detailed list of teas to try on page 49.

Here's something unusual that I do: I try not to drink water or anything else when I eat. My mother always encouraged my sisters and me to do this when we were young. Her theory was that the enzymes in our saliva and in our digestive system will be diluted by water if it is drunk along with solids, making digestion more difficult. She always pointed out that digestion starts in the mouth, which is why we were encouraged to chew our food forty times before swallowing. I didn't do so well on the chewing part of it! But I'm much better at abstaining from water during meals.

- **Dressings** (pages 220–28): Store-bought dressings are full of sugar, GMO oils, and all sorts of preservatives and fillers, so I make my own! We usually have a dressing or two already mixed in mason jars in the fridge at all times. Throughout the week, all you need do is shake it a bit, then use it on salads or even as a dip. Some dressings are good beyond salads, like Tamari Dressing (page 228) in a stir-fry or Dad's Honey-Mustard Dressing (page 220) as a glaze for grilled chicken.

- **Seeded bread:** Having my favorite Nut and Seed Bread (page 92) in the fridge means I'm only moments away from my favorite avocado toast or a quick toast with some almond butter and honey. Making two loaves at the same time is hardly more trouble, and they freeze beautifully.

- **Granolas** (pages 76 and 79): Grain-free or oat granola is my favorite sprinkle on an Acai Bowl (page 58).

- **Chia pudding:** The Coconut–Chia Seed Pudding (page 80) has to be made ahead, but takes only a few minutes to assemble. If you store the puddings in small lidded jars, you can easily take one with you for a breakfast on the go.

- **Wild rice salad:** Made ahead, the Warm Wild Rice Salad (page 116) can be stored in the fridge for at least 2 days. You can eat it plain, or top it with lentils, or serve it as a side with Fish Baked in Parchment (page 188).

- **Roasted vegetables:** Nothing disappears faster in our house than Roasted Vegetables (page 144) hot out of the oven, just before dinner. We all pick them right off the baking tray. So doubling the recipe means you will have enough for the meal as well! Plus, leftovers of these roasted veggies can be the base for so many last-minute soups, salads, frittatas (see page 87), and tacos (see pages 202–203), or are an easy side for Chicken Meatballs (page 194) or Pan-Fried Falafel (page 177). Lunch or dinner can be ready in the time it takes you to heat some broth or to toss everything with a little dressing.

- **Raw or blanched vegetables:** Prepping some raw celery, carrots, or green beans and blanching (see page 155) some broccoli or sugar snap peas so they are ready to eat or cook with is more than a huge timesaver—it's a lifestyle. It makes me so happy to see jars of these beautiful prepped veggies lined up in my fridge. Make your meal prep attractive and accessible, and it will get eaten. I promise!

FIVE TIPS FOR MAKING NUTRITIOUS CHOICES

When you're changing the way you eat, cooking for kids or family members with different tastes, traveling, or navigating work obligations or dinners with friends can make it hard to be consistent. Here are a few things to help you be intentional about making healthier choices, no matter the circumstances.

Always be prepared • Just as you dress for a change in the weather, make it routine to think ahead to the next meal—and have a plan.

Shop for groceries after you've eaten a healthy meal • Don't shop when you're hungry.

Stock your kitchen with only the nutritious food you want to eat • If you want to avoid certain foods, don't have them around!

Prep ahead recipe elements like roasted veggies or grilled chicken • These will be helpful to pull together last-minute meals.

Wash and dry raw vegetables when you buy them • Wrap them in dishtowels or put in glass containers, and keep them in the fridge for simple soups and salads. Likewise, fruit can be washed, cut, and refrigerated or frozen, if you like.

- **Hummus:** Prepare Hummus (page 180) and serve with blanched or raw veggies to eat anytime.

- **A veg-heavy legume dish:** Making a dish like French Lentil and Mushroom Ragout (page 183) or Sheet-Pan Squash and Chickpeas (page 151) is so flexible: eat it hot, top with an egg, or add leftovers to a salad or a bowl.

- **A blended soup:** Creamy Cauliflower Soup (page 131) or Butternut Squash Soup (page 132) can be made entirely ahead, frozen if you like, and heated up when you're ready to eat.

- **Seeded crackers:** The Seed Crackers (page 218) are excellent to have on hand for nibbling on their own, or for crumbling into soups or salads for some crispy texture.

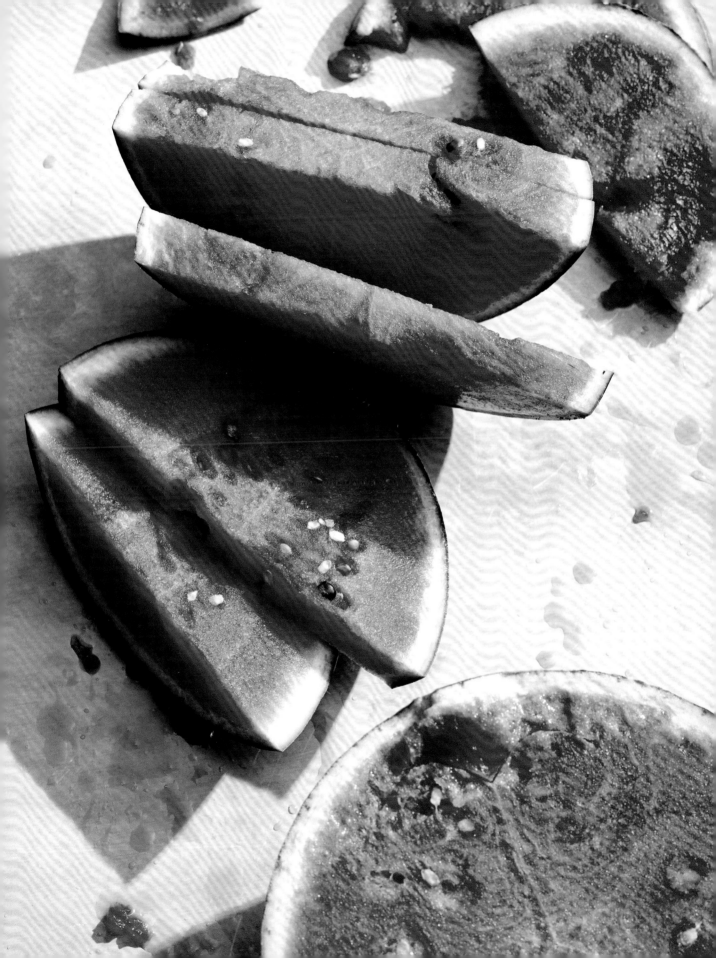

FOUR WEEKS OF MEAL PREP

Prepping a few things at the start of the week is always a good idea. Of course, you can mix and match any of the recipes in this book (especially the items on the make-ahead list on page 39), but here are four weeks' worth of meal prep ideas that include some of my favorites. Discover a favorite set that can become your new routine, or do the four weeks in a row for a month of variety. In each case, a few hours of work at the beginning of the week, much of which is hands-off, gives you at least a few meals that are ready to pull together with little to no additional effort.

Week 1	Week 2	Week 3	Week 4
Make chicken broth • make double batch, freeze half	**Make vegetable broth** • make double batch, freeze half	**Make granola**	**Bake frittata muffins**
Marinate chicken breasts • you can use the ones removed from the whole chicken in the broth	**Prep raw veggies** • put the scraps in broth	**Make butternut squash or cauliflower soup**	**Make seeded bread** • make double batch, freeze one
Blanch veggies • use scraps in broth	**Soak, cook, and peel chickpeas** • make double batch, half for hummus and half for salads/soups	**Prep shaved salad** and prep some extra raw or blanched veggies	**Cook roasted veggies** • could use some on frozen pizza dough from week 1
Make pizza dough • freeze one and make the other for dinner	**Prepare vegetable-quinoa cakes**	**Prepare lentil and mushroom ragu**	**Marinate a steak**
Prepare pesto • use in lettuce wraps, zucchini noodles, or pizza	**Mix tahini dressing**	**Stir together ginger-cashew sauce** • for spring rolls	**Make chimichurri**
Make chia pudding	**Bake baru nut bars**	**Make rosemary almonds**	**Prep and freeze fruit for smoothies** • use some for ice pops

- **Baru Nut Bars** (page 233) are a homemade version of a granola bar that gives you lots of energy, without any additives or refined sugar. They are easily made in advance, wrapped in parchment, and refrigerated, so they are ready to grab on the way out the door.

- **Marinated chicken or steak:** Marinating your protein is always done in advance. If you marinate chicken or beef, it will taste better, will be more tender, and will be ready to go for a meal. Then, all you need do is grill, bake, or sauté.

- **Vegetable-Quinoa Cakes** (page 159) or **Pan-Fried Falafel** (page 177): When made ahead, these are great to reheat, even when frozen. They can be eaten on their own or added to a salad, bowl, or wrap.

- **A sweet:** My kids and I love to have an ice pop (see page 62) in the afternoon or a cookie (see pages 241 and 249) on a special occasion.

Minimizing Waste

I am so grateful for the time and energy that is spent growing the food I eat, and I feel it's my responsibility to honor that achievement.

My aversion to waste began when I was a kid. In my family, we ate *everything* and threw away nothing. Growing up as a gaúcha meant we often had churrasco on Sundays, which was a big meal of grilled meats, plus salads, vegetables, and potato salad, which we ate with family and friends. We used every part of the animals, both as an economy measure and out of respect. My mom always made sure there was never any waste. Any leftover grilled meat was always made into *arroz con carretero* on Mondays. Using up everything was a way of life. My sisters and I were aware of how hard my parents had to work to give us a good life, and we were taught to honor and be grateful for whatever was on our plates. This is something I still do and I teach my kids.

Here are a few ways to combat waste in the kitchen:

- **Shop carefully.** Have a plan for the week that accounts for everything you bought. Because organic produce goes bad faster, shopping twice a week might be better than once a week.

- **Make the recipes work for you, not the other way around.** When it comes to amounts of vegetables, fruits, and proteins, the measurements given in these recipes are for guidance. Feel free to add a little bit more or less, depending on what you have, so you aren't left with little scraps that will go to waste. Most recipes in this book call for whole vegetables, like a whole cauliflower, so there is some wiggle room here, as not all vegetables are the same size.

- **Proactively make a clean-out-the-fridge recipe** (see page 160) once or twice a week to use up any ingredients that are ready to eat.

- **Plan more dishes around leftovers.** Leftover cooked vegetables, beans, and meats can be made into impromptu soups or salads. They are also a great addition to Egg and Cheese

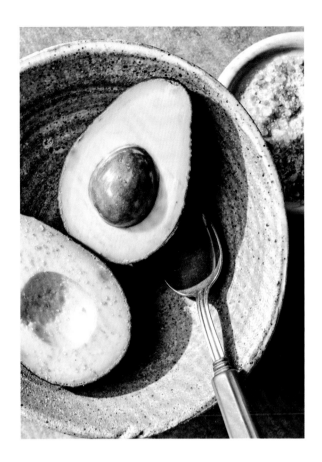

Quesadillas (page 84), a Veggie Frittata (page 87), or tacos (see page 202). Leftovers don't have the sexiest reputation, but they can really make a meal more delicious!

- **Freeze your fruit.** When your fruit is about to get too ripe, make it into ice pops (page 62) or freeze it and add it later to smoothies (see pages 55–57).

Making Recipes Work for Your Household

Many of the recipes in this book are not typical "square meals," as in a big serving of animal protein, plus a starch and a vegetable. First off, I don't eat meat or fish at every meal, and when I do eat animal protein, it is usually a small portion and not the focus of the meal (unless it is churrasco!). And for me, starches and carbs are more often an accent (like rice paper in a spring roll, or grain-free granola), not a base—though I do love starchy plants like butternut squash, sweet potatoes, and lentils. Instead, most of my meals focus purely on some particular vegetables and fruits that can then be rounded out with a salad, contrasting roasted vegetables, or some sautéed greens. Think of it as vegetables on vegetables! And sometimes I mix and match recipes with others to create a more complex meal.

To show the variety of ways you can assemble these recipes into meals, I sometimes include a feature called "Make It Yours," which lists a few suggestions on pairing them with other foods.

- **Light Pairings:** super straightforward combinations, which is how I most often eat.

- **Hearty Pairings:** vegetables or sides to bulk up the main recipe, when you want a more substantial meal.

- **For the Kids:** suggestions for making meals especially kid friendly (based on my children's preferences!).

- **Simple Swaps:** ideas for adjusting recipes according to the season, by using different ingredients, or by making variations.

My family is probably a lot like yours—we all have our individual food preferences. My kids like all the recipes in this book and in general are good eaters, but adding a favorite component—like cheese, noodles, or rice—means they are extra happy about whatever is on their plate (this is a great way to introduce new foods too!). Likewise, keeping meals varied by changing the same salad or stir-fry with a different sauce or dressing, making salads into wraps, and accommodating different dietary needs (like my vegetarian friends, or my sister's preference for meat) means everyone is happy when sitting down to eat. Keeping the ingredients in most recipes simple also makes it easy to customize the meal as desired.

KEEPING A SENSE OF SELF WHILE NAVIGATING PARENTHOOD

To be honest, being a parent can make it difficult to create and maintain a healthy routine. My kids are always my highest priority, so it is sometimes hard to balance their lives and my own. When my children were very little, I did lose myself for a while. Being the mother I wanted to be—breastfeeding for years, being closely involved—was a choice and a privilege, and the result was simply that my needs were not the biggest priority anymore.

I needed to find a way to keep my sense of self. So, I started to wake up extra early to ensure I had some time to myself before everyone was up. Having time to check in with myself and address my own needs was so important, especially in the morning, because it set my mood for the whole day. A little meditation and yoga made me feel like myself again, and having that daily reminder and personal space was a lifeline.

Also, I found that relaxing into this new role of motherhood helped me realize that this special time was part of a larger picture. Life has cycles, just as nature does. There are times when we need to be more outward, when we are ambitious and our own goals are prioritized, and there are times when it's important to prioritize others' needs. Sometimes we need to go inward and find our center to recharge. Like trees losing their leaves in winter and then blossoming in spring, I placed my pursuits on hold for a while, knowing that I'd be able to return to them when my children became more independent.

Now that my kids are older and much more able to take care of themselves, I can ask myself who I am *now*, what are the things I want to explore, what else I want to learn and create. I sometimes fall back into earlier patterns of being a pleaser and forgetting about my needs, but I am working on that. I had to learn that my yes answer meant nothing if I didn't also know how to say no, and that saying no wasn't selfish but, rather, an act of self-love. Not only is it important to find balance again and pursue some of my own goals, but it's also important for my kids to see me fulfilled and happy.

Becoming a mother was such a big transition; it changed my identity. I have learned so much with my kids and I continue to do so every day.

Vitamins and Supplements

I am a big believer in getting my nutrients from the purest source possible, meaning organic vegetables and fruits, and occasional proteins. With the variety of foods that I eat, I don't need to look elsewhere for most vitamins and minerals. But after I went through my healing journey, my doctor prescribed a few tinctures and supplements to balance my hormones, to support my adrenal health, and to reduce inflammation. A lot of these supplements give me support and benefits for my overall health that I can't always find in food, so I've been taking them ever since, now for twenty years.

As with the food I buy, when it comes to sourcing supplements, quality is nonnegotiable. As with organic produce, I buy the highest-quality supplements for the biggest impact. Low-quality versions can include things that are actually detrimental to your health, and they get absorbed directly into your system. I've found Gaia brand to be the best; I've been using them for 20 years and recently joined their team as a wellness ambassador. Unfortunately my grandmother is no longer here to teach me all she knew about plants, but I am grateful that now I get to work closely with the Gaia herbalists and learn from them. They test their products like crazy and are so transparent. Pure brand is good, too. You only have one body in this life, and you can't replace it like an old car; put premium gas in and it'll run much better and longer.

Daily Supplements

Adrenal supplements • I've taken these for the last twenty years, since my adrenals burned out (see page 16).

Ashwagandha • Helpful for stress relief.

Cranberry capsules • For urinary tract support.

Digestive enzymes • Helps digestion and reduces bloating.

Elderberry syrup (or gummies) • Great for immune support; I give this to my kids as a cold tonic every day in the winter. (In thirteen years of living in Boston, my kids got sick maybe once—amazing! I take it too.)

Lion's mane mushroom powder • Helps with brain fogginess and memory.

Lysine • Important for bones, skin, and immune function.

Turmeric • Anti-inflammatory and helpful for anxiety.

Vitamin C • Good for so many bodily functions, and helps with iron absorption.

Vitamin D₃ and K₂ • These are necessary for me in the winter, when I'm exposed to less sunlight; when I lived in Boston, these were a lifesaver. They are also helpful for calcium absorption.

As-Needed Supplements

Echinacea spray • For when I have a sore throat.

Ginger • Helps relieve occasional nausea and supports digestion.

Golden milk powder (which includes turmeric, ashwagandha, and dates) • You can make a hot drink by combining it with almond milk, honey, and cinnamon, or try adding it to cookies (Oatmeal Golden Milk Cookies, page 249).

Holy basil leaves (capsule) • Helpful for stress relief.

Magnesium powder • Aids digestion and sleep; I sometimes mix this with lukewarm water and drink it right before bed.

Oil of oregano • An antioxidant, anti-inflammatory, and antimicrobial; I credit this for keeping me healthy when in a rural town with no toilets for the UN's Energy Poverty summit in Africa. (Everyone got sick but me.)

Selenium • I take as needed when I'm sick.

Zinc • For a healthy immune system.

As always, be sure to check with your doctor before starting any new health routines.

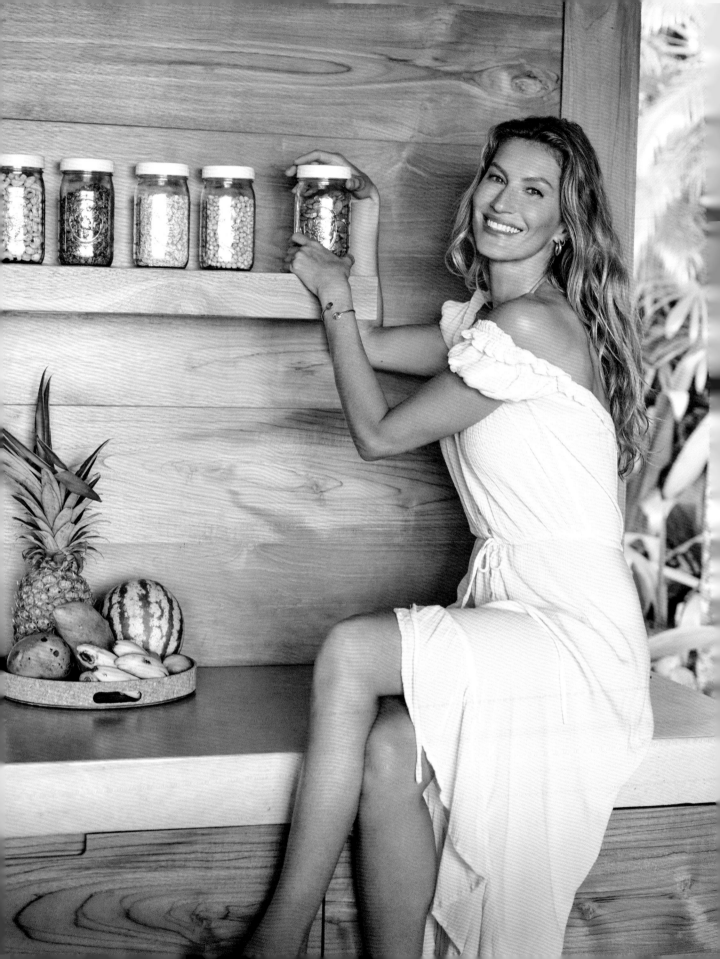

Pantry List

Keeping my kitchen filled with the best-quality foods is a way to invest in my and my family's health, as I believe wholeheartedly that our health is our wealth and that food is medicine. Having delicious, nutritious things to eat in my fridge and fruit bowl means I am less likely to deviate from those foods; as long as they are available, there is no way I'd want to eat anything else! Everything listed here is organic, whenever possible.

Oils and Vinegars

Extra-virgin olive oil · One of my favorite brands is Hygeia. I don't usually cook with it, as heat will degrade the quality, but I keep it on the table so I can drizzle it on almost everything.

Unrefined virgin coconut oil · I like Dr. Bronner's. This oil is my favorite for sweet potatoes and some desserts.

Avocado oil · This is a great neutral oil I use for cooking, since it has a high smoke point.

Ghee · I love the sweet, strong flavor of this kind of clarified butter, and I use it for many cooking applications. Coconut oil or avocado oil is a good substitute.

Good-quality butter

Apple cider vinegar

Balsamic vinegar

Almond oil · I really like its rich, aromatic flavor in salad dressings and drizzled on soup or fish.

Gluten-Free Grains

Note: When measuring any flours, I spoon the flour into a measuring cup, then level it off.

Wild rice · I prefer pure wild rice to a blend with other types of rice and grains. Avoid blends if you are sensitive to gluten.

Brown or white rice wrappers · For summer rolls, see page 156.

Rice noodles

Gluten-free pasta · I like Jovial brand.

Millet or brown rice noodles/ramen · I love the Lotus Foods brand.

Gluten-free flour mix · I like Bob's Red Mill (I use this brand for most of my flours).

Almond flour · I use it for making a crispy crust on pan-seared goat cheese (see page 106).

Coconut flour

Oatmeal · Be sure whatever you buy is certified gluten free, if that matters to you, as some oats are processed in factories that process wheat as well.

Tapioca flour/starch

Tapioca hidratada · This is a type of tapioca starch that I buy in Brazilian stores. It is granular and cannot be substituted with regular tapioca starch. I love the Da Terrinha brand, but it can be hard to find. It makes excellent tapioca "tortillas" that I like to fill with cheese and oregano, like a Brazilian quesadilla.

Rice crackers

Almond crackers

Nuts, Seeds, Beans, and Dried Fruits

Baru nuts · These Brazilian nuts, which taste like a cashew crossed with a peanut, are a new favorite. Barùkas brand is my favorite; I use them for my nut bars (see page 233).

Almonds, cashews, pecans, and walnuts · I always buy raw.

Pine nuts

Almond butter

Tahini

Corn nuts

Pumpkin seeds (pepitas) · I buy these raw for my Nut and Seed Bread (page 92).

Hemp seeds · Great to sprinkle on a salad.

Flax seeds · I usually buy milled flax seeds.

Unhulled sesame seeds

Chia seeds · Chia seeds need to be soaked before ingesting. This is why I love combining them with coconut milk in Coconut–Chia Seed Pudding (page 80).

Shelled sunflower seeds · I buy these raw for my Nut and Seed Bread (page 92).

Psyllium husk powder · For Nut and Seed Bread (page 92) and homemade pizza dough (see page 173).

Popcorn kernels

Dried beans and lentils · This includes chickpeas, white beans, brown lentils, and more.

Spirulina

Medjool dates · If your dates are very dry and you are blending them, soak them to make them soft again.

Dried goji berries

Teas (see page 49)

Dandelion tea • I love Dandy Blend brand, the organic type. Since giving up coffee, I've been enjoying this instead. It's strong tasting, so I like it with a little honey and sometimes a date on the side.

Golden milk • A blend of turmeric, ashwagandha, dates, and cardamom; Gaia Brand is the best.

Ayurvedic teas • From Banyan brand, I love the CCF tea (cumin, coriander, and fennel) and Ayurvedic Herbs tea.

Herbal and green teas • In the United States, I like the Traditional Medicinals brand; in Brazil, I like the blends from Iamaní Orgânicos brand.

Jarred, Canned, and Packaged Items

Jarred tuna • Tonnino brand is the best; I prefer to get it packed in water and add my own olive oil.

Tomato puree • Vivi loves tomatoes on pasta and pizza, and the Mutti brand jarred *passata* is made of only tomatoes and salt.

Canned salmon • Good for a quick salad; I like Vital Choice brand.

Cooked beans • I usually choose those packed in a Tetra Pak carton or a jar, since they'll definitely be BPA free.

Coconut milk/cream • I don't usually buy a lot of canned foods, but cartons of coconut milk contain all sorts of stabilizers and flavorings I don't want to ingest. Plus, the cans (I buy organic and full fat) have a higher fat content, which is more delicious and helpful for making Coconut Whipped Cream (page 237).

Unsweetened coconut water

Roasted seaweed snacks

Seasonings and Sauces

Fine sea salt • I often use Himalayan pink salt, as there are many trace minerals and nutrients found in it, plus it is minimally processed and has no additives. If you are replacing fine sea salt with Diamond Kosher Salt in these recipes, use approximately two times the amount called for.

Coarse/Kosher salt • An all-purpose salt that is my favorite for marinating meats.

Flaky salt (like Maldon) • This is my favorite to sprinkle on top of finished food.

Black pepper • I use freshly ground; I don't use a lot of pepper, except to activate the benefits of turmeric (see pages 45 and 48).

Onion powder

Garlic powder

Ground cinnamon

Paprika

Turmeric • Fresh turmeric root is the best, but can be hard to find. Ground turmeric works as well, and is great for fighting inflammation and is a powerful antioxidant. I use it in soups (like Sneeze-Be-Gone, page 127) and in my Oatmeal Golden Milk Cookies (page 249).

Dried herbs • I love fresh herbs, especially if I grow them myself, but you can also use dried herbs if you can't find fresh. I use dried rosemary and thyme most often.

Dried herb/spice blends • These are great for perking up plain roasted vegetables or soups. My go-tos are Italian blends, Moroccan blends, and herbes de Provence. Beware of salted versions, as they can include additives.

Fresh ginger

Harissa paste • I love this for my Maple Harissa Cashews (page 208).

Mustard

Yuzu juice • Yuzu is a Japanese citrus fruit, and the juice is available bottled. Fresh lemon juice can be substituted if you have trouble finding it.

Tamari

Maple syrup

Honey • I love honey, either locally bottled or Manuka honey, which is expensive but worth it to use in tea (page 75) when anyone is feeling sick.

For Baking

Coconut sugar

Coconut nectar

Unsweetened dried coconut/coconut chips

Dark chocolate • I used to be a real chocoholic, but I rarely crave it these days, I believe because of the amount of naturally sweet fruit, smoothies, and Acai Bowls (page 58) that I eat. When I do have it, I buy organic dark chocolate that is free of refined sugar, cane sugar, sugar alcohols, additives, dairy, palm oil, lecithin, and emulsifiers. And I wouldn't hand out any chocolate or candies for Halloween other than Unreal Candy; I trade my kids' junky Halloween candy for Unreal brand, and everyone is happy.

Unsweetened cacao powder

Vanilla extract

Frozen and Refrigerated Products

Frozen acai • Always buy unsweetened. I like Tambor brand.

Eggs • I like to buy from the farmer's market if possible, and always those from chickens that are humanely raised.

Coconut or almond milk–based yogurt

Cheese • I like goat and sheep's milk cheeses, as they are easier for my body to digest than pasteurized cow's milk cheese. Some of my favorites are manchego and soft goat cheese like Midnight Moon. I also like Brazilian cheeses when I can find them; my favorites are queijo qualho and queijo minas.

Almond flour tortillas • I like Siete brand. They freeze great, too (just let them come to room temperature before toasting in a pan), so stock up.

Chickpea flour tortillas

Hero bread • This contains gluten, but it's been processed in a way that eliminates any carbs. This brand also makes nice tortillas for wraps and a delicious croissant that the kids love.

Ezekiel flourless bread

MY FAVORITE TEAS

I love sipping hot drinks throughout the day. Since I don't drink coffee, when I want something warm to drink I make tea. Here are a few of my favorites (see brand recommendations on page 48).

Dandelion • I drink this in the morning or after lunch. It's my coffee replacement, and I take it sweetened with honey, so one cup a day is usually sufficient for me.

Mint • I drink this anytime, but usually after a meal. Peppermint tea can help ease a variety of digestive issues, including bloating and gas. This is owing to its menthol content, which can relax the muscles in the digestive tract. I also love the refreshing scent of this plant!

Raspberry leaf • Raspberry leaf tea is considered the "best-friend plant for women," as it is traditionally used for women's health at different stages of life (during periods, postpartum, and menopause). It's rich in iron, an important nutrient especially in the menstrual period, when women lose blood. It is also a source of potassium, a mineral that promotes relaxation of the arteries, favoring blood circulation, and maintaining healthy blood pressure.

Hibiscus • If you menstruate, this super-red tea is good to drink when you have your period because it has anti-inflammatory properties that may help reduce inflammation in the body. Hibiscus tea also contains iron, an essential mineral that supports blood production, which is important during heavy menstrual bleeding! (And why not eat a few extra dates for the iron, while you are at it.)

Fennel • Fennel is a medicinal herb which can help relieve abdominal pain and cramping. It's also helpful for digestion and bloating.

Lemon-ginger • Great for digestion, as well as when I feel I am getting a cold—I drink it all day and it works miracles! (Store-bought is good—but even better, make your own; see page 75.)

Lemongrass • This store-bought tea is one of my favorites, as it reminds me of my childhood. My mom used to make some fresh every day right from the plant in our backyard—I think I drank it more than plain water. If you have access to garden-fresh lemongrass, cut a handful of the plant's tips, add water to cover, and boil for a few minutes, then let steep until the strength of flavor is right for you. Drink this warm, at room temperature, or iced.

Yerba mate • As a Brazilian and gaúcha (from Rio Grande do Sul), I grew up drinking a lot of chimarrão—a traditional drink made from yerba mate. Chimarrão has its roots in indigenous culture, especially among Guarani communities in South America, who consumed yerba mate and developed their own techniques for growing, drying, and preparing the herb. Nowadays I avoid caffeinated drinks, but every now and then, when I'm with my family in Brazil or when I want to remember my roots, I love to prepare a chimarrão! The combination of caffeine and other compounds in yerba mate can improve cognitive function, helping to sharpen focus and enhance concentration. (It's the only caffeine I would drink, these days.) But for me, chimarrão's main superpower is that it brings people together, because the essence of this drink is that of sharing it with family and friends.

Chamomile • I love having a chamomile tea an hour or so before bed. It's the perfect soothing ritual to wind down after the day. My kids like it with a little manuka honey.

Kitchen Equipment

The following is what I use most in my kitchen. Some of these items are expensive, but they will often outlast their less pricey counterpoints, so they are actually better in the long run (for your wallet and the environment). This is not an exhaustive list; it's just the things that might need more explanation.

Appliances

Vitamix (or other high-power blender) • A Vitamix is pricey, but there is no question that it is worth the money if you can afford it. Mine has been going strong for *years* and I know it will be around for many more (plus, the brand will actually service your blender should it need it! So much better than ending up in a landfill). It makes the smoothest smoothies and nut milks, blended soups, Hummus (page 180), and my favorite Ginger-Cashew Sauce (page 223), among many other things. I bought two jars and labeled them so I can keep one for just smoothies.

Champion juicer (or other high-quality juicer) • I got a Champion juicer on eBay and I think it is the best juicer ever made. For making most of my smoothies (see pages 55–57), this is a very helpful piece of equipment. I also use it to make amazing banana "ice cream" (see page 65).

Waffle maker • My kids love waffles (see page 83) on the weekends.

Air-fryer • This is great for cooking veggies and making my favorite crunchy chickpeas (see page 213)! Buy the largest that you can comfortably fit in your kitchen, and be sure it has a stainless-steel interior.

Multicooker • I am just starting to experiment with this combination pressure cooker/slow cooker, but like everyone says, it is pretty amazing for cooking beans and making broths.

Cookware and Utensils

Mandoline • A mandoline cuts evenly and quickly, and I love playing with textures of vegetables using this easy, inexpensive tool. A simple cucumber salad (see page 98) is made special when the cucumbers are just the right thinness. Just be careful—the blades are sharp!

Meat mallet • You can substitute a rolling pin.

Nut milk bag • A fine-mesh nut milk bag is helpful if you are making nut milks on a regular basis. Just don't throw out the remaining nut solids—they can be used in all my smoothies (see pages 55–57).

Nonstick skillet • In general, I use stainless-steel or ceramic-coated pans for almost all my cooking, but I do have high-quality nonstick pans from GreenPan for pancakes and eggs. Be sure to use only silicone or wooden implements; a metal utensil will scrape and compromise the pan's surface.

Outdoor grill and/or a grill pan • Grilling outside is great, but I use a grill pan too (see Rosemary-Lemon Chicken Paillards, page 197).

Kitchen Organization

Label maker • I could go on and on about this: I love organizing with this little machine. Since we have so much homemade food in the house, every jar and container is labeled with the contents and the date it was made. This helps prevent waste, as I can track what food is oldest and needs to get eaten first.

Mason jars and other glass storage containers • I have so many glass containers, as I use them to store all the food we make ahead for the week—dressings, cut-up vegetables, and more—as well as leftovers. I also use them in my pantry, decanting all the bulk items I buy (see label maker, previous entry). One trick is to buy a variety of shapes and sizes, to best accommodate what you use them for. In addition to keeping food fresher than in their original bags or boxes, mason jars also look so uniform and pretty! When I make homemade broth, I refrigerate it in mason jars if I'm using it in the next few days, or I freeze it in a combination of large and small freezer bags, so I can easily defrost only what I need.

Plastic • I avoid plastic containers and bags as much as possible, but freezer bags are helpful to freeze cut-up fruit, broth, or bread. You can easily wash and reuse the bags for the same items (though I wouldn't reuse bags used for meat).

Parchment paper • I try to avoid foil, as studies have shown that foil can leach aluminum into your food when exposed to high heat. Instead, I use parchment under roasting vegetables, to steam fish, or to wrap up baru nut bars or other food on the go.

Reusable waxed cloths • Since I don't use plastic wrap, these are convenient for wrapping up cheese and bread or anything you don't want to dry out in the fridge.

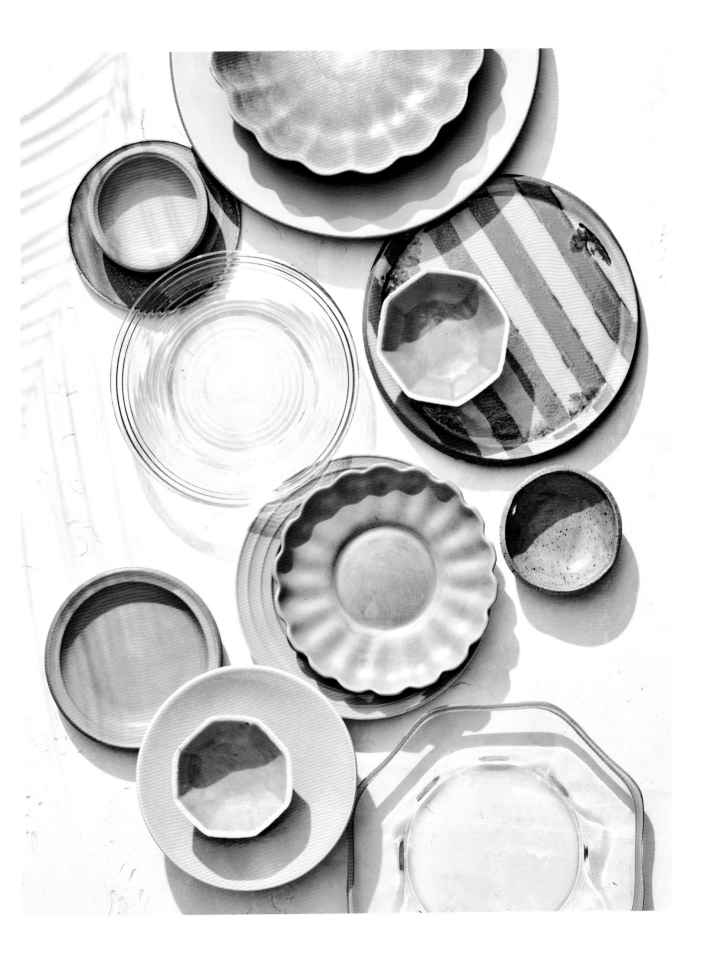

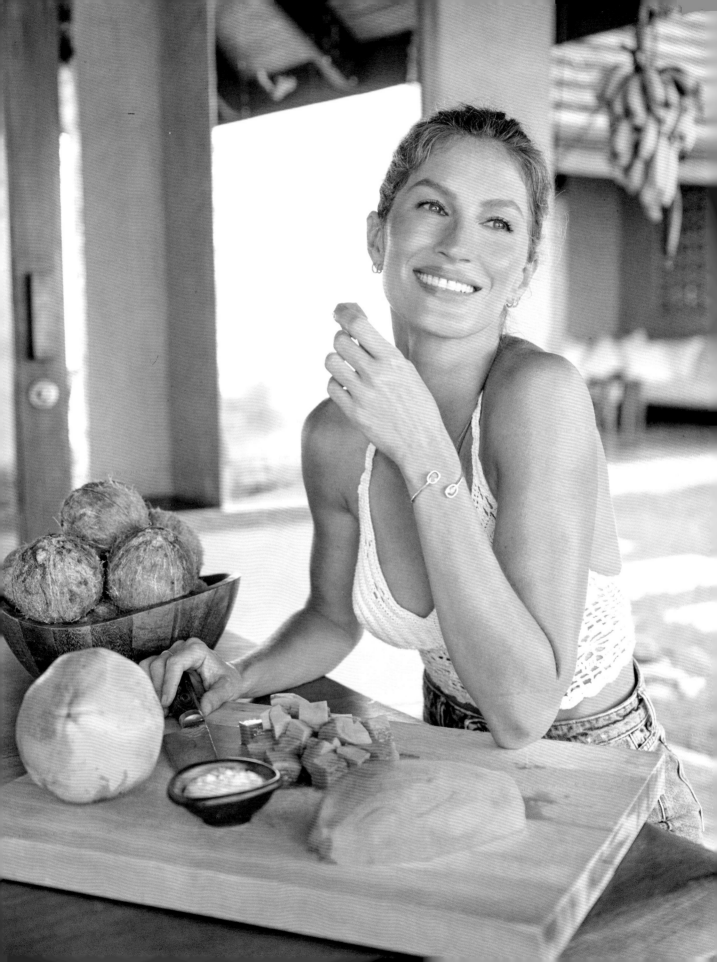

Everyday Fruits

Fruit might be my favorite food. Yes, it is full of natural sugars,
but also tons of vitamins and fiber. And there are so many varieties!
It is an accessible whole food that requires no cooking and is easy
to digest—plus, it makes me feel so energized and fulfilled.
I just love these fruit-driven meals; they feel like a treat, and
I usually eat at least one a day.

Daily Smoothie

I used to do cleanses when I was run down (see page 23), but I've found a new routine that gives me tons of energy, has overhauled my gut health, satisfies my sweet tooth, and is easier to execute: drinking a daily smoothie made with sweet fruit.

As I learned from the Valente Brothers (see page 58), different types of food take different amounts of time and enzymes to be processed by our bodies. Therefore, simplifying food combinations can help to simplify digestion. So these smoothies include only three or four ingredients: one "solid" sweet fruit for bulk, the juice of one "liquid" sweet fruit, and sometimes dates for sweetness. This combination blends easily without water, which keeps it nutritionally dense. I also add almonds or unflavored protein powder to make a complete meal. Since I use frozen fruit, the texture is super thick, a bit like ice cream, which my kids and I love.

The following recipes are three of my favorite combinations, but experiment using the list of "liquid" and "solid" fruits (see page 54). While these smoothies are designed to be digested easily and quickly, you can always deconstruct them and eat the fruit and nuts unprocessed, if you would rather chew your meal—this gives all the same health benefits with just a bit more time needed to digest. (Note: eating these ingredients unprocessed will likely mean you will eat less than the amounts called for.)

"SOLID" AND "LIQUID" FRUITS FOR SMOOTHIES

The Valentes categorize sweet fruits as "solid" fruits and "liquid" fruits. Every smoothie requires frozen "solid" fruit to bulk up the smoothie, "liquid" fruit to aid in the processing of the solid fruit, and other additions (almonds, dates, etc.). The exact recipes include some of my favorite fruit combinations—experiment to find your favorites.

"Liquid" Fruits

Other than coconut water and apple juice, these "liquid" fruits need to be put through a juicer to remove seeds and fibers. If you do not have a juicer, you can process these in the blender until very smooth, then strain using a fine sieve.

Honeydew

Cantaloupe

Watermelon

Apples • not green (see Note)

Unsweetened coconut water

Unsweetened pure apple juice • fruits processed at home are best, but purchased organic juice is fine in a pinch

"Solid" Fruits

All the "solid" fruits are frozen for the best smoothie texture

Pears • cored, roughly chopped

Papayas • seeded, pulp scooped from the skin

Bananas • peeled

Apples • not green (see Note), cored, roughly chopped

Red guava • halved, peeled

Jackfruit • interior flesh only

Coconut meat

Acai

Note: Sweet red apples can function as a "liquid" or "solid" fruit, depending on whether you need liquid to aid in the blending process or want the fiber and texture.

Banana Smoothie

SERVES 2 OR 3

About 4 cups frozen peeled, halved bananas (about 4 large bananas)

About 3 cups juice from a "liquid" fruit (see page 54)

¼ cup soaked and peeled almonds (page 69), blanched almonds, almond cream (page 57), or ground almond solids (from making almond milk, page 69); or 1 scoop unflavored protein powder

I like drinking these banana smoothies in the daytime, as the banana tends to be more binding. My favorite "liquid" fruits for this smoothie are watermelon, honeydew, or unsweetened coconut water.

Place the bananas in the blender with the juice and almonds. (Or you can prepare the juice ahead of time and store in the fridge for up to 24 hours, then quickly blend with the remaining ingredients the next morning.)

Blend until creamy and smooth. If desired, strain through a fine-mesh sieve to remove the tiny banana seeds for easier digestion. Enjoy!

QUICKEST SMOOTHIE

The fastest and simplest smoothie is a banana smoothie made with unsweetened coconut water and blanched almonds. I strain the smoothie for optimal digestion, but you don't have to. This smoothie requires no juicer or other prep ahead of time—perfect for the last minute.

Pear Smoothie

SERVES 2 OR 3

About 4 cups frozen roughly chopped pears (about 3 pears)

About 3 cups juice from "liquid" fruit (see page 54)

¼ cup soaked and peeled almonds (page 69), blanched almonds, almond cream (page 57), or ground almond solids (from making almond milk, page 69); or 1 scoop unflavored protein powder

2 pitted Medjool dates (peeled ideally, see page 57), to taste

My favorite juice for this smoothie is honeydew.

Place the pears in the blender with the juice, almonds, and dates. (Or you can prepare the juice ahead of time and store in the fridge for up to 24 hours, then quickly blend with the remaining ingredients the next morning.)

Blend until smooth. Enjoy!

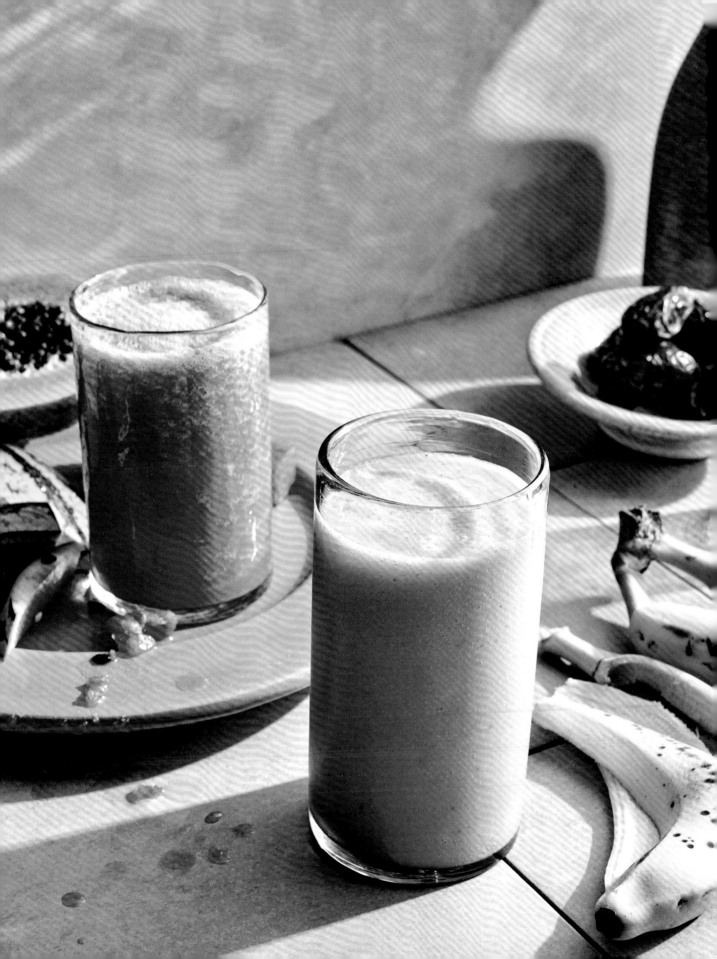

Papaya Smoothie

SERVES 2 OR 3

About 4 cups frozen papaya, peeled, seeds removed

About 3 cups juice from "liquid" fruit (see page 54)

¼ cup soaked and peeled almonds (page 69), blanched almonds, almond cream (page 57), or ground almond solids (from making almond milk, page 69); or 1 scoop unflavored protein powder

1 to 3 pitted Medjool dates (peeled ideally; see below), to taste

This smoothie is best for nighttime, as papayas tend to loosen up your digestion. My favorite juice for this smoothie is watermelon.

Place the papaya in the blender with the juice, almonds, and dates. (Or you can prepare the juice ahead of time and store in the fridge for up to 24 hours, then quickly blend with the remaining ingredients the next morning.)

Blend until smooth. Enjoy!

PEELING DATES

I rehydrate and peel the dates for my smoothies and acai bowls because it makes for a smoother, creamier consistency. To do this, place the dates in a small bowl and cover with warm water to soak for 15 minutes. Drain and then slip off the skins with your fingers. Remove the pit.

You can refrigerate the peeled, pitted dates in a covered glass container for up to 2 weeks, so I prep a bunch at a time so they're ready when I need them.

MAKING ALMOND CREAM

Almonds are vital for my daily smoothies. They add heft, body, and protein, and are what make these smoothies a full meal. (Almond butter, which is made from roasted almonds with their skins, is not a good replacement.)

While you can easily just blend in soaked and peeled almonds, blanched almonds, or leftover almond pulp (from making almond milk) as directed in the recipes, I often make a simple almond cream to keep in the fridge, because it's easy to use and it makes the almonds extra smooth and silky. There are two ways to make almond cream: making it from soaked whole almonds or using leftover ground almonds from making Almond Milk (page 69).

To make almond cream from scratch, soak unpeeled raw almonds in water overnight. In the morning, rinse, peel (discard or compost the peels), and grind the almonds in a blender with just enough filtered water to blend and make a thick paste (texture should be similar to oatmeal).

To make almond cream using remains from almond milk, mix the strained almond pulp with just enough water to make a similarly thick paste. Refrigerate the almond cream in a covered container for up to 4 days.

FRUITS AND DIGESTION

A couple of years ago, I started taking self-defense classes in Florida, and met the Valente Brothers. Born in Brazil and third-generation jiujitsu practitioners, Pedro, Gui, and Joaquim Valente have taught me so much that goes beyond the sport—including how to live a lifestyle that is intentional and thoughtful, centered on health and wellness. One thing that has really stuck with me these last few years is the Valente Brothers' philosophy about consuming food to prioritize gut health. They believe that digesting efficiently helps utilize all the nutrients that food has to offer, so they consider how best to combine foods to achieve that ideal digestion, as well as optimizing how your body will process foods—especially when it comes to fruits.

The Valentes divide fruits into two categories: sweet and acidic. This categorization is not based on the pH value of the fruit prior to eating; instead, it is based on how these two groups of fruits interact with each other and with the body while being digested. Combining acidic fruits—like oranges or blueberries—with other types of food in the same meal can be taxing on the body's

digestion. They recommend eating acidic fruits on their own. But sweet fruits, like melons and bananas, don't conflict with the digestion of other sweet fruits, nuts, or starches. I often combine sweet fruits with each other, sometimes with almonds or granola. That said, ingesting fewer ingredients at the same time always makes it easier for your body to digest everything—which is why I try to keep my smoothie and acai recipes to just a few ingredients. Having followed these guidelines, I can tell you I feel great and my digestion is working better than it ever has!

My favorite way to consume acidic fruits is to cut up a single type, ripe and in season ideally, and enjoy it on its own: a few mangoes, a whole pineapple, a bowl of berries, cut-up citrus, or pomegranate seeds. You can also make fresh juice, like orange or tangerine. Freezing acidic fruit is also delicious: try the Mango "Ice Cream" (page 65) or the Pineapple-Spirulina Pops (page 62). I try not to snack, but if I do, I love frozen green grapes and blueberries, which are so delicious.

Though it's not ideal to mix an acidic fruit with other foods, I occasionally make exceptions (life is about

balance, right?). I love to make strawberry and chia ice pops with coconut water (see page 62), to top Coconut–Chia Seed Pudding (page 80) with frozen blueberries, or to add strawberries to one of my favorite desserts, Coconut Heaven (page 246). Rules are sometimes meant to be broken, as long as they won't hurt anyone!

Here is a list of some sweet and acidic fruits (just my favorites—this is not complete):

Sweet Fruits	Acidic Fruits
Honeydew	Mangoes
Cantaloupe	Pineapples
Watermelon	Oranges
Red apples	Tangerines
Pears	Lemons
Papayas	Limes
Bananas	Strawberries
Red guavas	Raspberries
Jackfruit	Blueberries
Coconuts (both meat and water)	Green apples
	Green grapes
Acai	Pomegranates
Custard apples	Kiwis
	Cherries
	Peaches
	Nectarines
	Plums

Acai Bowls

SERVES 2

About 4 cups fresh papaya (peeled, seeds removed) or peeled bananas

4 or 5 pitted Medjool dates (peeled ideally; see page 57)

6 (3½-ounce) packages unsweetened frozen acai (see Note)

Sliced or chopped sweet fruit, for topping

Granola (page 76 or 79), for topping

An acai bowl is one of my go-to meals—especially a quick lunch. Naturally sweet and semi-frozen, it tastes like a dessert but makes my body feel so energized and fulfilled. Unlike the acai bowls you can get in a shop, this one is not diluted with water or ice, or sweetened with sugar—it's pure fruit. Like my smoothies (pages 55–57), this acai bowl is heavily influenced by the Valente Brothers' digestion philosophy of not mixing acidic fruits with sweet ones (see page 54). Since acai is a sweet fruit, I use only sweet fruits in my acai bowl, like banana or papaya, or my kids' favorite, Red Delicious apples—plus some dates or honey to sweeten. Because I love crunchy things, I often sprinkle granola over the top. Sometimes I cut up more of whatever fruit I'm using in the bowl, or another sweet fruit, and add it on top for more texture. This may seem like a large amount to feed only two people, but remember this is a whole meal—and it takes a lot to fill me up! And if you have any left over, use it to make ice pops (page 62)—so good on a hot day!

Place the papaya and dates in a blender. Blend until smooth.

Rinse the acai packages under running water long enough so the acai releases from the bags. Massage the bags to break up the contents, then cut them open. Add the acai to the blender and blend again until smooth.

Pour the mixture into 2 serving bowls and sprinkle with the fruit and/or granola, if using. Enjoy immediately.

APPLE ACAI BOWL

This is a thinner, lighter acai bowl. Substitute 1½ cups apple juice (from 3 to 5 small Red Delicious apples, or use store-bought organic, unsweetened apple juice) for the papaya. Add 1 to 2 tablespoons honey instead of the dates, then add the acai and blend until smooth. Serve topped with sweet fruit, if desired.

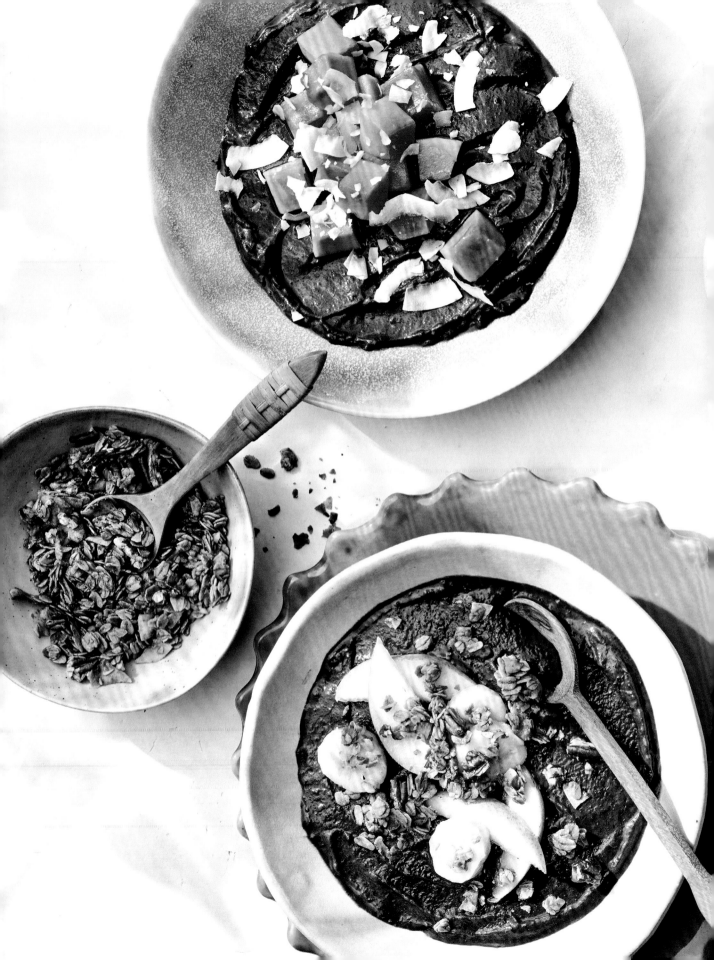

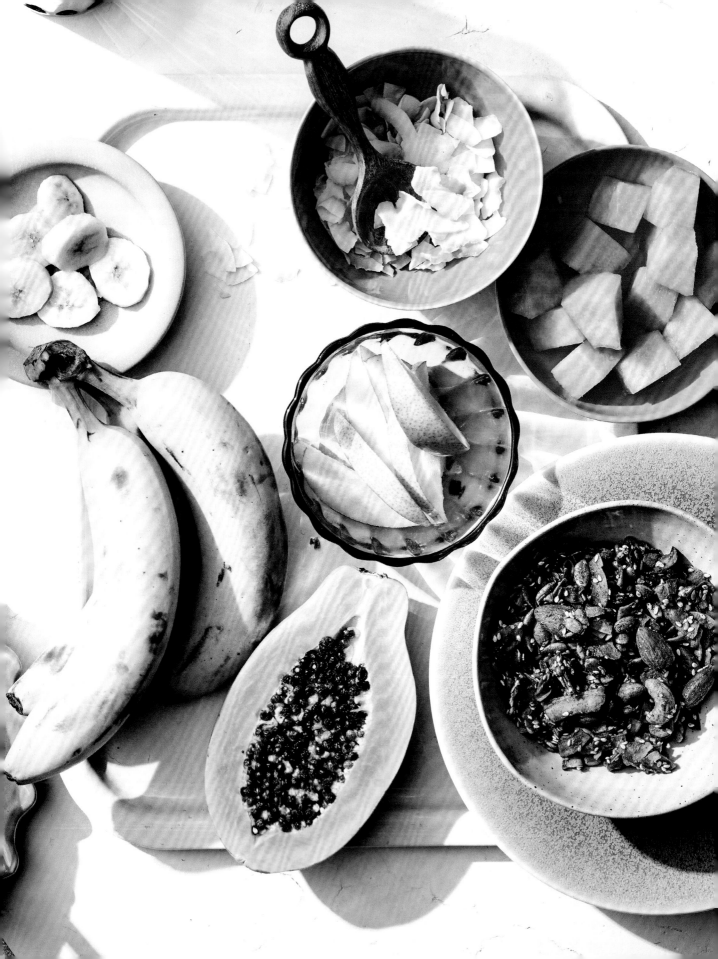

Pineapple-Spirulina Pops

MAKES 6 POPS

½ very ripe pineapple, peeled, cored, and cut into chunks (about 3½ cups), defrosted if frozen

1 tablespoon spirulina powder

2 tablespoons honey or to taste (optional)

Ice pops are the perfect way to capture ripe fruit at its best. Whenever I have ready-to-eat fruit, or even a leftover smoothie or acai bowl, I just turn it into an ice pop! To add extra nutrition to these easy treats, James Kelly, who is an incredible chef, taught me to incorporate superfoods like spirulina (which is full of antioxidants and nutrients, and has anti-inflammatory properties) with sweet juicy pineapple, or to combine chia seeds (full of fiber and omega-3 fatty acids) with strawberry and coconut water (the chia also gives a fun texture). Experiment—it's hard to go wrong!

Place the pineapple and spirulina in a blender and process on high until very smooth. Taste for sweetness; the mixture will be less sweet once frozen, so add honey as needed. Divide the mixture among 6 (3-ounce) silicone ice pop molds. Gently tap the molds on the counter so the filling settles evenly (you don't want air bubbles). Freeze according to the manufacturer's instructions; it will usually take 6 hours. If you have reusable sticks, you can usually insert them right away, but if using wood sticks, you'll want to freeze the mixture for 1 or 2 hours to firm up before inserting them, so that they stay centered in the pops.

Since the silicone molds aren't airtight, remove the pops from the molds once frozen, place between layers of parchment in an airtight container, and store in the freezer. If your popsicle molds form an airtight seal, just leave the pops in the molds until you're ready to eat them.

MORE POPS!

STRAWBERRY-CHIA POPS

Place 2 cups halved fresh strawberries and ½ cup unsweetened coconut water in a blender. Blend until smooth, then taste for sweetness, adding 3 tablespoons honey if desired. Add ¼ cup chia seeds and pulse to distribute. Let sit for 2 minutes so the chia can bloom. Divide and freeze as instructed for the recipe above.

ICE POPS MADE FROM OTHER RECIPES

Filling for Banana Dream Pie (page 247) • Apple Acai Bowl (page 59) • Banana Smoothie (page 55) • Papaya Smoothie (page 57) • Pear Smoothie (page 55).

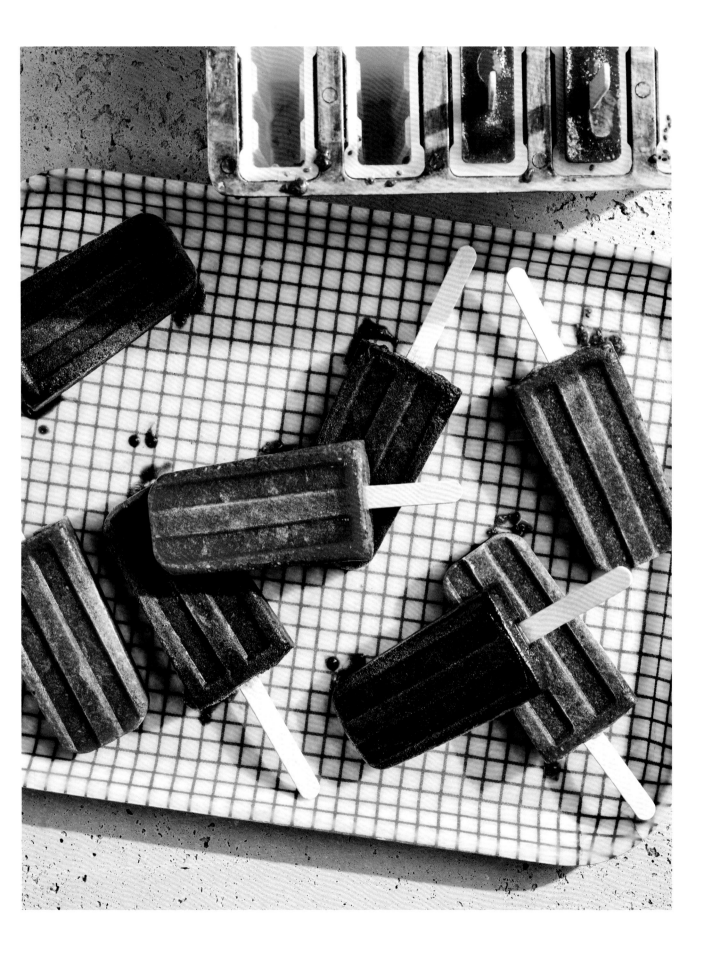

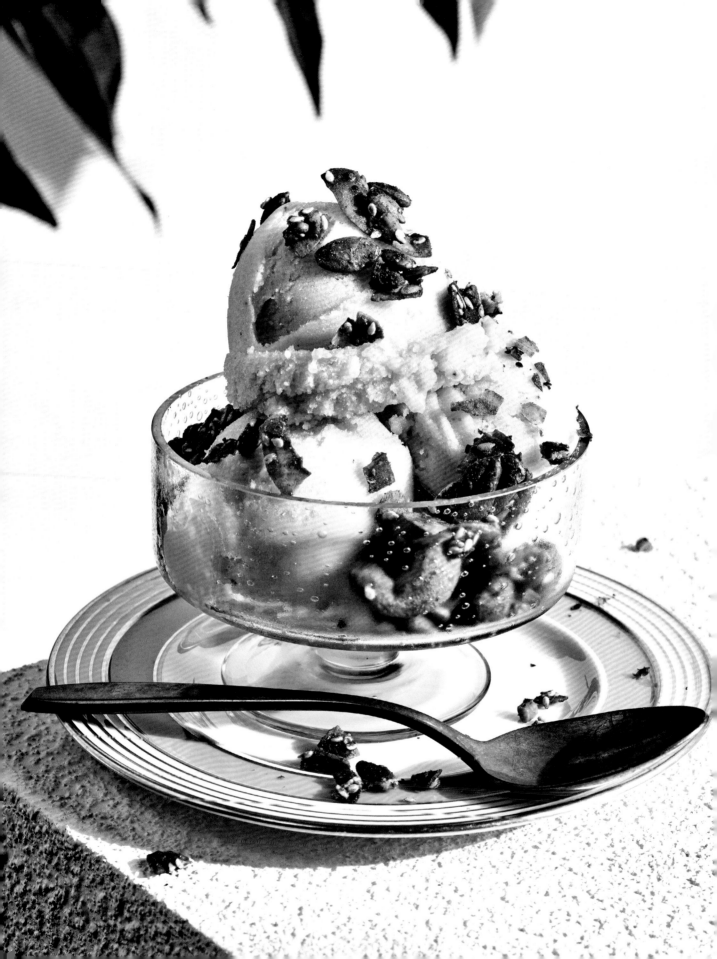

Frozen Banana "Ice Cream"

SERVES 1

2 frozen peeled bananas

Frozen bananas make an amazing ice cream when put through the juicer (or food processor)—the result is naturally sweet and has a smooth texture like soft-serve ice cream. No wonder Benny loves this for dessert (in our house, we usually have sweets as an afternoon treat, not after dinner). Feel free to top this with a sprinkle of granola or coconut chips, or a drizzle of honey and some chopped sweet fruit.

Put the frozen banana through the juicer and enjoy right away! (Alternatively, chop the fruit prior to freezing it, then add it to a food processor and process it until smooth, scraping down the sides as needed; do not overprocess.)

MANGO "ICE CREAM"

Mangoes make delicious ice cream, too. It's even silkier than the banana. Peel and chop a mango and freeze the pieces until hard. Put the frozen mango through the juicer and enjoy right away! (Alternatively, add the mango pieces to a food processor and process until smooth, scraping down the sides as needed.) Because mango is an acidic fruit, I suggest enjoying this plain, not topped with anything.

THE POWER OF PREPARATION

Having a balanced and productive day is always my goal. But I cannot expect my day to always accommodate me. So, I try to prepare ahead of time, to make sure everything runs as smoothly as possible later on. It's why I wake up early to meditate, walk the dogs, and exercise. It's also why I often do some prep for myself and my family at night. When the kids are getting ready for bed, I often listen to an audiobook or my favorite playlist and make juice for a smoothie (pages 55–57), soak some nuts for milk or bread (pages 69–71 or 89), marinate some chicken, and/or prep some raw veggies for the fridge.

In addition to prepping some healthy food, I get a few minutes to listen to what I like (not what my kids want!). Seeing the blender of juice ready to go or the mason jars lined up with delicious wholesome food ready to eat fills me with joy. Everything worthwhile takes effort. That time isn't a task to be dreaded but, rather, a ritual of care, an opportunity to take a few minutes to help my future self. I sleep better knowing I've done everything I can to make my path as smooth as possible the next day.

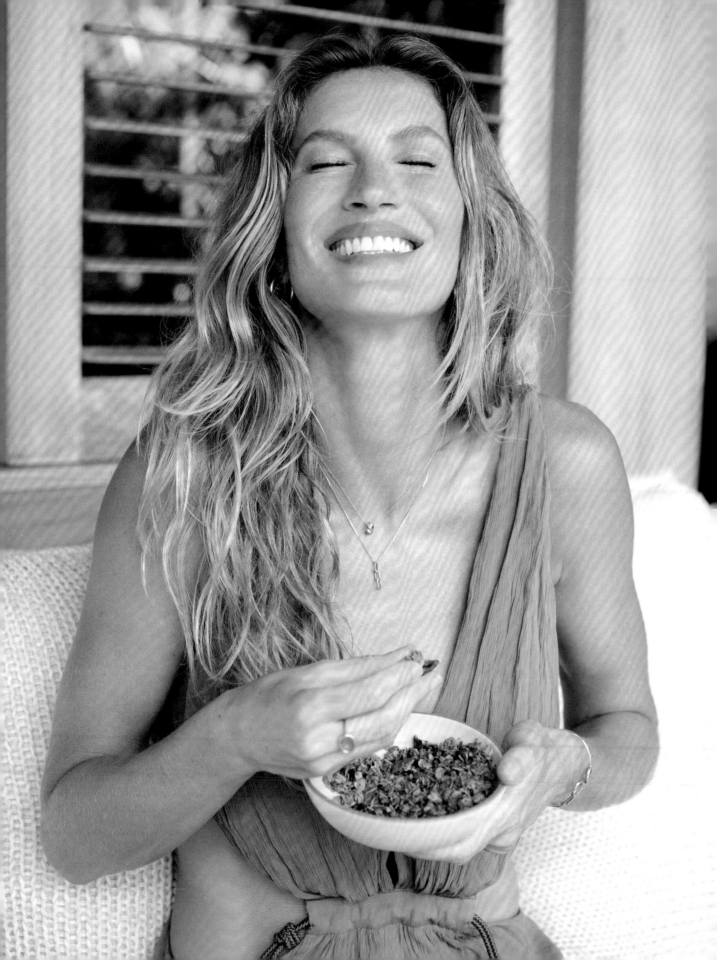

Breakfasts & Breads

———

Depending on what I have planned, breakfast can be as simple as a smoothie, as hearty as an egg and cheese quesadilla, as quick as a chia pudding (in a to-go jar), or as decadent as Sunday waffles with bananas and maple syrup (see page 83). Whatever I choose, it sets the mood for the whole day.

Plant-Based Milks

When I was a vegan in my twenties, I was introduced to a lot of foods I had never tried before. Plant-based milks weren't as popular as they are now; you could really only find them in health food stores. So, I didn't have much experience with milks made from cashews, almonds, or oats. It turns out that conventional, processed dairy was not great for my digestion, and swapping in a nut- or grain-based milk felt a whole lot better for my system.

Now I try to always make my own plant-based milk. Store-bought versions usually include fillers, thickeners, stabilizers, flavorings, and sweeteners that I prefer not to ingest, and homemade ones are easy to make as long as you have a high-power blender (definitely worth the investment!). I like adding dates and/or vanilla to sweeten them sometimes (feel free to use peeled dates from page 57, if you have them around). Note that fresh-made plant milks don't last forever like the store-bought—you should try to drink them within a few days.

Oat Milk

**MAKES APPROXIMATELY
3 CUPS**

1 cup old-fashioned rolled oats
(such as Bob's Red Mill)

4 cups very cold filtered water

2 pitted Medjool dates
or 1 tablespoon pure
maple syrup (optional)

½ teaspoon ground cinnamon
(optional)

½ teaspoon vanilla extract
(optional)

Oat milk is simple to make, but there are a few secrets to making a really good one. High-quality oats have less powdery debris, which makes the milk gummy. Using very cold water and blending the oats only until just blended yields a milk that will not be too viscous. Straining the milk two times through a nut-milk bag also helps create good texture.

This is my favorite milk for tea, and it's delicious with granola, as the oats are naturally a little sweet (plus I add some dates or maple syrup). I love the cinnamon and vanilla for extra flavor, but they can be left out if you want a plain version.

Place the oats, water, dates, cinnamon, and vanilla in a blender and blend on high just until the oats are broken down and smooth, about 30 seconds. Do not overblend.

Place a strainer over a large bowl and fit with a nut-milk bag. Pour the mixture into the bag and gently squeeze to strain out the liquid. (Do not squeeze too hard.) Remove the solids in the bag, then strain the milk a second time through the bag. Pour into a glass container or jar, cover with the lid, and refrigerate for up to 3 days.

Almond Milk

MAKES 2 CUPS

1 cup raw whole almonds

2 cups filtered water

2 or 3 pitted Medjool dates, peeled if you like (see page 57; optional)

½ teaspoon vanilla extract (optional)

Feel free to use blanched almonds instead of whole raw ones, which will save you the steps of soaking and peeling them.

Soak the almonds in a bowl of cold water for 8 hours or overnight.

Drain and rinse the almonds, then slip off the skins and compost them. Add the peeled nuts to a blender along with the filtered water and blend on high until very smooth.

Set a sieve over a medium bowl and line the sieve with a nut-milk bag. Pour the contents of the blender through the bag, collecting the strained milk in the bowl below, then wring the bag to extract as much milk as possible. (See page 71 for tips on how to re-use the nut solids.) Rinse the blender.

Return the strained milk to the blender and add the dates and vanilla, if using. Blend thoroughly on high for about 1 minute. Pour the milk into a glass container or jar, cover with the lid, and refrigerate. Shake before serving, as solids may collect at the bottom. The milk will last in the fridge for up to 3 days.

SKINNING ALMONDS

I find almond skins to be bitter and hard to digest, so I remove them after soaking (which makes the skins so easy to slip off!). Pinching the nuts free of their skins is totally worth the few minutes' work for the clean, buttery taste you get in return. Plus, I find that any repetitive kitchen task is an opportunity to clear my mind and have a moment of quiet reflection— you can think of it as a moving meditation!

THE BENEFITS OF SOAKING NUTS

You'll notice that many of the recipes in this book call for soaking nuts ahead of use. This is important for a few reasons. First, in the case of almonds, soaking allows you to easily remove the skins. Even with nuts that retain their skins after soaking (like walnuts), soaking is incredibly beneficial, as it removes dirt, tannins, and nutrient inhibitors (which protect the nuts from being eaten by insects), making the nutrients of the soaked nuts more accessible to whoever eats them. This soaking process also improves both the texture and the taste; the nuts become more buttery, smoother, and less bitter. For blended applications, as when you're making almond or cashew milk or cashew cream, the soaked nuts grind up much easier, with a more velvety, creamy result.

You'll see a few instances in this book where you can "power soak" the nuts by soaking them in boiling water for 1 hour. This is a good technique when you want to soften a nut for blending (like cashews for sauce), but note it may not be long enough to loosen the skins.

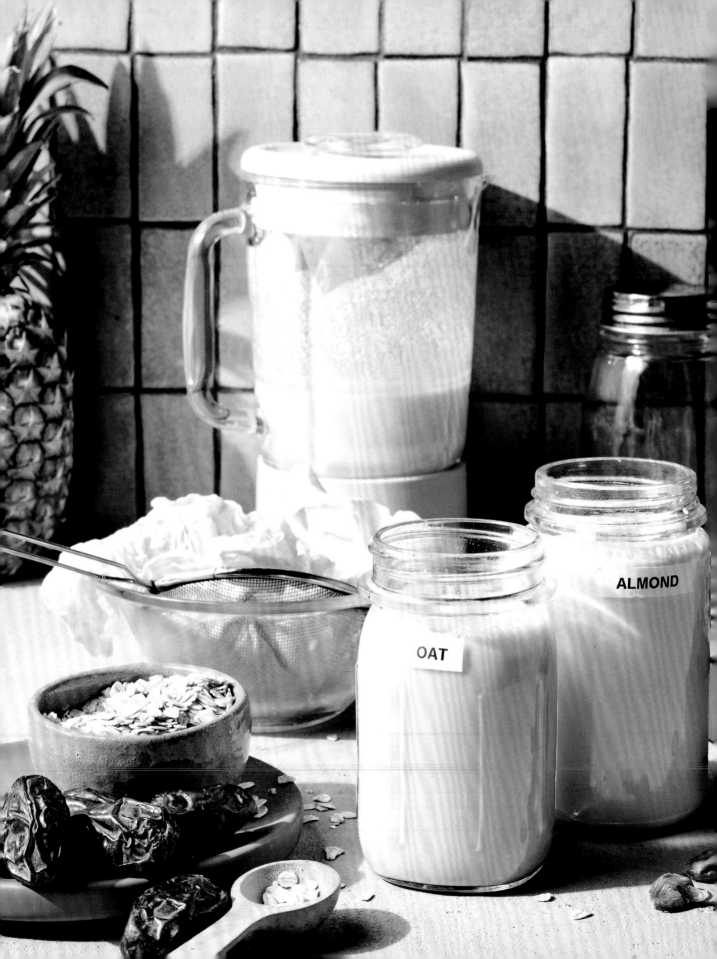

Cashew Milk

MAKES 2 CUPS

1 cup raw whole cashews

2 cups filtered water

2 or 3 pitted Medjool dates, peeled if you like (see page 57; optional)

½ teaspoon vanilla extract (optional)

Soak the cashews in a bowl of cold water for 30 minutes (or up to 24 hours). Drain and rinse the cashews, then place them in a blender and add the filtered water. Blend thoroughly on high until very smooth.

Set a sieve over a medium bowl and line the sieve with a nut-milk bag. Pour the contents of the blender through the bag, collecting the strained milk in the bowl below, then wring the bag to extract as much milk as possible. (See below for ways to reuse the nut milk solids.) Rinse the blender.

Place the strained milk in the blender again, then add the dates and vanilla, if using. Blend thoroughly on high until completely smooth. Pour into a glass container or jar, cover with the lid, and refrigerate. Shake before serving, as solids may collect at the bottom. The milk will last in the fridge for up to 3 days.

USING NUT SOLIDS

Please don't waste the residue from making nut milks! Those finely ground pieces of almonds or cashews are versatile and can boost the nutritional content and taste of whatever you put them in. Here are a few ideas:

Nut and Seed Bread (page 92) · Use ⅓ cup nut solids (what's usually left from making milk) in place of the almond flour.

Smoothies · Nut solids can be added directly to smoothies or see page 57 for how to make almond solids into a simple almond cream.

Seed Crackers (page 218) · Replace the 2 tablespoons almond flour with the same amount of almond solids.

Coconut Milk—Two Ways

In Costa Rica, I drink fresh coconut milk every day because we have coconuts everywhere. (Just blend the coconut water and the scooped coconut meat together.) But it's hard to find very fresh coconuts, and you never know what's inside. So here are two alternatives: make coconut milk with frozen coconut meat or with unsweetened dried coconut. Either way, the results are creamy and delicious. I sometimes mix coconut milk with oat milk—they taste great together.

Frozen Coconut Milk

**MAKES APPROXIMATELY
3 CUPS**

3 cups frozen coconut meat,
preferably defrosted

3 cups warm coconut water
or filtered water

This is a rich coconut milk—you can increase or decrease the liquid if you prefer.

Add the coconut meat and coconut water to a blender. Blend on high for about 1 minute, until completely smooth. Set a sieve over a medium bowl and line the sieve with a nut-milk bag. Pour the contents of the blender through the bag, collecting the strained milk in the bowl. Wring the bag to extract as much milk as possible.

Pour the milk into a glass jar, cover with the lid, and store in the refrigerator for up to 2 days. Shake before serving.

Dried Coconut Milk

MAKES 2 CUPS

1 cup unsweetened dried
coconut

2 cups warm filtered water

2 or 3 pitted Medjool dates,
peeled if you like (see page 57)

½ teaspoon vanilla extract

This is a thinner coconut milk. If you have high-quality coconut water, use that instead of the water.

Place the coconut and water into a blender. Blend on high for about 1 minute, until very smooth.

Set a sieve over a medium bowl and line the sieve with a nut-milk bag. Pour the contents of the blender through the bag, collecting the strained milk in the bowl. Wring the bag to extract as much milk as possible. Rinse the blender.

Return the strained milk to the blender and add the dates and vanilla. Blend on high for 1 minute. Pour into a glass jar, cover with the lid, and store in the refrigerator for up to 3 days. Shake before serving.

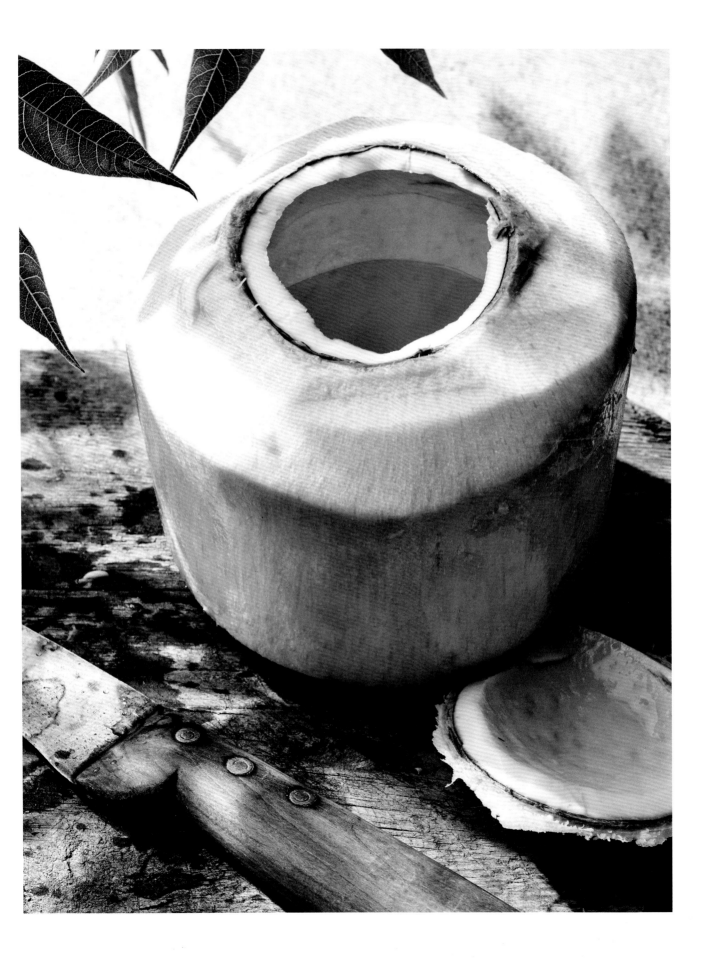

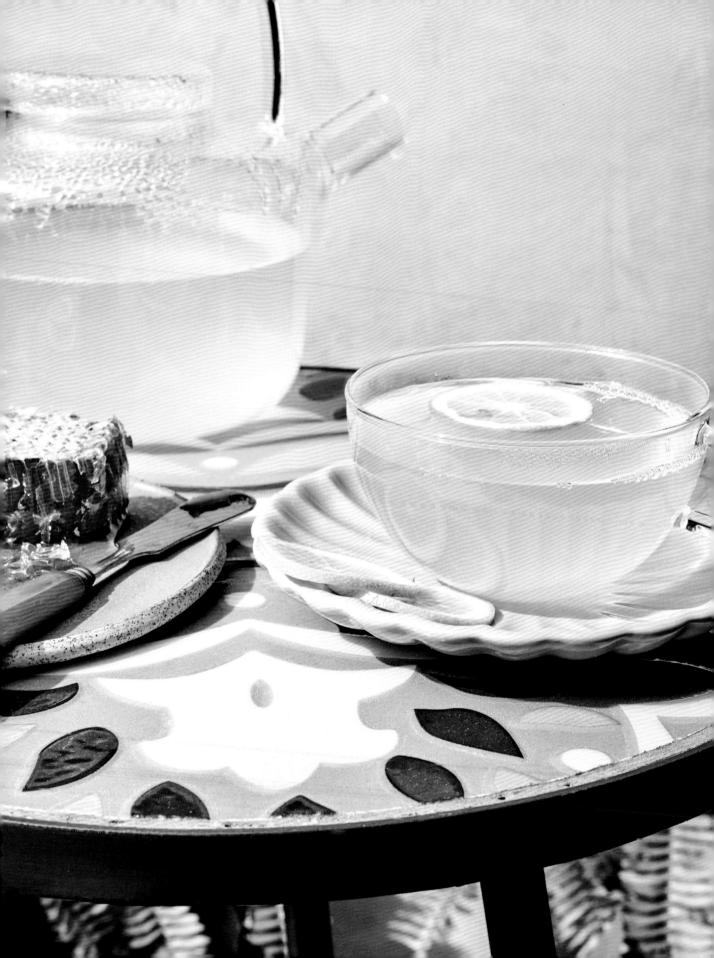

Ginger-Lemon Healing Tea

**MAKES ABOUT
4 SERVINGS**

3 large lemons, scrubbed

1 (2-inch) piece fresh ginger, peeled and finely chopped

6 cups filtered water

Handful of fresh mint (optional)

4 tablespoons honey (manuka is great, if you have it)

We have been drinking this healing tea in our home for years. It's delicious and is the perfect thing to drink when you are feeling sick. The combination of ginger, lemon, and honey is a classic for a reason—it's full of vitamin C and has other immune-boosting properties. You can peel the skin off the ginger using the edge of a spoon or scrape it off with a paring knife. This is great made in real time, or you can make it ahead and freeze it (if so, consider making a double or triple batch).

Using a vegetable peeler or small sharp knife, remove just the outside skin of the lemon (only the yellow part, not the white pith, which is bitter) and add it to a medium saucepan. Halve the lemons and, using a lemon juicer, squeeze the juice into the saucepan. Add the ginger and the water.

Bring the mixture to a boil over medium heat, then turn down to low and simmer for 5 minutes. Turn off the heat, add the mint, if using, cover the pan, and let the tea steep for 5 to 10 minutes.

Strain the tea through a fine-mesh sieve set over a medium bowl; compost the solids. Stir in the honey. Divide the tea among 4 serving mugs and enjoy.

EXERCISING

Body movement is huge in my life. I don't think I could live without it. It's a commitment I feel strongly about, for my mental state as well as the overall health of my body. If I'm short on time, I go for a fast walk with my dog. Even if I get off an overnight flight, I go to the gym in the morning—no excuses. I know I'll feel better afterwards, and that it is best for me in the long term, so I prioritize it.

I feel so different after I've exercised, which is why I build it into my day (multiple times, if I can). I meditate in the morning, I take two 30-minute walks with my dogs (in the morning and evening), and go to the gym on weekdays, where I warm up with 10 minutes of uphill cardio, then do weights or bands. On the weekend, I do more outdoor exercise, often with my kids, like going on the trampoline, kayaking, paddleboarding, and biking. I also love surfing and horseback riding.

Now that I'm in my forties, I've found that it's important to focus on retaining and building muscle mass. If I build strength now, it's like depositing money in the bank for when I'm older. I feel like exercise—and other things I have control over, like diet, rest, and good influences and relationships—is a way of taking responsibility for my body and my life. Through my past experiences with anxiety and depression, I have learned that no one—even my doctors, whom I credit for much of my good health—has as much influence on my well-being as I do. Life is a gift—nurture it!

Grain-Free Granola

MAKES ABOUT 6 CUPS

3 tablespoons melted ghee, unrefined virgin coconut oil, or avocado oil

3 tablespoons pure maple syrup

1 tablespoon coconut sugar

1½ teaspoons ground cinnamon

1 teaspoon ground ginger

½ teaspoon freshly grated nutmeg

½ teaspoon fine sea salt

1 cup mixed whole raw nuts, such as almonds, cashews, walnuts, skinned hazelnuts, or pecans (see Note)

2 cups unsweetened coconut chips

¾ cup raw pepitas (pumpkin seeds)

¾ cup raw sunflower seeds

¼ cup unhulled sesame seeds

2 tablespoons flax seeds

I love granola. If I have it in my kitchen, it's hard to stop myself from eating it. And this granola is my favorite kind: grain free and super crunchy, with clumps of nuts and seeds. (Many thanks to Chef Lukas Volger for creating it with me.) Use any raw nuts you like, including soaked nuts (which is my preference; see page 69), or a mix. The granola is lightly sweetened with maple syrup and coconut sugar, and is heavy on the naturally sweet coconut chips (do not use dried grated coconut). It is easy to make, as all the ingredients come right from the pantry, and it will stay crispy for a week in an airtight mason jar—but good luck keeping it around that long!

Preheat the oven to 300°F. Line a baking sheet with parchment.

In a large bowl, stir together the ghee, maple syrup, coconut sugar, cinnamon, ginger, nutmeg, and salt. Add the nuts, coconut chips, pepitas, sunflower seeds, sesame seeds, and flax seeds and stir until everything is evenly and thoroughly coated.

Spread the mixture evenly onto the baking sheet. Bake, flipping carefully every 15 minutes, until evenly browned and very fragrant, about 45 minutes. (Refrain from stirring too vigorously, as it will break up the delicious clumps!) After 45 minutes, remove a small spoonful or clump of granola and let it cool for 3 or 4 minutes to test that it hardens; if it doesn't, keep baking for another 5 to 10 minutes, then test again.

Let the granola cool completely and then transfer to an airtight container and cover with the lid. Granola will keep crisp for up to 1 week.

Note: If you'd like to use soaked nuts to increase digestibility and other benefits, soak the raw nuts for a few hours or overnight, depending on type, at room temperature in cold water. Drain, rinse, and drain again. Spread out on a baking sheet and bake for 15 to 20 minutes, just until dry to the touch. Let cool, then combine with the remaining ingredients and proceed with the recipe.

MAKE IT YOURS

Light Pairings: Sprinkle the granola on cut-up fruit or serve with a splash of nut or oat milk and a spoon.

Hearty Pairings: Granola makes a great topping for an Acai Bowl (page 58), Coconut–Chia Seed Pudding (page 80), Frozen Banana "Ice Cream" (page 65), or your favorite yogurt and fruit.

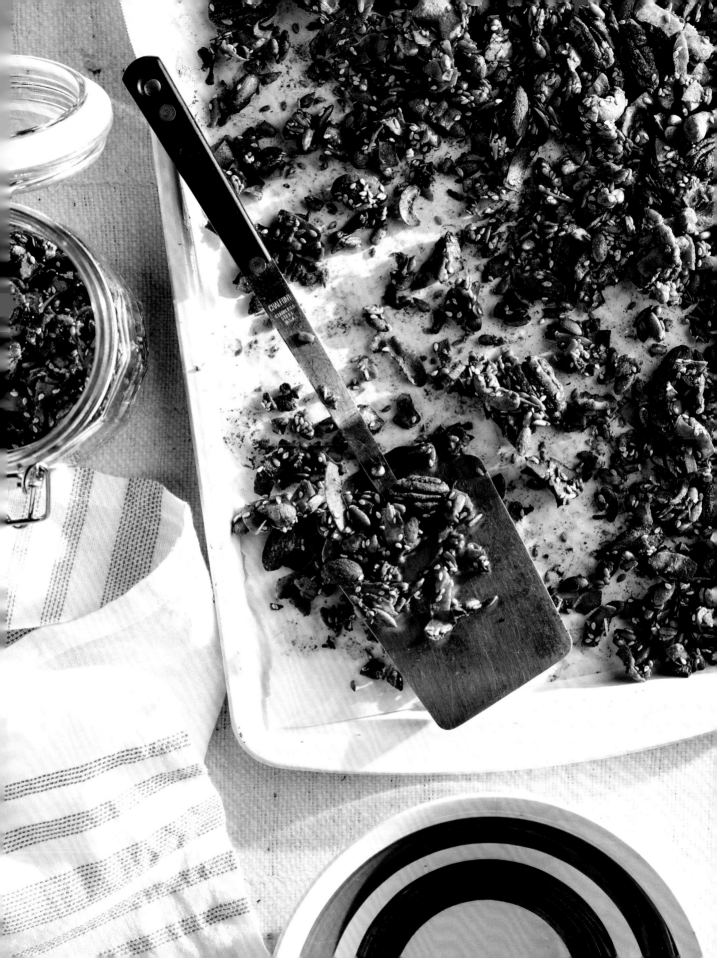

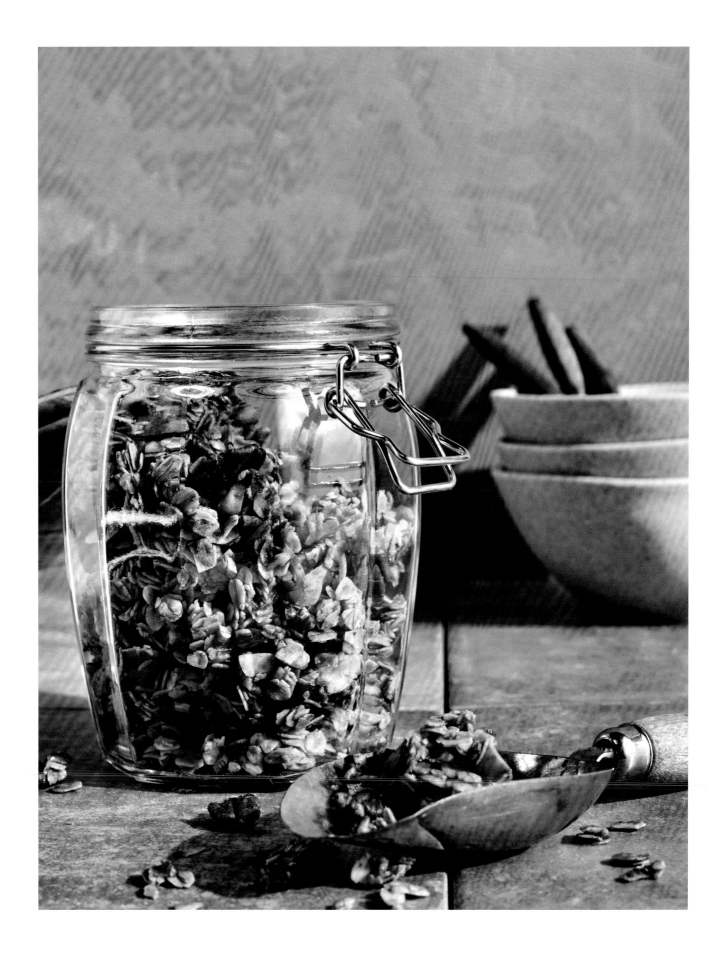

Oat Granola with Pecans

MAKES APPROXIMATELY 6 CUPS

⅔ cup unrefined virgin coconut oil or ghee, plus some for the pan

⅔ cup runny honey

1 teaspoon vanilla extract

1 teaspoon fine sea salt

½ teaspoon ground cinnamon

4 cups old-fashioned rolled oats (gluten free, if necessary)

2 cups raw pecans, chopped

1 cup unsweetened dried coconut

I am so into granola that I had to include a second recipe as well. It's oat-based, flavored simply with honey, vanilla, and cinnamon. It's a little sweet and super crispy—perfect for sprinkling on an Acai Bowl (page 58). I love it because of the pecans, which are so crunchy and rich.

Preheat the oven to 325°F. Line two baking sheets with parchment and very lightly brush with some coconut oil.

In a large bowl, whisk together the coconut oil, honey, vanilla, salt, and cinnamon until well combined. Fold in the oats, pecans, and coconut until everything is evenly coated.

Press the oat mixture into a thin, even layer on the baking sheets. Bake for 15 to 20 minutes, then flip over, using a spatula. If it breaks apart just spread out the mixture and press it again into a thin, even layer. Bake for an additional 15 to 20 minutes, until golden and nicely toasted. Remove from the oven and allow to cool completely.

When the granola is cool, transfer to an airtight container, cover with the lid, and set aside, where it will keep crisp for up to 1 week.

MAKE IT YOURS

For the kids: When the granola has cooled, mix in up to 1 cup of goji berries or other bite-sized dried fruit your kids like.

Coconut–Chia Seed Pudding

SERVES 4 TO 6

1 (13½-ounce) can organic
full-fat coconut milk
or 1¾ cups Coconut Milk
(page 72)

2 tablespoons honey or pure
maple syrup, plus more
for drizzling

1 teaspoon vanilla extract

½ cup chia seeds

Optional toppings

Fresh or frozen blueberries,
raspberries, or strawberries

Slices of banana or mango

Spoonful of cultured coconut
yogurt and coconut chips

The array of health benefits from chia seeds is nothing new. And when I pull one of these rich, creamy puddings out of the fridge (they set overnight—see also the overnight oat variation below), I am just so happy that nutritious food like this can also be so easy and delicious! Naturally gluten free, sweetened only with a little honey or syrup, and flavored with vanilla, these little puddings are so good. Bananas are delicious on top, as are a dollop of coconut yogurt, a drizzle of honey, and a few coconut chips. Though I try not to mix acidic fruits with other foods for ideal digestibility (see page 58 for more on this), I do still love to top these with berries occasionally—I aim to be conscientious with my food choices, but rigidity creates stress. Plus what other breakfast is so high in fiber, is antioxidant rich, can be made ahead, and can be topped so many ways? Let me know if you find one—I'll be eating one of these in the meantime.

In a medium bowl, whisk together the coconut milk, honey, and vanilla. Add the chia seeds and whisk until thoroughly combined.

Divide the pudding among 4 to 6 ramekins or ½-pint jars (if you would like the pudding pre-portioned and/or ready to take on the go) or in a 1-quart glass jar or container. Then cover or seal and refrigerate overnight or up to 3 days (it will thicken the longer it sits).

Eat directly from the ramekins or spoon from the large container into individual bowls to serve. Drizzle with honey or maple syrup, or add other toppings, if you like.

OVERNIGHT OATS

In a medium bowl, combine 2 cups of a plant-based milk (like almond, page 69; cashew, page 71; or coconut, page 72) and 1 cup of old-fashioned rolled oats. Sweeten with ½ teaspoon vanilla extract, if you like. Place in a medium container or divide among 4 ramekins or ½-pint jars. Cover and refrigerate overnight. In the morning, top with some sliced apples, a little ground cinnamon, and a drizzle of honey, if you like. Makes 4 servings.

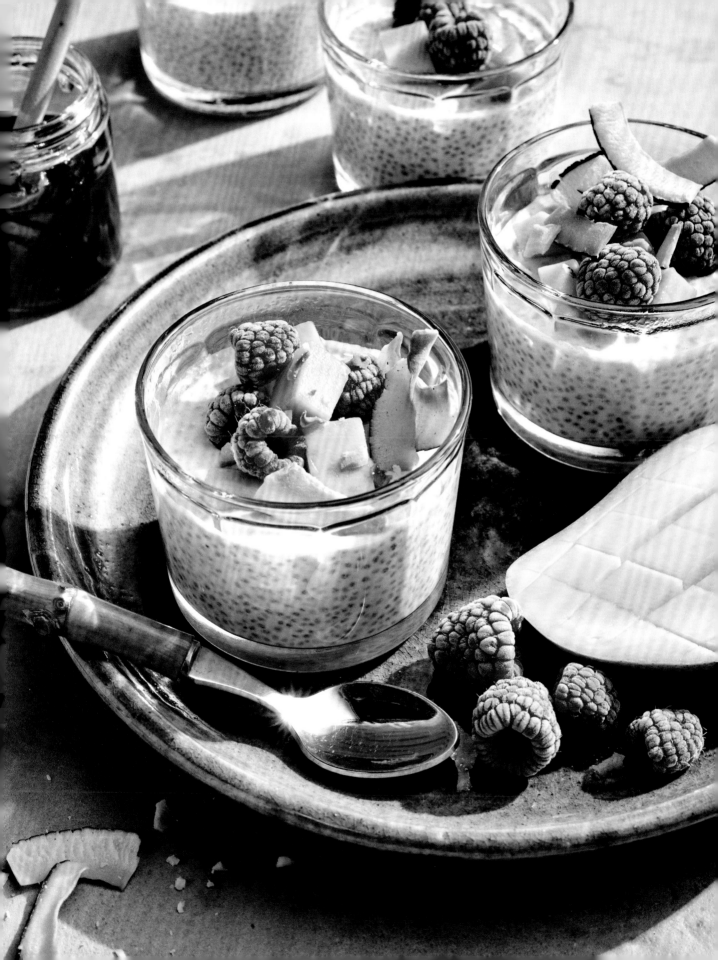

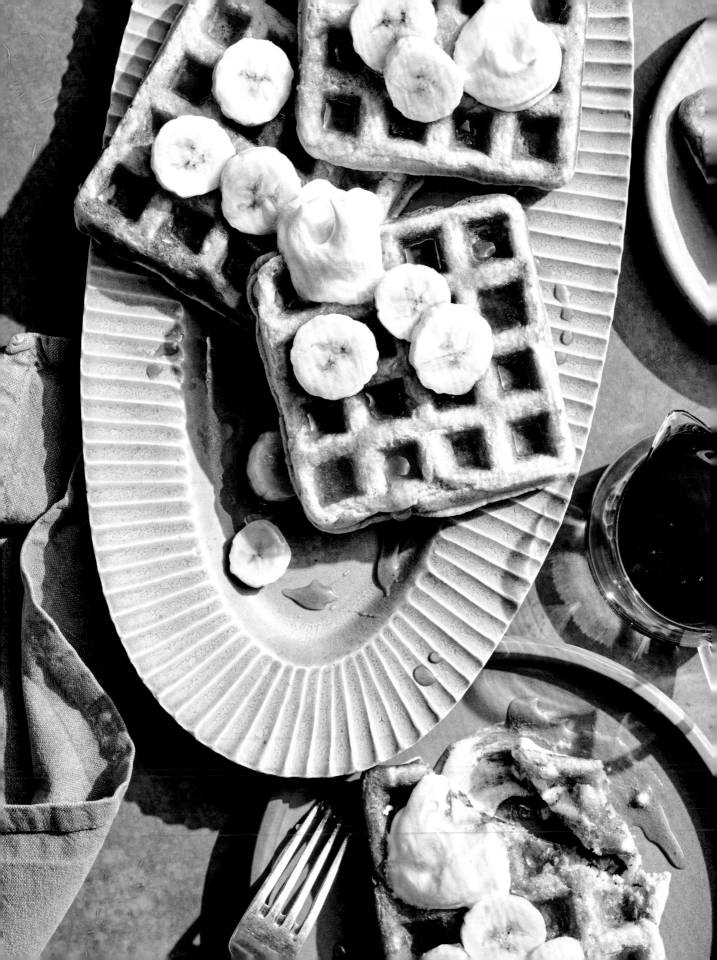

Sunday Banana Waffles

MAKES 8 TO 10 SMALL
WAFFLES

1 ripe banana

½ cup filtered water

2 large eggs

¼ cup pure maple syrup

1 tablespoon flax meal

1½ teaspoons vanilla extract

¾ cup almond flour

¾ cup oat flour

2 tablespoons arrowroot
powder or tapioca flour

1 tablespoon baking powder

Fine sea salt

3 tablespoons melted
unrefined virgin coconut oil,
plus more for greasing

Honey, for serving

TIP: I measure flours by
spooning them into the cup
measure until heaping full, then
leveling with a straight edge.

MORE TOPPING IDEAS

Banana Flambé: Combine
1 sliced banana and 2 to
3 tablespoons maple syrup
in a small skillet, and heat
until just warmed through.
Spoon over the waffles and
top with Coconut Whipped
Cream (page 237).

**Coconut Sugar and
Cinnamon Sprinkle:** Stir
together 3 parts coconut
sugar with 1 part cinnamon
and sprinkle over hot
pancakes.

My kids and I spend a lot of time together on the weekends, and a fun breakfast is always a good way to start the day. Sometimes I make a frittata (see page 87) and sometimes we grab Baru Nut Bars (page 233) to take in the car on our way to an adventure, but more often than not, it's waffles or pancakes we enjoy while still in our pajamas. A mix of healthy flours makes these waffles more nutritious than the usual: my current favorite is a combination of almond flour, oat flour, and flax meal, flavored with banana and vanilla, and with coconut oil for richness and crunch. I like them simply drizzled with honey, but if I'm going all out, I'll do "banana flambé," which in my house doesn't actually include anything set on fire; rather, it's just a warm sauce (maple syrup and sliced bananas), topped with homemade whipped cream. This time with my kids is so special, so I like to treat us to something a bit over the top.

In a medium bowl, use a fork to smash the banana to a paste. Whisk in the water, eggs, maple syrup, flax meal, and vanilla. Set aside for about 5 minutes to allow the flax to hydrate.

Preheat a waffle iron on its hottest setting. Preheat the oven to 250°F. Place an oven-safe wire cooling rack in a sheet pan.

In another medium bowl, combine the almond flour, oat flour, arrowroot powder, baking powder, and a pinch of salt. Add the flour mixture to the egg mixture and stir until just combined. Stir in the coconut oil.

When the waffle iron is hot, brush lightly with a bit of coconut oil and add enough batter to fill the iron (mine takes ¼ cup per waffle). Following manufacturer's directions, cook until waffle is well browned and crisp, usually 4 to 6 minutes (if they are browning too quickly, lower the heat). Transfer the waffle to the rack and set the sheet pan in the warm oven.

Make more waffles with the remaining batter, adding a bit more coconut oil to the iron as needed.

Drizzle the waffles with honey, if you like, and serve.

BANANA PANCAKES

Omit the 3 tablespoons coconut oil from the waffle batter. Warm a large nonstick skillet or griddle over medium heat, and when hot, brush with a bit of coconut oil. Dollop the batter in ¼ cup portions into the skillet without crowding, and cook until well browned, 2 to 4 minutes per side.

Egg and Cheese Quesadilla

SERVES 1

2 large eggs

Fine sea salt

1 teaspoon ghee or avocado oil

¼ cup chopped Roasted Vegetables (page 144; optional)

1 large or 2 small almond, chickpea, or gluten-free flour tortillas

¼ to ⅓ cup grated manchego and/or Midnight Moon cheese

Vivi is so full of energy. She is fast at almost everything she does, but when it comes to eating, she slows down and savors every bite, even when her brother has long been excused and left the table. Eggs are one of her favorite breakfasts—and mine, too (especially if I've lifted weights at the gym that morning). After 8-minute hard-boiled eggs (they are the best!), her second most requested breakfast is this simple, flexible quesadilla. I always use my favorite cheeses—manchego and/or Midnight Moon—which are assertive enough to need only a light scattering. I also add chopped roasted veggies, if I have any left over, especially cauliflower, green beans, and broccoli. This comes together in a single pan in less than 5 minutes, which is nice because I treasure these moments with my girl, sitting around the table. I know she'll speed off soon, so for now we slow down together.

In a small bowl, whisk the eggs with a pinch of salt.

Preheat a medium nonstick sauté pan over medium-low heat. When hot, add the ghee, then pour in the eggs and allow to set for 15 to 30 seconds, then add the veggies, if using. Scramble until the eggs are set but still soft, about 2 minutes. Transfer to a plate. Wipe out the pan.

Return the pan to the heat and add the tortillas. Warm on one side for 10 to 15 seconds, until slightly softened, then flip and scatter the cheese evenly over the surface (you don't need a lot). After less than a minute, scoop the cooked eggs into the center of the tortillas and use a spatula to fold the tortillas over the eggs.

STUFFED QUESADILLA

Omit the eggs and instead scatter the cheese over the warmed tortilla. When it starts to melt, arrange shredded or diced leftover meat and/or roasted vegetables over one half of the tortilla. Fold the other half over the filling and gently compress the quesadilla with a spatula. Carefully flip it over to crisp the tortilla on both sides (some gluten-free tortillas burn quickly, so adjust the heat as needed). When the cheese is melted and the fillings are heated through, transfer the quesadilla to a plate, slice into quarters, and serve.

For the filling, consider Rosemary-Lemon Chicken Paillards (page 197), Grilled Rib Eye (pages 199), or blanched or roasted veggies (see pages 155 and 144).

MAKE IT YOURS

Hearty Pairings: Add crumbled cooked turkey bacon to the egg mixture prior to cooking; or serve some roasted potatoes on the side. (I like to heat them in the air-fryer until they're extra crispy, sprinkled with some finely chopped rosemary.)

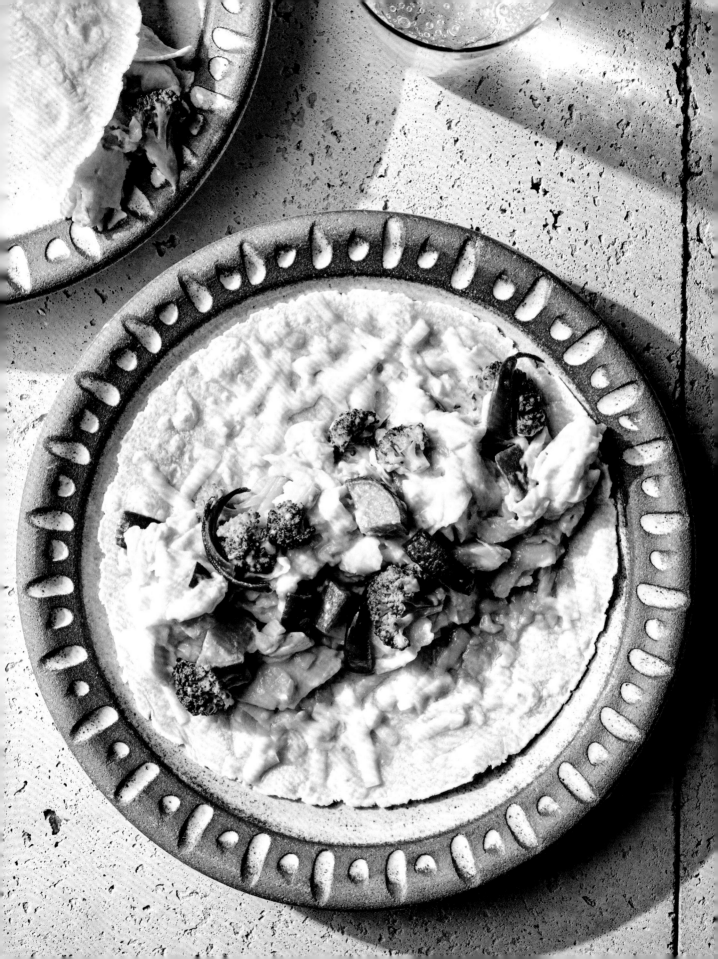

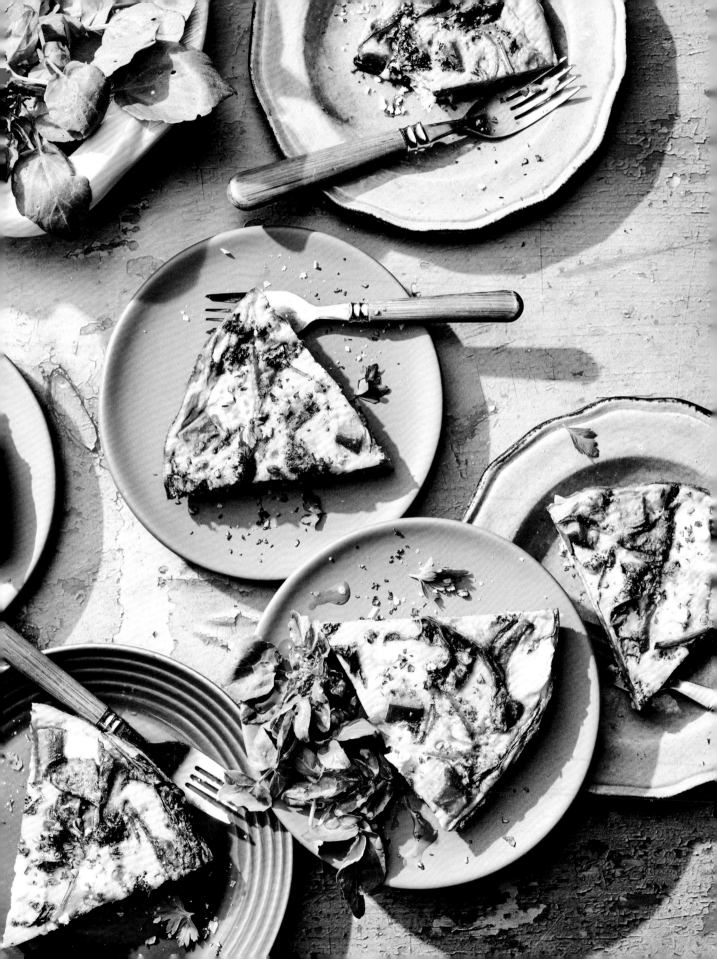

Veggie Frittata

SERVES 4 TO 6

4 teaspoons melted ghee
or avocado oil

About 5 cups trimmed and
chopped fresh greens, such as
kale or spinach

Fine sea salt

8 large eggs

½ medium white or red onion,
diced or sliced; or 1 bunch
scallions, white and light green
parts diced or sliced

1½ to 2 cups chopped roasted
or blanched vegetables
(see pages 144 and 155)

¼ cup crumbled soft goat
cheese or shavings of hard
goat cheese (optional)

I keep glass containers or mason jars of blanched vegetables, roasted vegetables, and herbs in my fridge all the time. That way, I always have veggies ready to eat as is or to use for a quick meal. Here, I take some of those veggies (such as sweet potatoes, winter squash, cauliflower, broccoli, zucchini, green beans, and/or peas) and add them to beaten eggs to make the simplest anytime dish: a frittata. I make this for friends who come for brunch or keep it handy in my fridge for easy lunches. Benny and Vivi especially love the muffin version (see page 88), which is also great when you are in a rush and need to grab and go.

Preheat the oven to 350°F.

Place a 10-inch oven-safe nonstick skillet or a seasoned cast-iron skillet on medium heat. When hot, add 1 teaspoon of ghee, then add the greens and a pinch of salt. Sauté until softened and wilted, stirring often, then transfer to a plate to cool somewhat. When cool enough to handle, give the greens a gentle squeeze to extract any excess liquid, then coarsely chop them on a cutting board.

In a medium bowl, whisk together the eggs and ¼ teaspoon salt.

Return the skillet to medium heat and swirl in the remaining 3 teaspoons ghee, followed by the onion and a big pinch of salt. Cook until the onions are soft and translucent, 4 to 7 minutes (or until they begin to caramelize and get jammy, another 10 minutes). Stir in the roasted or blanched vegetables to warm them, followed by the sautéed greens.

(recipe continues)

MAKE IT YOURS

Light Pairings: Top with Chimichurri (page 224) or Pesto (page 224), or serve with any green salad.

Hearty Pairings: Sliced Chicken Meatballs (page 194) or plain zucchini noodles would be great added to the pan prior to adding the eggs. Eat alongside Warm Wild Rice Salad (page 116) or Beet and Arugula Salad (page 105).

Simple Swaps: Chopped Favorite Sautéed Leafy Greens (page 152) can replace the raw greens—just add along with the roasted vegetables.

Pour the eggs over the mixture, scraping out every last bit from the bowl. Without stirring, allow the eggs to set in the bottom to the sides of the pan. Then, after a minute or so, use a flexible spatula to lift the edges of the eggs, gently tilting the pan to allow any uncooked egg to flow underneath. Repeat until the edges of the frittata are mostly set, 3 to 5 minutes. Gently nudge the fillings so they're evenly distributed, then scatter the cheese over the surface, if using.

Transfer the skillet to the oven and bake until the top is firm and the frittata is just set in the center, 12 minutes. Allow to cool for about 10 minutes in the pan (which will make it release more easily), then slide onto a cutting board or plate to slice into wedges. Serve hot, warm, or at room temperature. (Stored in an airtight glass container, the frittata will keep for up to 3 days.)

FRITTATA WRAP

Tuck a slice of frittata into a cauliflower or almond tortilla or another gluten-free wrap, or even a couple leaves of Bibb lettuce. Add shredded cabbage or Simple Cabbage Slaw (page 101), and a drizzle of the sauce of your choice (I love Cashew Ranch, page 227).

FRITTATA MUFFINS

Brush the cups of a muffin tin lightly with oil and fit with liners (the oil is just a bit of insurance in case the filling spills over). Prepare the filling as described, but instead of adding the eggs, divide the vegetables among the muffin cups. Then transfer the beaten eggs into a tall measuring glass with a spout and carefully pour over the fillings, up to about ½ inch from the rim. Bake for 20 to 25 minutes, until puffed slightly and set. Serve warm or at room temperature.

Brazilian Cheese Bread
(Pão de Queijo)

MAKES ABOUT 16 ROLLS

2 cups tapioca starch

1 teaspoon fine sea salt

¼ cup unsweetened milk of choice

¼ cup avocado oil or ghee

1 large egg, beaten

1½ cups coarsely grated Parmesan

½ cup grated or crumbled soft cheese, like Gruyère

About ⅓ cup Requeijão, Catupiry, or soft goat cheese, for stuffing (optional)

When I was a 15-year-old model living on my own in São Paulo, I was hungry all the time. Not for the reason one might expect in my industry—dieting—but because I had a strong metabolism and absolutely no money to spare for extra food. Lucky for me, a few fancy restaurants in town had deals with modeling agencies to hold a prominent table for models and feed whoever showed up for free. I just had to call my agent in the morning, and they would put me on the list. So you better believe that's what I did most days.

The first thing those restaurants did was bring over a basket full of hot pão de queijo. I knew about this traditional, naturally gluten-free bread—chewy on the inside and crisp on the outside—from birthday parties and other special occasions when I was growing up, but at these restaurants, the cheese bread was even fancier and was stuffed with creamy, flavorful Brazilian cream cheese like Requeijão or Catupiry. It was so delicious I would eat baskets full (endless refills!) and would barely have room to eat anything else. Now, I love to make pão de queijo for special occasions because my kids love it as much as I do.

These are best hot out of the oven; they are not nearly as good cold or the next day. So I usually make the full recipe but freeze half, unbaked, for another time; see the Note following.

Preheat the oven to 375°F. Line a baking sheet with parchment.

In a large bowl, stir together the tapioca starch and salt.

In a small saucepan, combine the milk and oil. Bring to a simmer over medium heat, then pour over the tapioca. Use a sturdy spoon or spatula to combine—the mixture will be dry and will almost look like cheese curds; it won't be smooth. Allow to cool for about 5 minutes.

Add the egg, Parmesan, and grated soft cheese to the milk mixture. Stir a few times with a spoon to distribute, then switch to your hands and knead the dough right in the bowl for 2 to 3 minutes, until a soft, smooth, and barely sticky dough forms.

(recipe continues)

Use your hands to roll the dough into approximately 16 smooth balls. If you want to stuff the balls, flatten each one into a disc in your palm, then place a heaping ½ teaspoon (or more!) of the Requeijão cheese in the center. Wrap the dough around the cheese, pinch the edges to close completely, and reroll into a smooth ball.

Arrange the dough balls, stuffed or plain, on the baking sheet, spacing them 1 inch apart. Bake on the middle rack until puffed on top and lightly browned on the bottom, 20 to 25 minutes, rotating the pan halfway through. Serve immediately.

Note: The unbaked dough balls can be frozen and baked later. Quick-freeze them on a sheet pan for about 30 minutes, then transfer to an airtight container. There's no need to thaw before baking; just place the frozen dough balls on a parchment-lined baking sheet and add 5 minutes to the baking time.

MINDFULNESS WHILE WORKING OUT

I try to bring my focus and full attention to whatever it is I am doing, from a conversation with a friend, to being a parent, to my work, to organizing my pantry. It's just how I am—and exercise is no exception. Being fully present while working out means that instead of getting lost in the number of reps or trying to distract myself, I lean into the impact and purpose of every exercise. I focus on my breath and on every muscle: What can I contract tighter? Extend further? Hold even one second longer? Can I adjust my form to be better? Can I use my breath better to help give me more fuel? Of course, this is not always easy, but it's what I strive for. Aiming high is a mindset that helps make the absolute most of every moment. We are not guaranteed another day, so I want this one— and every minute—to count.

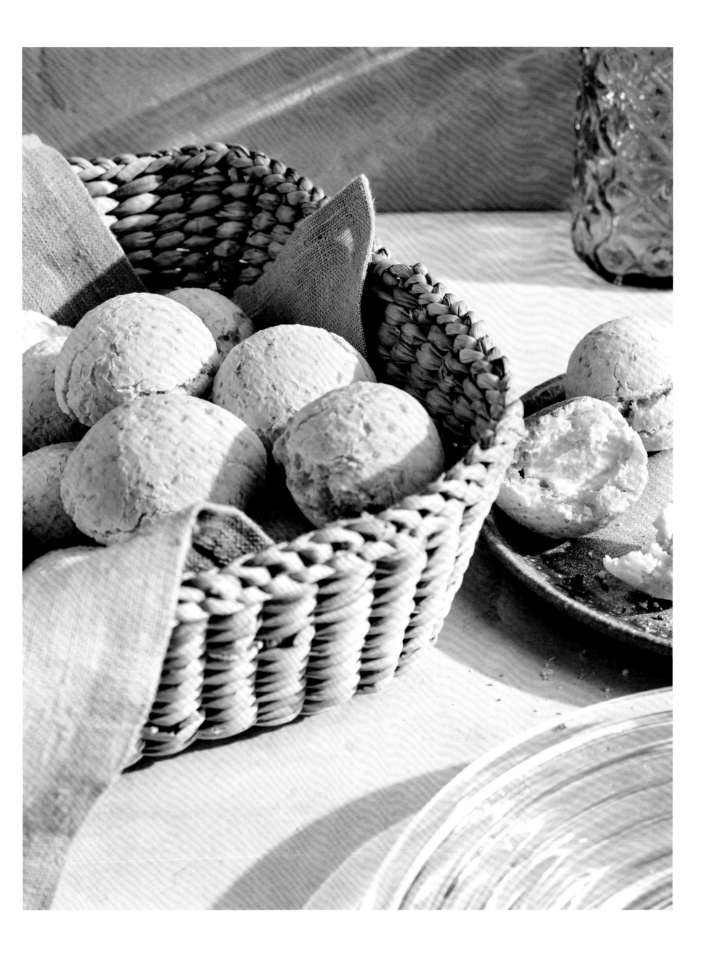

Nut and Seed Bread

MAKES 1 LOAF

3 tablespoons melted unrefined virgin coconut oil, ghee, or avocado oil, plus some for the pan

½ cup flax meal

¼ cup unhulled raw sesame seeds

2 tablespoons chia seeds

½ cup shelled raw sunflower seeds

½ cup shelled raw pumpkin seeds

½ cup raw walnuts, almonds, or skinned hazelnuts

¾ cup old-fashioned rolled oats (gluten free, if necessary)

¾ cup almond flour or ⅓ cup residual nut solids from making almond milk (page 69)

1 tablespoon psyllium husk powder

1 teaspoon fine sea salt

1½ cups unsweetened coconut water or filtered water

2 teaspoons honey or pure maple syrup

Why is bread so yummy? I love to dip it in olive oil, spread it with good butter, or dip a crusty chunk into soup. But as we know, most commercial bread is pretty devoid of nutrition; even the gluten-free type includes fillers and preservatives I'd rather not consume. Here I was influenced by Sarah Britton, of the My New Roots blog, who makes amazing gluten-free bread. This recipe satisfies my craving and is also nourishing and extra delicious. All you do to make it is stir together the various raw nuts and seeds (some of which need to be cracked in the blender), oats, and psyllium husk powder into your chosen liquid, let it hydrate for a few hours, then bake. A bit of almond flour gives the mix a more bready texture, but you can replace it with the ⅓ cup of almond pulp that remains from making a batch of Almond Milk (page 69).

While the bread doesn't rise (there's no yeast or baking powder), it does bake up dense, almost like a traditional dark rye. Thinly sliced and toasted until a little crunchy, it makes a yummy base that is delicious with avocado or nearly any other topping you can think of. Or, make croutons by cutting a slice into cubes, drizzling them with a little olive oil and salt, and baking until crisp.

Brush an 8½ by 4½-inch loaf pan with a little coconut oil, then line with parchment, with the 2 ends hanging over the longer sides of the pan like a sling. Brush the parchment with a little oil.

Place the flax meal, sesame seeds, and chia seeds in a blender and blend until a coarse powder. Transfer to a medium bowl and add the sunflower seeds, pumpkin seeds, nuts, and oats. Stir in the almond flour, psyllium husk powder, and salt. Stir well to distribute the psyllium evenly.

In a tall measuring glass, whisk together the coconut water, 3 tablespoons coconut oil, and honey, then pour over the dry ingredients. Stir thoroughly with a spatula—the mixture will be thick, and it will continue to thicken as you stir. Let stand for about 5 minutes to further thicken.

Scrape the batter into the loaf pan, packing it in tightly and compressing it into a dense, even layer with a flat, smooth surface. Drape a clean towel over the pan and allow to rest at room temperature for at least 6 hours, or overnight.

Preheat the oven to 350°F.

Bake the bread in the center of the oven for 60 to 70 minutes, until a tester inserted into the center comes out clean and the loaf sounds hollow when the top is tapped. Remove from the oven and run a thin knife or offset spatula along the edges of the loaf to loosen it from the pan, then lift out the bread, using the parchment overhang; let cool completely on a wire rack. (If the top surface of the bread remains raw, remove the loaf from the pan and place upside-down directly on the rack of the oven, and continue cooking until just cooked through.)

Wrapped in parchment or a reusable waxed food storage cloth the loaf will keep for about 5 days in the refrigerator. Or thinly slice, wrap in parchment or a waxed cloth, place in a zippered freezer bag, and keep in the freezer for about 2 months.

TOPPINGS FOR NUT AND SEED BREAD

Thinly sliced avocado, a fried egg, microgreens, and salt to taste, served with a simple green salad

Soft goat cheese with a drizzle of extra-virgin olive oil

Mashed avocado, a bit of salt, and extra-virgin olive oil

Your favorite nut butter and a drizzle of honey

A scoop of Tuna Salad with Olives (page 112)

A few thin slices of Veggie Frittata (page 87)

Hummus (page 180) and sliced cucumbers or microgreens

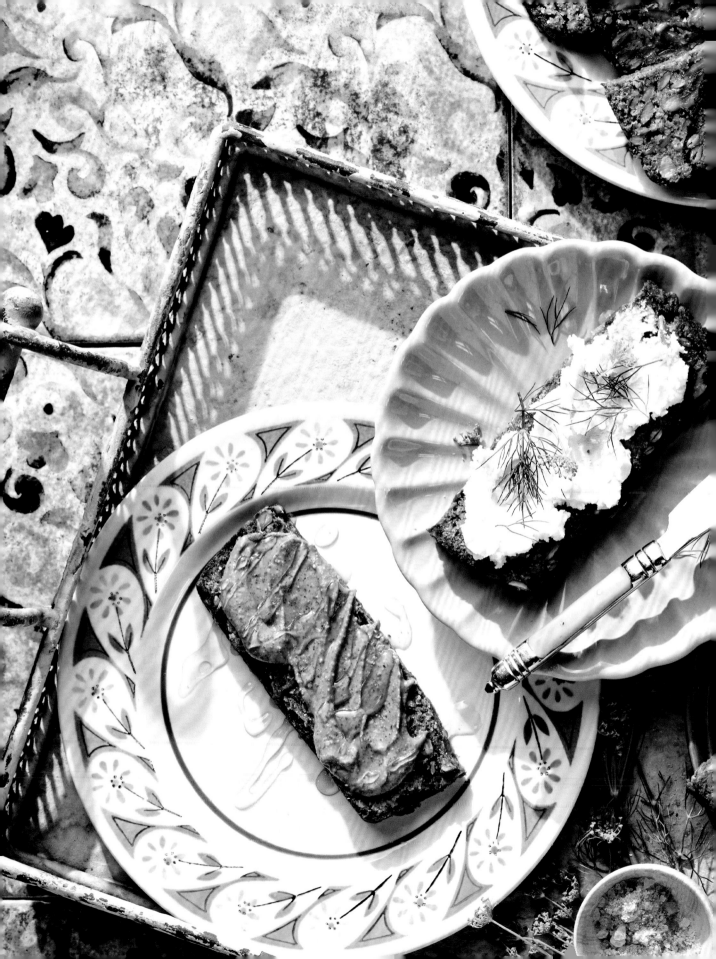

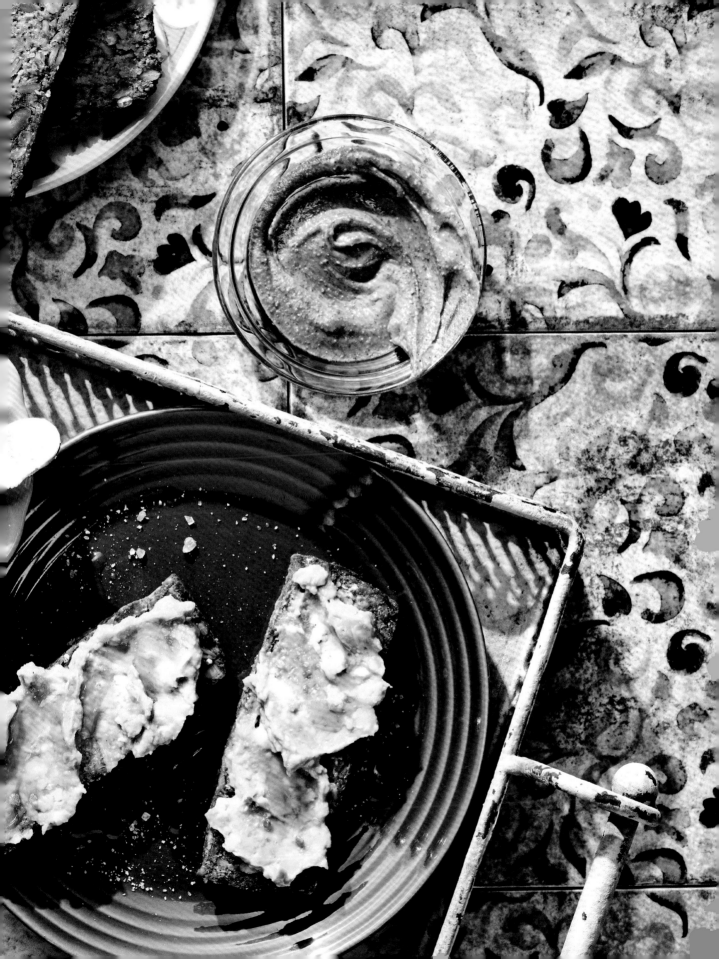

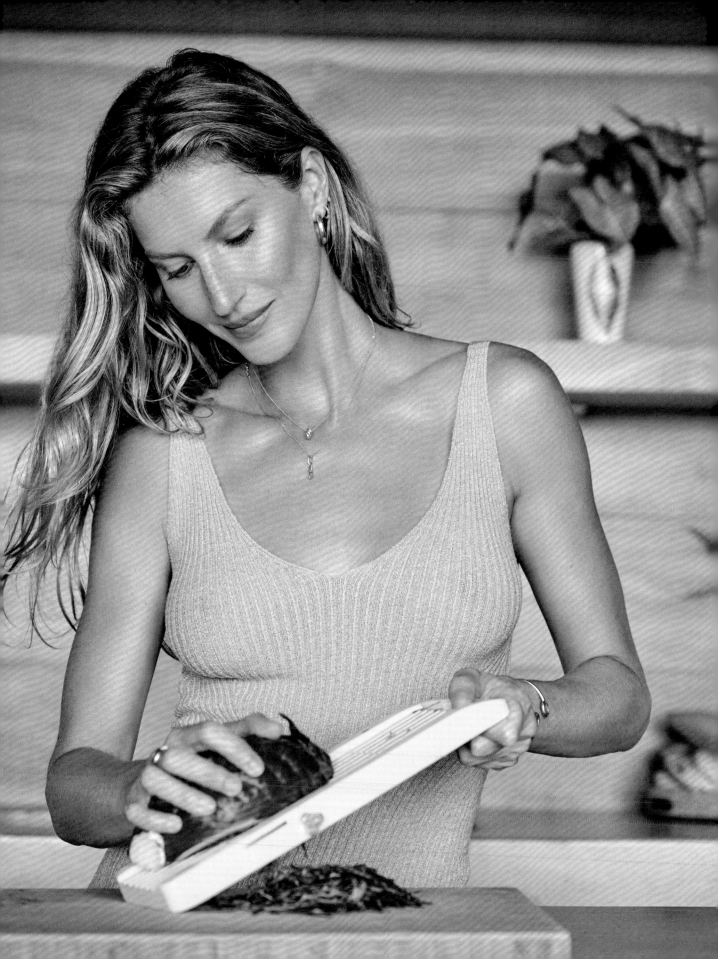

Salads

My favorite salads are simple, mostly raw dishes that focus on seasonal vegetables and proteins. They are nutritious, fast, and flexible. I love them for their natural crunch, of course, but most of all for how they make my body feel.

Hearts of Palm, Avocado, and Cucumber Salad

SERVES 2 TO 4

1 medium English cucumber, chopped

1 avocado, peeled, seeded, and sliced

1 (14-ounce) jar hearts of palm, rinsed and drained, sliced

1 lemon, halved

3 tablespoons extra-virgin olive oil

½ teaspoon fine sea salt, or more as needed

Canned hearts of palm, which are popular in Brazil and other parts of South America, make this otherwise super-simple salad a bit more dynamic. It is all about the textures: the soft bite of the hearts of palm, the creaminess of the avocado, and the crunch of the cucumber. Lemon, olive oil, and a pinch of salt finish it—so easy. It is the ideal side dish for a barbeque, as it goes well with any grilled protein, or just pile it on top of some lettuces and add a sprinkle of toasted pine nuts for a quick, elegant lunch.

Place the cucumbers, avocados, and hearts of palm in a large bowl. Squeeze half of the lemon over the vegetables, drizzle with the olive oil, and sprinkle with the salt, then gently toss. Taste, adding additional salt and lemon juice as needed.

MAKE IT YOURS

Hearty Pairings: Serve with any grilled meats or fish. Or, pile into a gluten-free wrap with a couple of Vegetable-Quinoa Cakes (page 159). Top with Rosemary Almonds (page 210) or toasted pine nuts for some protein, if you like.

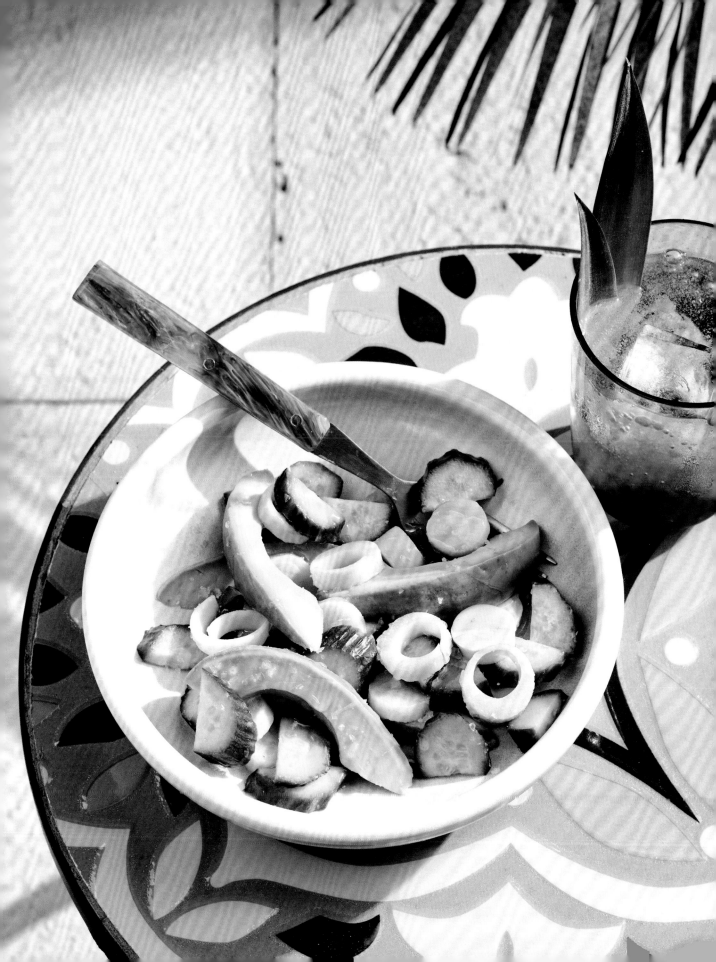

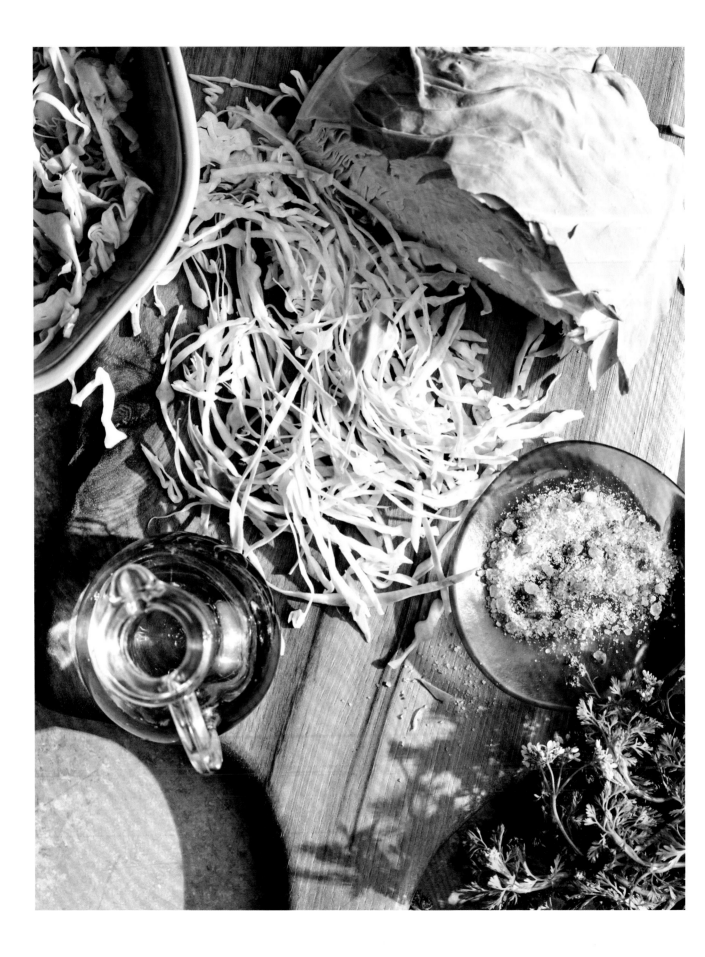

Simple Cabbage Slaw

SERVES 4

½ green cabbage,
finely shredded on a
mandoline (or thinly sliced)

4 teaspoons apple cider
vinegar

½ teaspoon fine sea salt, plus
more as needed

½ cup coarsely chopped
fresh cilantro or parsley
(optional)

You might be tempted to make this salad more complicated, but I recommend making it this way first—simple and pure. If you treat your ingredients well, they taste better, so shred the cabbage with a mandoline, if you have one, for uniform thickness. Then dress the slaw with the vinegar and salt (I don't even add oil!), and taste along the way—we have different preferences, so add more or less of each until it's just the way you like.

Freshly made, this salad is crisp and snappy; if it sits in the bowl for a few minutes, it will start to wilt—it's delicious either way.

In a large bowl, toss the cabbage with the vinegar and ½ teaspoon salt. Season to taste with additional salt, if desired. Just before serving, add the cilantro, if you like.

CHANGING AFTER ANXIETY

After I learned how to deal with my anxiety by changing my mindset and diet, I was left with a big question: How do I meet life's daily challenges in a positive and healthy way?

As mentioned elsewhere, I focused my energy on learning to observe my body and my mind. I invested in establishing positive practices: eating well, getting enough sleep, and journaling, for example. My moving meditation also helps me become more mindful of my physical and mental state. Exercise helps me relieve stress and makes me feel strong.

In short, my attitude changed. I thought less about what I had to do and more about the opportunities I had, every day, to make my life better. I now realize that every day is a gift. Good health is a gift.

MAKE IT YOURS

Hearty Pairings: Pile this slaw onto tacos (see page 202) or serve on the side of a stuffed quesadilla with chicken (see page 84), or in a bowl with Pan-Fried Falafel (page 177) and some Roasted Vegetables (page 144).

For the Kids: My kids love this with mandoline-sliced cucumbers instead of cabbage—delicious!

Simple Swap: Feel free to use different herbs or different varieties of cabbage, or swap out the vinegar for fresh lemon or lime juice.

Benny's Shaved Salad

SERVES 2 TO 4

1 small head of broccoli, including stalk

Fine sea salt

4 ounces fresh green beans, trimmed and cut into bite-size pieces (about 1½ cups)

1 tablespoon fine sea salt, or more as needed

½ green cabbage

½ to 1 cup chopped or sliced cooked chicken (such as from Rosemary-Lemon Chicken Paillards, page 197; optional)

⅓ cup Tamari Dressing (page 228) or Cilantro-Mint Dressing (page 221), or more as needed

½ cup coarsely chopped roasted cashews

½ cup Crispy Roasted Shiitake Mushrooms (page 214; optional)

¼ cup coarsely chopped fresh cilantro

My son, Benny, has always loved vegetables, and this nutrient-packed salad is one of his favorites. He loves the salty, delicious tamari dressing, but also the mix of textures: thin shreds of raw cabbage, crunchy bites of blanched broccoli and green beans, crispy roasted shiitakes, and chopped roasted cashews. Every bite feels and tastes different—so even if you are a 14-going-on-20-year-old boy, you'll never get bored.

This salad is also a great vehicle for any lingering vegetable odds and ends in your fridge—shaved celery, Brussels sprouts, carrots or radishes, or shredded spinach or arugula are all delicious additions.

Trim the broccoli, cutting small florets off the stalk. Use a vegetable peeler to remove the tough peel from the stalk, then thinly slice it.

Make an ice bath by filling a large bowl with ice cubes and water. Bring a saucepan of water to a boil. Season with 1 tablespoon salt, then add the broccoli and the green beans and blanch until bright green, about 1 minute—there should be plenty of crunch left. Using a slotted spoon or spider, transfer the vegetables to the ice bath. When they have cooled, drain them and blot dry.

Slice the cabbage in half through the core and remove the core. Working with one wedge at a time, carefully shave it into thin wisps, using a sharp chef's knife or a mandoline.

Place the cabbage shreds in a large bowl. Add the broccoli and beans, and the chicken (if using) until combined. Drizzle with the dressing.

Just before serving, taste and add a bit more dressing or salt to taste, then add the cashews, shiitakes (if using), and cilantro. Toss again and serve.

MAKE IT YOURS

Simple Swaps: Use 2 to 3 cups of blanched vegetables (see page 155) in place of the broccoli and green beans; replace the green cabbage with red cabbage or savoy cabbage; add a handful of thinly shaved raw brussels sprouts, carrots, or celery; swap in roasted almonds for the cashews.

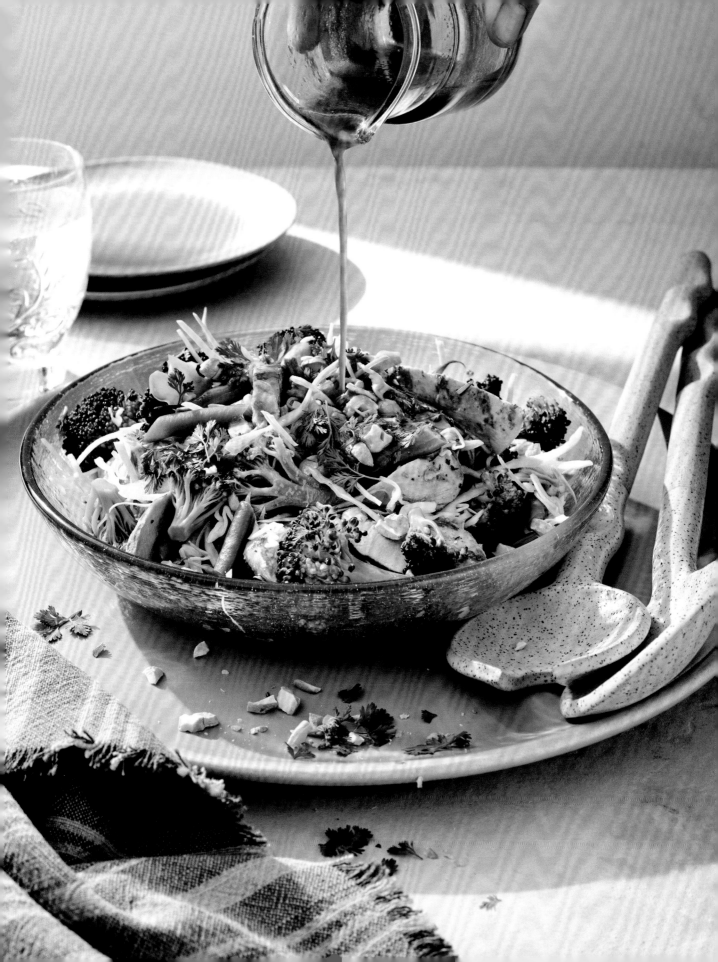

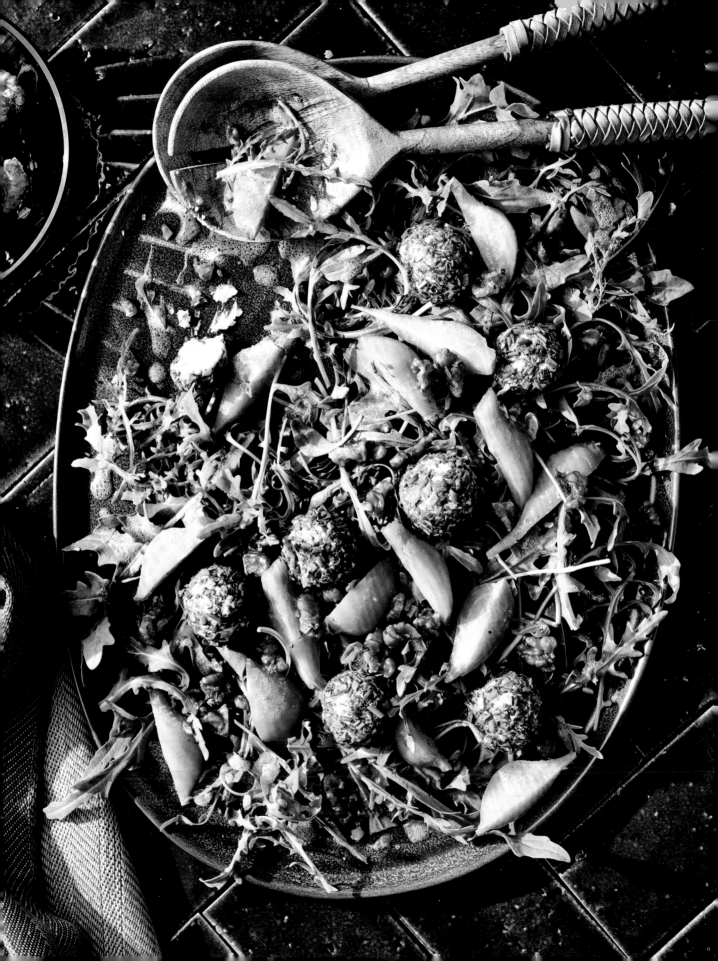

Beet and Arugula Salad
with Herby Goat Cheese

SERVES 4

2 medium or 4 small red and/or golden beets (about 8 ounces total), scrubbed (see Note)

Avocado oil, for drizzling

Fine sea salt

6 tablespoons extra-virgin olive oil

4 tablespoons balsamic vinegar or Champagne vinegar

Juice of ½ lemon

¼ cup chopped fresh parsley or cilantro

5 ounces soft goat cheese, cold

About 8 cups fresh arugula

½ cup rosemary walnuts (see page 210) or toasted walnuts

MAKE IT YOURS

Hearty Pairings: Add slices of roasted or grilled chicken (like Rosemary-Lemon Chicken Paillards, page 197) to the salad; or serve the salad with Seed Crackers (page 218) or a slice of toasted Nut and Seed Bread (page 92) spread with avocado.

Simple Swaps: Use spinach, watercress, or a blend of tender salad greens instead of the arugula. Replace the walnuts with Rosemary Almonds (page 210).

Beets, with their natural sweetness and earthiness, are one of my favorite vegetables. I like a mix of red and golden ones here, roasted until tender and gorgeous—the vibrant range of colors reminds me of the sunset. The goat cheese is rolled into balls and coated with fresh herbs for extra flavor and nutrition. Paired with peppery arugula and crunchy homemade rosemary walnuts, this is a salad worth staining your fingers for—though you can wear gloves while handling the beets, if you prefer.

Preheat the oven to 350°F and line a small baking dish with parchment.

Add the beets to the baking dish and rub all over with a small bit of avocado oil and a few pinches of salt. Sprinkle with about 2 tablespoons of water, then fold the parchment over the beets and crimp the edges to form a pouch; this helps the beets steam evenly. Roast until the beets are tender and easily pierced with a small knife, from 30 to 60 minutes depending on beet size. Allow the beets to cool, then gently rub off the skins (wear gloves to prevent staining, and be careful of your cutting board and countertop). Cut the beets into wedges or slices.

Add the olive oil, vinegar, lemon juice, and a pinch of salt to a glass jar, cover, and shake to emulsify (or whisk together in a small bowl).

Spread the parsley on a small plate. Using a chef's knife, divide the goat cheese into 8 equal portions and roll each portion into a ball. Roll the balls in the parsley to coat, then set on a clean plate. (You can do this up to a few hours in advance and store in the refrigerator.)

Pile the arugula on a large serving platter. Drop the goat cheese balls and beets on top, then drizzle with the dressing. Using your hands, crumble the walnuts over the salad, sprinkle with a pinch or two of salt, and serve right away.

Note: Beets can be cooked at any temperature from 300° to 400°F, so add them to the oven along with whatever else you might be baking and check them occasionally to see if they are tender. They can be roasted in advance and refrigerated for up to 2 days.

Spinach Salad with
Almond-Crusted Goat Cheese Medallions

SERVES 2 TO 4

¼ cup almond flour

¼ cup coarsely chopped blanched almonds

¼ teaspoon fine sea salt, plus more to taste

1 large egg

1 (5-ounce) log goat cheese, cold

1 tablespoon extra-virgin olive oil

1 tablespoon unsalted butter

About 8 cups (8 ounces) baby spinach

4 to 6 radishes, trimmed and thinly sliced (optional)

Dad's Honey Mustard Dressing (page 220)

½ cup coarsely chopped Rosemary Almonds (page 210) or roasted almonds

MAKE IT YOURS

Hearty Pairings: Roasted beets (see page 144) are a delicious addition to the salad.

Simple Swaps: Use hazelnuts and hazelnut meal instead of the blanched almonds and almond flour to coat the cheese rounds. Use arugula, watercress, or a blend of tender salad greens instead of the spinach. Replace the almonds with rosemary walnuts (see page 210).

When I was 17, I went to Paris for the first time. It was a whole new world for me, and the food was so yummy—I never imagined that just bread and butter could taste that good. I don't usually eat gluten, but when I visit France now, even just for a layover, you better believe I have a baguette in the airport lounge!

That trip was also where I first tried a chèvre chaud salad—a big pile of fresh frisée and baby lettuces, with two discs of goat cheese wrapped in flaky pastry. I didn't speak French, so I didn't exactly know what I was ordering, but I was so happy when I cut open the pastry and there was warm goat cheese inside. Now I make this salad my own way at home, rolling the cheese in almond flour and chopped almonds for crunch, and pan-frying it in butter until browned on the outside and molten on the inside. It's not the same as in France, but it still tastes delicious!

Combine the almond flour, blanched almonds, and salt on a plate or in a shallow bowl.

Lightly whisk the egg in a small bowl.

Using a sharp knife, cut the goat cheese into 8 rounds. (To make smooth, clean cuts, dip the knife in hot water and wipe it dry with a paper towel between each slice.) Working with one piece at a time, dip each cheese round into the egg and then dredge it in the almond mixture, coating all sides and gently reshaping each piece into a round disc, if necessary. Arrange the cheese rounds on a plate or small baking sheet and refrigerate for at least 30 minutes.

Heat a medium skillet over medium-low heat. When hot, add the olive oil and the butter to the pan. Swirl until the butter is melted, then carefully add the cheese rounds, quickly pan-frying them until golden brown on the top and bottom, just 1 to 2 minutes per side.

Place the spinach and radishes, if using, in a large bowl and toss with the dressing to taste. Pile onto a serving platter. Place the warm cheese on the greens, and sprinkle with a little salt. Garnish with the almonds and serve immediately.

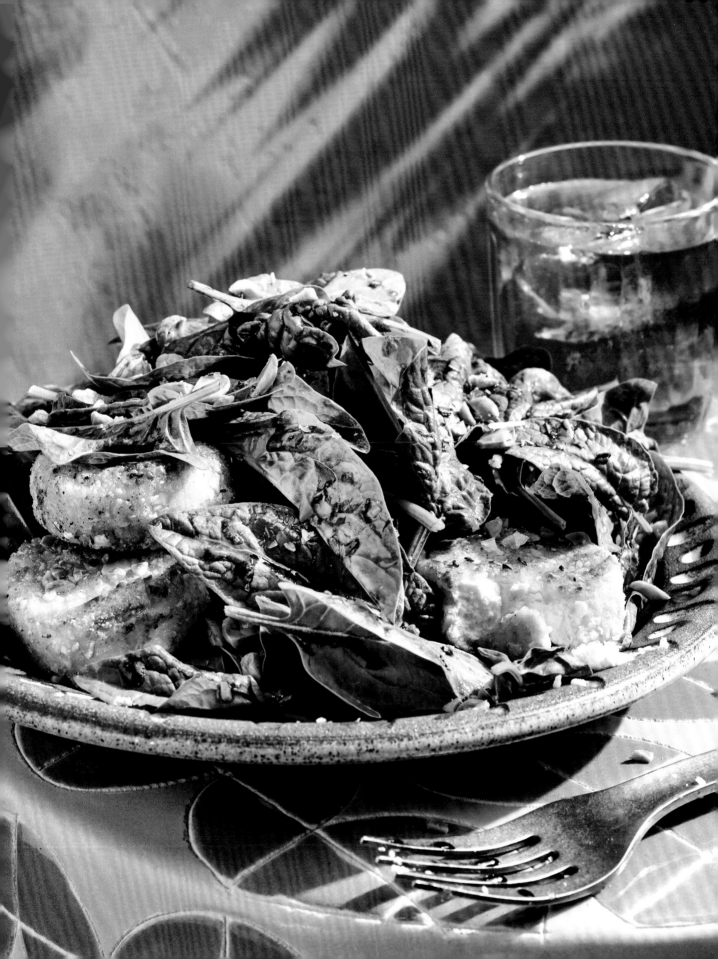

Steak Salad

SERVES 4

1½ to 2 pounds boneless
skirt steak

1 or 2 teaspoons coarse salt,
or more as needed

Avocado oil, as needed

About 10 cups mixed salad
greens

1 to 2 avocados, halved, pitted,
and cubed

A few very thin slices of
red onion

Extra-virgin olive oil,
for drizzling

Flaky salt

Lemon wedges (optional)

Being from the south of Brazil, I grew up eating steak. I don't eat it nearly as much today as I did then, usually only a few times a month. But after becoming anemic when I was on a vegetarian diet, I was glad to reintroduce it into my diet. I am grateful for the iron that red meat provides. Using an excellent-quality grass-fed skirt steak makes a big difference in this simple but delicious salad. The steak is so rich and juicy that you don't even need to dress the greens—just drizzle the whole thing with a little olive oil and sprinkle with salt, and you're done.

Pat the steak dry, then cut it crosswise into 4 pieces. Arrange them on a sheet pan or in a shallow baking dish in a single layer. Sprinkle evenly with coarse salt and massage it into the meat with your fingers. Cover the dish and set aside to marinate for 30 to 45 minutes at room temperature.

To cook the steak in a grill pan, place a large grill pan over high heat for about 5 minutes. Brush lightly with avocado oil, then add the steak, arranging the pieces in a single layer (you may need to cook in 2 batches; take care not to overcrowd the pan, or the steaks will steam, not sear). Cook, flipping once, until well seared on each side, 3 to 5 minutes per side (for medium-rare to medium), or more or less time depending on how thick the steak is and how you like it cooked.

To cook the steak on an outdoor grill, preheat the grill to very hot direct heat. Brush the pan or grates very lightly with avocado oil, then using tongs, add the steak, arranging the pieces in a single layer on the grate. Cook, flipping once, until well seared on each side, 3 to 5 minutes per side (for medium-rare to medium), or more or less time depending on how thick the steak is and how you like it cooked. To check for doneness, make a small cut with a paring knife into the thickest part. Transfer the steak to a cutting board to rest for at least 5 minutes while you prepare the salad.

MAKE IT YOURS

Light Pairing: If you have some Chimichurri (page 224) or Cilantro-Mint Dressing (page 221), use it for an extra boost of flavor.

Simple Swap: Leftover rib eye (page 199) or flank steak (page 203) works great instead of cooking the skirt steak from scratch. Balsamic vinaigrette (like the one on page 112) is delicious instead of olive oil and lemon.

Arrange the salad greens on a large serving platter and scatter the avocados and onion on top. Drizzle lightly with the olive oil and sprinkle with a pinch of flaky salt.

Slice the steak pieces against the grain into ½-inch-thick strips and arrange over the greens. If you like, add a spritz of lemon juice over the steak and salad at the table.

PERFECT FOODS

There are a few foods I consider perfect; not only do they taste amazing but they are nutritional bombs. For me, it doesn't get any better than the combination of good and good for you—it's what I base my lifestyle on!

Avocados • These are full of healthy fats, as well as fiber, potassium, and immune-boosting vitamins. I love them spread on toast (see Nut and Seed Bread on page 92), cubed into a salad (see Steak Salad, opposite), or whipped up into dessert (see page 244).

Coconuts • Versatile and delicious, coconuts are packed with nutrition, as they are high in magnesium, zinc, copper, iron, potassium, fatty acids, and minerals. I make my own coconut milk (page 72), which I then use in Coconut-Curry Vegetable Soup (page 140), one of my favorite wintertime soups. Canned coconut milk can also be cooked down to make a dessert drizzle similar to dulce de leche (see page 239). You can also use coconut sugar as a 1:1 replacement for granulated sugar, which is a much better choice for balancing blood sugar. Coconut flakes add body and chew to Baru Nut Bars (page 233). And unsweetened coconut water is delicious in a smoothie (see page 55). Is there anything a coconut can't do?

Dates • What can I say? I love dates. They add sweetness to smoothies (see pages 55–57), non-dairy milks (see page 68), and baked goods like Pecan Bars (page 234). Plus, dates may be my all-time favorite simple pick-me-up, especially with an almond or two stuffed inside.

Almonds • I eat almonds almost every day. Full of protein and endlessly versatile, almonds are always in my house, often in various states of being soaked, peeled, toasted, or ground. When I make Almond Milk (page 69), I then use the leftover pulp for my smoothies (see pages 55–57). Rosemary Almonds (page 210) are delicious as a garnish with most salads and soups. And using more almond flour in my cooking has been a bit of a revelation—it makes things both more delicious and more nutritious. Among many others, see Sunday Banana Waffles (page 83), Chicken Meatballs (page 194), and an extra-special Spinach Salad (page 106), with medallions of tangy goat cheese rolled in almond flour—I pan-fry them to get them crisp—so good!

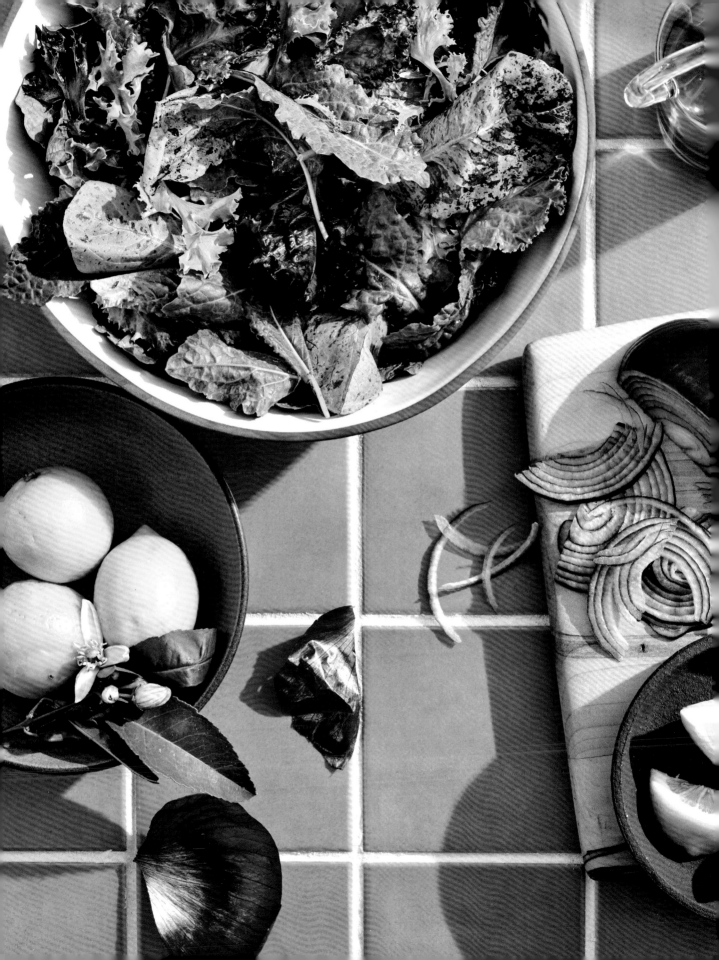

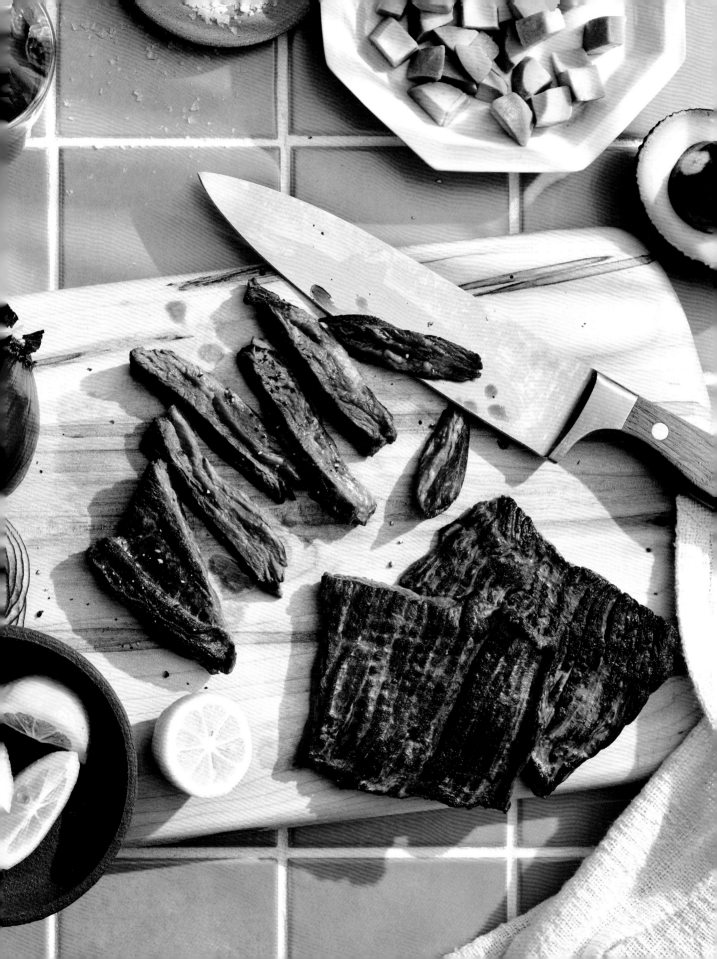

Tuna Salad with Olives

SERVES 2 TO 4

7 tablespoons extra-virgin
olive oil

3 tablespoons balsamic
vinegar

Fine sea salt

2 (6.7-ounce) jars water-
packed tuna (see Note)

About 8 cups baby arugula
or baby lettuce

1 (9-ounce) jar whole
artichoke hearts, drained and
rinsed, then quartered

½ cup good-quality green
or black olives, rinsed

1 medium carrot, thinly sliced
with a mandoline or shaved
with a vegetable peeler

About 1 cup blanched
and chilled green beans
or asparagus (see page 155)

When you use the best ingredients, you don't need to make complicated dishes. That's what I learned when I started cooking for myself. This salad is really just an assemblage of high-quality jarred tuna, jarred artichokes, black or green olives, and a few fresh vegetables. Like everything else, but perhaps most important here, buy the best olive oil you can afford.

In a 1-pint glass jar, combine 6 tablespoons of the olive oil, the balsamic vinegar, and a pinch of salt, then shake to emulsify.

Drain the tuna and add to a small bowl. Use a fork to break up the tuna and then add the remaining tablespoon of olive oil and mix well.

Arrange the arugula in a wide bowl or on a serving platter. Mound the tuna in the center, then arrange the artichokes, olives, carrot, and green beans around the tuna.

At the table, spoon the dressing over the salad, and add more salt to taste. Serve.

Note: I like to buy Tonnino tuna packed in water, as I can then dress it with my favorite olive oil. If you prefer olive oil–packed tuna, simply lift it from the oil and break it up, and skip adding the remaining olive oil.

MAKE IT YOURS

Light Pairing: Chopped baby cucumbers are a great addition to the salad.

Hearty Pairing: Add a hard-boiled egg or a piece of toasted Nut and Seed Bread (page 02) with avocado.

For the Kids: Make tuna lettuce wraps. prepare the tuna as directed (mixing it with 1 tablespoon of either olivo oil or mayonnaise, Benny's favorite), then scoop it into Bibb or romaine lettuce leaves; the carrot and green beans can be served on the side.

Simple Swap: High-quality canned salmon works great instead of the tuna (I like Vital Choice brand).

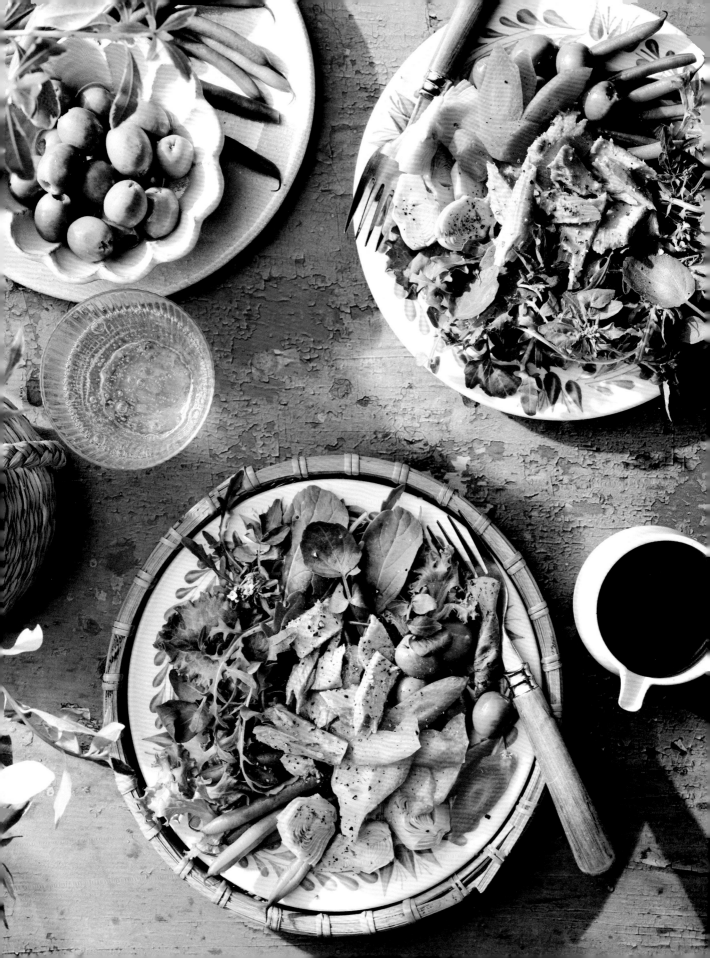

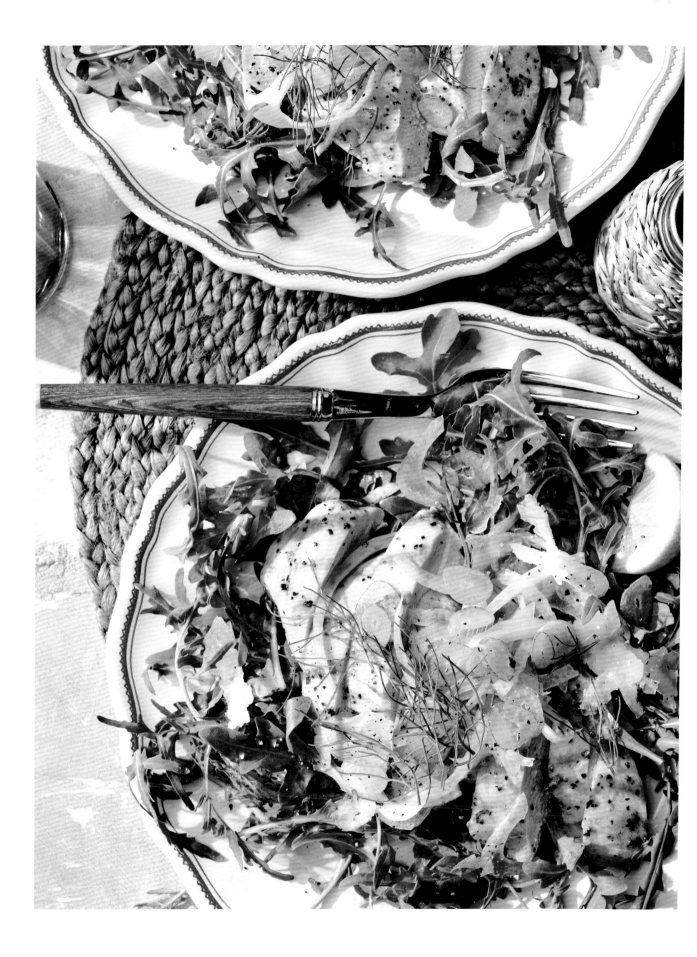

Arugula and Chicken Salad

SERVES 2

2 boneless, skinless chicken breasts (about 1 pound)

¼ cup olive oil, plus more for drizzling

1 lemon, halved

Fine sea salt

Freshly ground black pepper

Avocado oil

About 6 cups baby arugula

1 small or ½ medium fennel bulb, trimmed, cored, and thinly sliced (preferably on a mandoline)

Shavings of manchego or parmesan cheese (optional)

MAKE IT YOURS

Hearty Pairings: Top with Rosemary Almonds (page 210) or Maple Harissa Cashews (page 208).

Simple Swaps: Use cooked chicken or skip the chicken altogether and add a scoop of Sheet-Pan Squash and Chickpeas (page 151) with a drizzle of Cilantro-Mint Dressing (page 221). Tender baby lettuces would be a great replacement or addition to the arugula. Tamari Dressing (page 228) or Tahini Dressing (page 220) is excellent on this as well, instead of the lemon and olive oil.

When pounded very thin and simply marinated in lemon, olive oil, and salt, chicken breasts cook in moments and are a delicious, juicy centerpiece for this quick and easy salad, which I make all the time. Arugula and thinly sliced fennel make a fresh, peppery base. I often like to shave a thin layer of manchego or parmesan over the top for some extra richness.

Blot the chicken breasts dry with paper towels. Working one at a time, use a sharp knife to horizontally slice each breast into 2 cutlets so that you have 4 thin, even pieces. Working one at a time, place the chicken pieces between 2 sheets of parchment and, using the smooth side of a meat mallet, pound them to an even thinness of ¼ inch.

In a shallow bowl, whisk together the ¼ cup olive oil and the juice from half of the lemon, then add the chicken cutlets, turning to coat evenly. Cover and let marinate at room temperature for 30 to 45 minutes.

Set a grill pan or large heavy skillet over high heat and preheat for 3 to 5 minutes. When hot, lift the chicken cutlets from the marinade and gently blot excess marinade with a paper towel. Sprinkle on both sides with a few pinches of salt and pepper. Brush the pan lightly with avocado oil, then add the breasts (cooking two at a time if necessary so the pan isn't overcrowded) and cook until the chicken has developed some color and easily releases from the pan, 90 seconds to 3 minutes. Flip and cook on the opposite side until the chicken is lightly browned and just cooked through, another 2 to 3 minutes. Transfer to a plate.

Divide the arugula and fennel between two plates and dress with a squeeze of lemon, a drizzle of olive oil, and salt to taste. Lay two cooked chicken cutlets on each plate. Garnish with cheese, if using.

TWO RECIPES IN ONE

When I make chicken broth (page 124), which we do at least once a week, I always remove the breast meat from the whole chicken before cooking, since the breasts don't add much flavor to the broth—the leanness of that light meat makes it much better suited to quick cooking. This is the perfect lunch to make on the day I make broth!

Warm Wild Rice Salad

SERVES 4

1½ cups wild rice

6 cups filtered water

Fine sea salt

¼ cup extra-virgin olive oil

2 large garlic cloves,
finely minced or grated

1 medium shallot
or ¼ red onion, diced

1 lemon, halved

2 medium carrots, diced
or coarsely grated

2 celery stalks, diced

Freshly ground black pepper

¼ cup coarsely chopped
flat-leaf parsley

½ cup toasted pecans
(see Note)

Most of the time I eat gluten free, so wild rice, which is actually a grass and does not contain gluten, is a nice side dish for when I want something starchy but with extra dietary fiber and antioxidants. The sweet, herbaceous fragrance and hearty texture of wild rice go well with fresh, vibrant parsley leaves, specks of carrots and celery, and lightly pickled shallots in the dressing. The toasted pecans add richness and crunch—my favorite part. Be sure to look for pure wild rice, not a blend.

Rinse the rice in a fine-mesh colander, then place in a medium saucepan and add the water. Bring to a boil over medium-high heat, then add 2 teaspoons salt. Reduce the heat to medium-low, partially cover the pan, and simmer until the rice is tender and begins to open up, 50 to 60 minutes. Strain the rice (there might be extra liquid) and return it to the pot. Stir in the olive oil and garlic, and cover the pan to keep the rice warm.

Place the shallot in a medium bowl and add the juice from half of the lemon and a big pinch of salt; let sit for a few minutes to soften and lightly pickle. Then add the carrots and celery, the warm rice, and a few grinds of black pepper. Stir to combine. Taste, adding a few extra spritzes of lemon, if desired, and more salt to taste. Lastly, stir in the parsley and scatter on the pecans. Serve warm.

Note: To toast the pecans, place them in a small oven-safe skillet and bake at 350°F until they're light brown and fragrant, 10 to 15 minutes, stirring midway through cooking.

MAKE IT YOURS

Light Pairings: Serve along with Favorite Sautéed Leafy Greens (page 152) or Easy Sautéed Veggies with Garlic (page 165).

Hearty Pairings: Serve with a poached or boiled egg on top; or use the salad as a base for a bowl with Roasted Vegetables (page 144).

For the Kids: Serve with Rosemary-Lemon Chicken Paillards (page 197).

Simple Swap: Instead of pecans, use toasted almonds or walnuts.

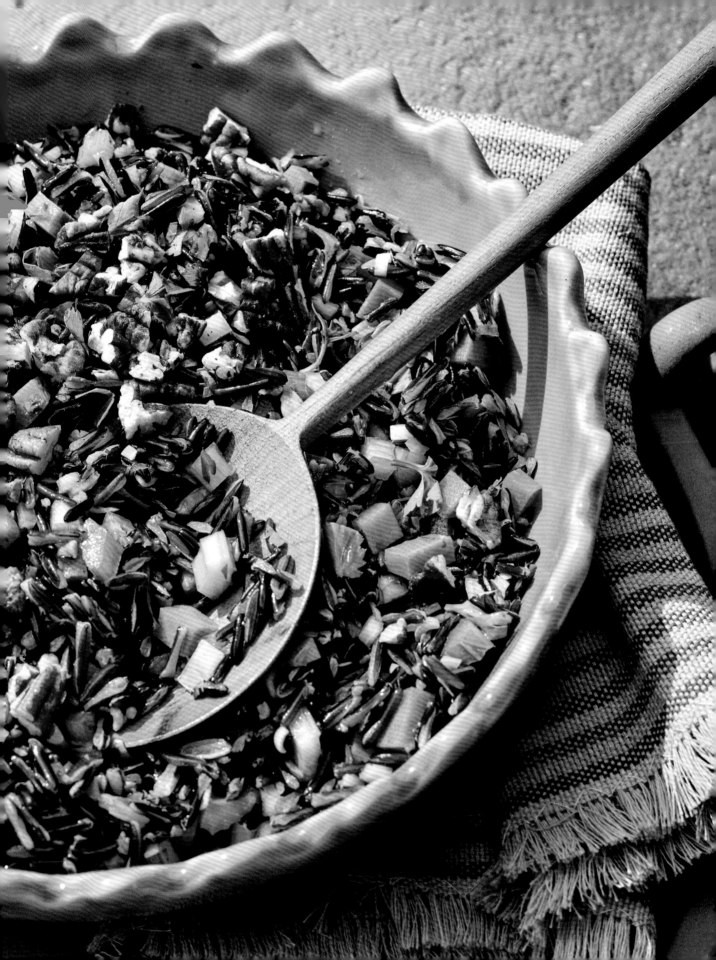

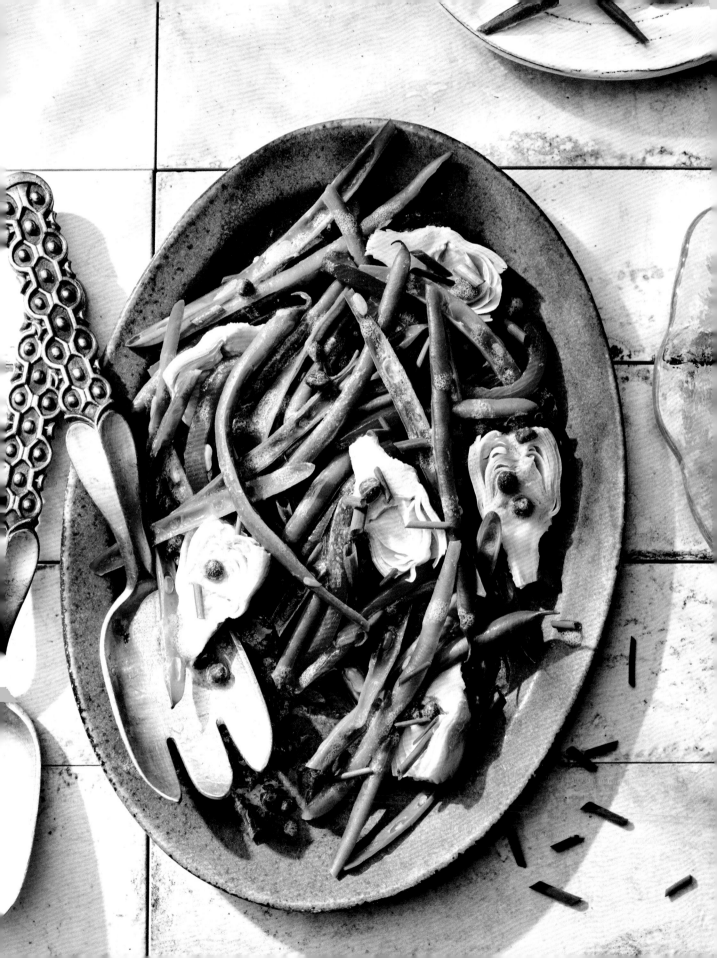

Green Bean Salad

SERVES 4

1 pound green beans, trimmed

1 small roasted red pepper (see page 144)

1 cup rinsed and drained jarred whole artichoke hearts

Tahini Dressing (page 220) or Dad's Honey Mustard Dressing (page 220)

2 tablespoons minced fresh chives

Capers, to garnish (optional)

Vivi loves green beans, even raw, so I am constantly trying to find new ways to serve them. In fact, she loves them so much that any time I am making this salad I have to make sure she isn't in the kitchen, as the beans will all be gone before I complete the dish!

I like this salad because the green beans, when blanched and cut lengthwise, have a flexible texture that almost resembles noodles. Add a slivered roasted pepper and artichoke hearts, and this salad starts to feel a lot more fun than everyday leafy greens.

Fill a medium bowl with ice cubes and cold water. Bring a large saucepan of salted water to a boil. Add the beans and blanch for 90 seconds, until tender but still retaining a bit of crunch. Use a slotted spoon to transfer the beans to the ice bath to cool them, then drain in a colander.

Working carefully, slice the beans in half lengthwise to make long, noodle-like strips. Pile the beans in a serving bowl.

Slice the red pepper into long strips. Slice the artichoke hearts in half lengthwise and add both to the bowl with the beans. Add the mixture to a large skillet over medium heat to just warm through, about 1 minute. (This is also delicious served cold.)

Gently stir the dressing into the vegetables, using only as much as desired, and place in a serving bowl. Garnish with the chives and capers, if using, and serve immediately.

MAKE IT YOURS

Hearty Pairings: Add 1 (6-ounce) can water-packed tuna, drained, or a few big spoonfuls of cooked chickpeas (see page 179) to the salad. Topping with Rosemary Almonds (page 210) or Maple Harissa Cashews (page 208) adds a little crunch.

Simple Swap: Use Cilantro-Mint Dressing (page 221) instead of the Tahini Dressing.

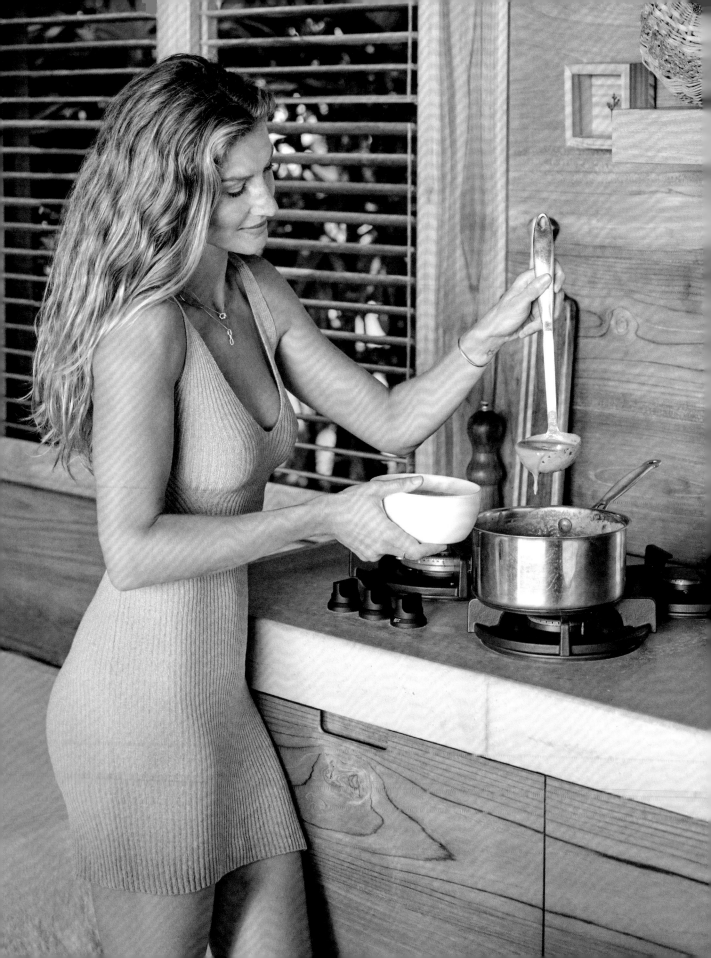

Soups

Soup and broth are super nutritious and easy to digest, which is why they are among my favorite dinners. Plus, they are flexible to cook and easy to reheat for a last-minute meal. My mom's homemade broth might be my most treasured recipe; I always have some in the house—it feels so nourishing.

Vegetable Broth

**MAKES ABOUT
2 ½ QUARTS**

3 celery stalks, roughly chopped

2 large carrots, roughly chopped

1 medium onion, quartered

1 bunch scallions, green and white parts roughly chopped

1 head of garlic, cut in half crosswise

2 dried bay leaves

Several bushy sprigs of fresh parsley or thyme

Up to 4 cups vegetable trimmings (such as squash skins, leek trimmings, mushroom stems, fennel or cabbage cores, parsnip peels, kale stems)

Fine sea salt

You could say that I have an obsession about not wasting food; I think this is why making vegetable broth gives me so much satisfaction. Every week, I gather all of my saved vegetable trimmings: the stems, tops, skins, and cores, plus any vegetables that aren't quite salad worthy anymore. (I sometimes freeze these bits and pieces in a glass container until I'm ready to cook.) They all get added to a pot along with the usual suspects of carrots, celery, onions, and garlic—no need to peel any of them. The end result is a fully flavored, fortified, rich broth that has extracted everything from the vegetables, making something delicious out of what could easily just have been thrown away. Vegetable broth is delicious and nutritious, and the process of not wasting is the cherry on top.

In a stockpot or Dutch oven, combine all the ingredients except the salt and add enough filtered water to submerge the vegetables, with plenty of room for them to float around—about 3 quarts. Bring to a boil over medium-high heat, then lower the heat and partially cover the pot with a lid. Simmer for 90 minutes to 2 hours, checking periodically and skimming off any foam that collects on the surface, until the broth is rich and rounded with vegetable flavor. Uncover and let cool. (Alternatively, combine all the ingredients except the salt in a slow cooker. Add 10 cups of water, or enough to almost reach the maximum fill line. Set on low heat and cook for 8 hours.)

Carefully strain the broth through a fine-mesh sieve into a large bowl. Gently press on the solids to extract a bit more broth; compost the solids. Taste the broth and add salt to taste.

Divide the broth among airtight glass containers, add the lids, and refrigerate, or let cool and freeze in freezer bags. The broth will keep for 4 to 5 days in the refrigerator, or up to 2 months in the freezer.

Note: Fennel scraps add an especially distinct taste. Other interesting additions include onion peels, trimmings from green beans or asparagus, stem ends of zucchini, or chard stems.

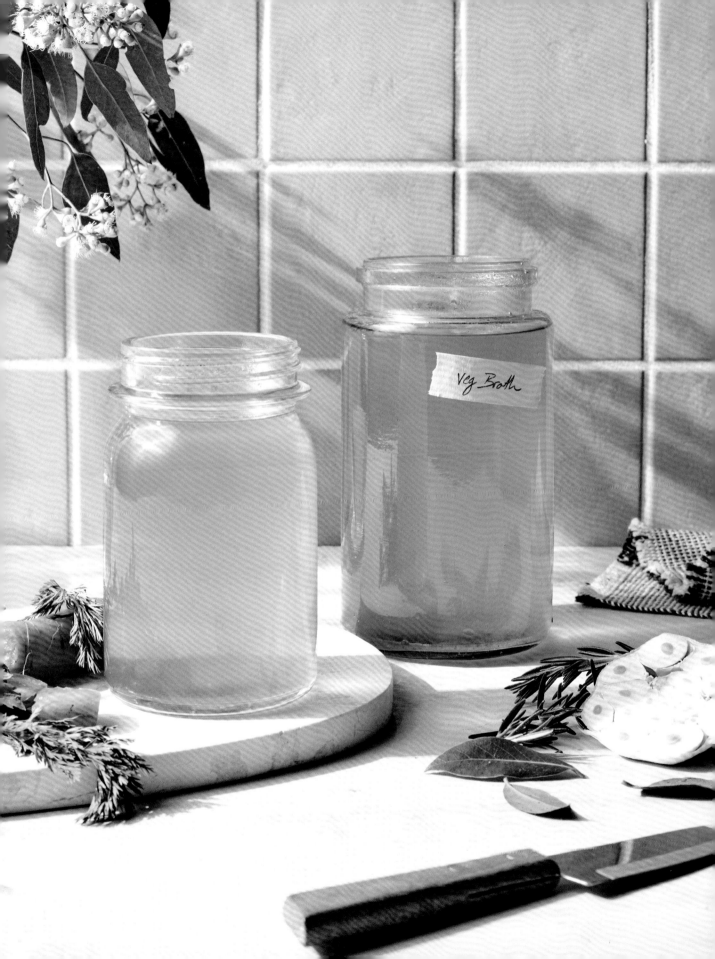

Mom's Chicken Broth

**MAKES ABOUT
2½ QUARTS**

1 (3- to 4-pound) chicken
or equivalent in chicken legs,
thighs, backs, and/or wings

2 celery stalks, roughly
chopped

1 large carrot, roughly chopped

1 medium white onion,
quartered

1 bunch scallions, white and
green parts, trimmed and
roughly chopped

1 head of garlic, halved
crosswise

2 dried bay leaves

Several bushy sprigs of
fresh parsley or thyme

Up to 4 cups vegetable
trimmings (squash skins, leek
trimmings, mushroom stems,
fennel or cabbage cores,
parsnip peels, kale stems; see
Note, page 122)

Fine sea salt

When people ask me about my beauty routine, they usually want to know what brands of face cream and cosmetics I use. But honestly, the most impactful thing I do to maintain my skin has not as much to do with beauty products as with how I eat. I consume collagen, which is found naturally in bone broth. I have been eating this chicken broth forever, as my mom has been making a version of this since I was little. Today this broth is the base for pretty much all my soups, like the Beans and Greens (page 135) and Sneeze-Be-Gone (page 127), as well as the weekly improvisations incorporating whatever leftovers I have in the fridge. (Some broth, shredded chicken, and a couple of random vegetables can make a quick and cozy meal in minutes.) I also sip on this broth all the time. Plus, if I want to add more flavor to a dish, I just add some broth and voilà! In short, making a pot of my mom's broth is one of those slow, worthwhile tasks that pays dividends, inside and out.

I often go through a whole batch in one week, and so I sometimes make a double batch, freezing half, so I always have some on hand. One thing I always do is remove the breasts from the chicken before cooking—the lightly flavored meat is best grilled or sautéed.

If working with a whole chicken, use a sharp knife to remove the chicken breasts, making deep slices on each side of the breastbone and then tracing the knife smoothly against the rib cage to carefully detach the breasts. Refrigerate or freeze the chicken breasts for another use. Cut the rest of the carcass into pieces, separating the legs and wings.

Place the chicken pieces in a stockpot or Dutch oven and add the remaining ingredients except the salt. Add enough filtered water to cover the meat and vegetables, with plenty of room for them to float around—about 3 quarts. Bring to a boil over high heat, then lower the heat and partially cover the pot with a lid. Simmer for 4 hours, skimming off any

MAKE IT YOURS

Light Pairings: Simmer chopped raw vegetables in the broth until tender for a simple and nutritious lunch or dinner. My mom makes a particularly good version with carrots, sliced broccoli stems, celery, and bay leaves and cooks just until the vegetables are fork-tender. Or, add leftover roasted or blanched veggies (see pages 144 or 155) to the broth and simply reheat, or puree the mix for a rich, smooth, and creamy (but creamless!) result.

foam that collects on the surface and adding more water as needed to keep the solids submerged, until the broth tastes rich and full flavored. (Alternatively, place ingredients, except the salt, in a slow cooker and add 10 cups of filtered water. Set on low heat and cook for 12 hours.)

Remove the lid and let cool. Using a spider or slotted spoon, carefully remove the chicken from the broth and set it on a plate. Strain the remaining broth through a fine-mesh sieve set over a large bowl.

Remove and discard the chicken skin, then pull the meat from the bones (it will fall right off) and reserve for another use, if you like (see Note). Pour any collected juices from the plate through the sieve into the broth. Taste the broth and add salt to taste.

Divide the broth among airtight glass containers, add the lids, and refrigerate, or let cool and freeze in freezer bags. The broth will keep for 3 days in the refrigerator, or up to 2 months in the freezer. The fat in the broth will harden at the top of the containers; when you reheat it, that fat will melt back into the broth and make it extra rich—delicious!

Note: Though most of the flavor has been transferred to the broth, the chicken meat is still fine to eat, if you like. Just shred it and fry in a couple tablespoons of butter with a little garlic and salt to add some flavor back in.

SICKNESS, WELLNESS, AND FOOD

When I'm sick, my preference is to use herbal and homeopathic remedies before anything I'd get over the counter, as I often have positive results with none of the misgivings. There are all sorts of ways to treat and heal with food, and if you can avoid putting chemicals into your body and instead reach for something natural, why not try it?

Ginger-Lemon Healing Tea (page 74) with some manuka honey is a go-to when my kids or I are feeling sick. Vegetables and homemade broth are nutrient packed, so a recipe like Sneeze-Be-Gone Soup (page 127) is beneficial for a cold or sore throat. To proactively boost our immune systems and gain overall wellness, we eat superfoods like ginger, turmeric, and herbs daily. I take my herbal supplements most days (I like Gaia herbs the best), including elderberry syrup for the kids (see page 45 for more information).

Lastly, I make sure we consume a variety of produce to gain the full spectrum of vitamins and minerals; I remind the kids to "eat the rainbow," which helps them be more conscious of all the types of nutrients they are eating every day. This is another way of ensuring I am doing all I can to protect my biggest asset: my own and my family's health.

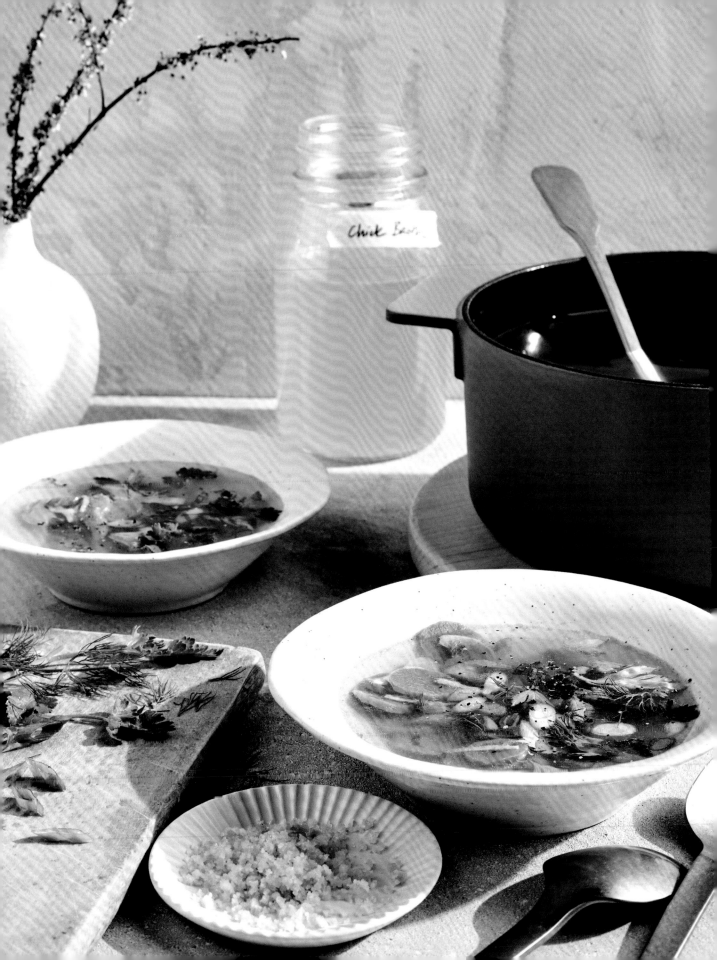

Sneeze-Be-Gone Soup

SERVES 4

1 tablespoon ghee or avocado oil

3 medium carrots, thinly sliced

2 celery stalks, thinly sliced, plus a handful of celery leaves

4 garlic cloves, thinly sliced

1 thumb-sized piece of fresh ginger, peeled and finely grated or cut into thin matchsticks

½ teaspoon ground turmeric or 1-inch fresh turmeric, thinly sliced

½ teaspoon fine sea salt, or more as desired

6 cups Mom's Chicken Broth (page 124)

1 scallion, green and white parts thinly sliced

Handful of fresh parsley leaves and/or dill, coarsely chopped

Freshly ground black pepper

Flaky sea salt (optional)

Obviously, I am a great believer in the healing power of food. And when you are sick, it is even more important to give your body lots of healthful, easy-to-digest foods. Despite its mild, soothing effect, this simple soup is a nutritional powerhouse, with antioxidant-rich ginger, garlic, and turmeric (be sure to add black pepper here, as it helps activate the turmeric), vitamin-packed carrots and celery, and revitalizing fresh dill and parsley. And most important of all, the chicken broth—loaded with zinc and other minerals extracted from the bones—addresses the generic symptoms of a cold. Straight broth is easiest to digest when sick, but Vivi, my meat eater, often asks for this soup even when she is her regular happy, healthy self, so I often throw in some chicken for her.

Place a soup pot or Dutch oven over medium-low heat, and when hot, add the ghee. Then add the carrots, celery, garlic, ginger, turmeric, and sea salt, stirring to coat. Cook for a few minutes, allowing the vegetables to soften, then pour in the broth and bring to a boil. Reduce the heat to low and simmer gently until the vegetables are just tender, 10 to 15 minutes. Taste, adding a few extra pinches of sea salt, if needed.

To serve, ladle into soup bowls and garnish with the scallion, parsley, a few grinds of black pepper, and a pinch of flaky salt, if you like.

MAKE IT YOURS

Light Pairing: Add a peeled and chopped chayote squash and a handful of fresh spinach.

Hearty Pairings: Serve over cooked wild rice; or stir a beaten egg into the simmering broth right before serving.

For the Kids: To each serving, add a handful of shredded cooked chicken. Or sauté some uncooked chicken pieces in a little avocado oil, with chopped garlic and a pinch of salt, then add to the soup. Cooked udon noodles are also a favorite addition to this soup.

Simple Swaps: Use up to 2 cups of Best Blanched Vegetables (page 155) instead of the carrots and celery, and cook only 5 to 10 minutes. Other fresh herbs, like cilantro, are also delicious here.

Fresh Pea Soup
with Crispy Sweet Potatoes

SERVES 4 TO 6

2 leeks, white and light green parts, trimmed

2 tablespoons unrefined virgin coconut oil or avocado oil, plus more for drizzling

3 garlic cloves, smashed

1 teaspoon fine sea salt

1 small zucchini, chopped

4½ cups Mom's Chicken Broth (page 124) or Vegetable Broth (page 122), or more as needed

1 pound fresh peas in their pods, shelled (about 2 cups), or 2 (10-ounce) bags frozen petite peas (see Note)

Roasted Sweet Potato Cubes (page 147)

Extra-virgin olive oil

Peas are one of the best vegetables to showcase the benefits of seasonal eating. In the spring, when I can still feel the echo of winter's browns and grays, the farmer's market showcases bright green, vibrant peas still in their pods. This simple symbol of the season is so inspiring. Their sweet green flavor is like sunshine.

After a long, dark winter, especially when I lived in Boston, fresh green produce was all I wanted to consume. This simple soup, which comes together quickly in the blender and can be garnished with crispy cubes of sweet potato, is a wonderful way to welcome spring.

Halve the leeks and slice them into half moons. Place the pieces in a fine-mesh strainer and rinse well under running water, and then drain.

Place a Dutch oven over medium heat and when hot, add the oil. Then add the leeks, garlic, and ¼ teaspoon of the salt. Cover and cook until soft and tender, stirring periodically, 7 to 10 minutes.

Stir in the zucchini, then add the broth. Bring to a boil and add the remaining ¾ teaspoon salt, then cover partially and simmer until the zucchini is tender, 10 to 15 minutes.

Add the peas to the soup and cook until just tender, 3 to 5 minutes (usually as long as it takes for the liquid to return to a simmer).

Remove the Dutch oven from the heat. Working in batches, add the soup to the blender and puree until very smooth. (Be sure to fill the blender only halfway and process with the lid vented.) Return the soup to the pot and gently reheat. Add additional broth to thin the consistency, if desired. Taste for salt.

Serve hot, garnished with the sweet potato cubes and a drizzle of olive oil, if desired.

Note: If fresh peas are out of season, use frozen peas, ideally the organic petite variety. There's no need to defrost them prior to adding to the soup.

MAKE IT YOURS

Light Pairing: A sprinkling of roasted pumpkin seeds makes a great topping and adds a little crunch.

Hearty Pairings: Leftover roasted vegetables, like carrots or winter squash, are excellent additions to the soup.

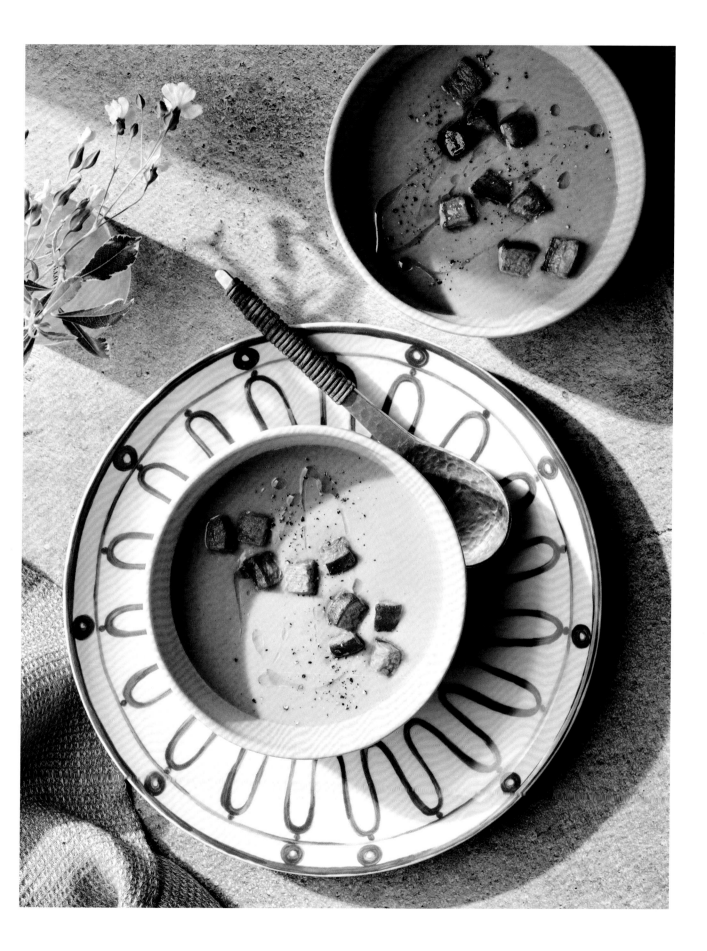

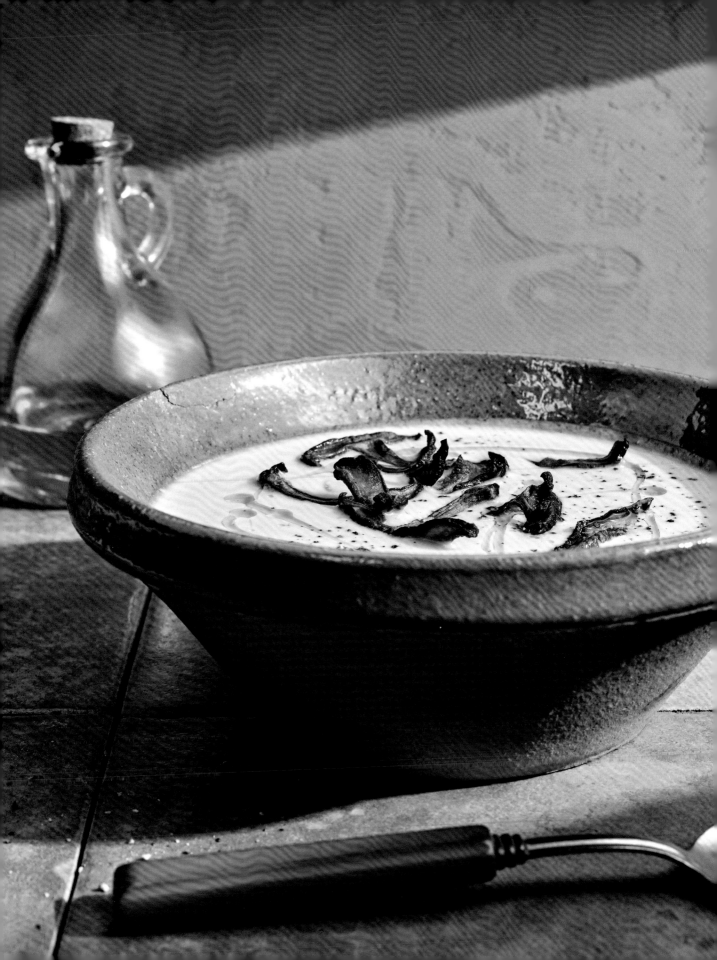

Creamy Cauliflower Soup

SERVES 4 TO 6

2 leeks, white and pale green parts only, trimmed (see Note); or 1 large white or yellow onion, chopped

2 tablespoons avocado oil or ghee

3 garlic cloves, smashed

1 teaspoon fine sea salt

Freshly ground black pepper

1 large cauliflower (about 2 pounds), broken into florets, core chopped

1 medium zucchini, diced

6 cups Mom's Chicken Broth (page 124) or Vegetable Broth (page 122)

½ cup raw cashews

Extra-virgin olive oil

Crispy Roasted Shiitake Mushrooms (page 214)

I don't eat a ton of conventional dairy, but I still love creamy foods, so this soup is very satisfying. There are two special ingredients for achieving this effect: cashews and zucchini. The cashews are simmered in the broth, which helps them blend up smooth, while the zucchini adds body. But neither is a distraction from the sweet, pure cauliflower flavor here. Try it topped with roasted shiitakes, whose crispy texture contrasts so well with the velvety, creamy-without-cream soup.

Halve the leeks and slice them into half moons. Place the pieces in a fine-mesh strainer and rinse well under running water, and then drain.

Place a soup pot or Dutch oven over medium heat, and when hot, swirl in the avocado oil. Then add the leeks, garlic, and ½ teaspoon of the salt. Cook, stirring often, until soft and translucent, and the garlic is beginning to brown, 6 to 8 minutes. Stir in the cauliflower and zucchini, and lightly sauté, stirring often, for about 3 minutes.

Add the broth, the cashews, and the remaining ½ teaspoon salt. Bring to a boil, then reduce the heat to low, and simmer, partially covered, until the cauliflower is tender, 10 to 15 minutes.

Working in batches, carefully add the soup to a blender and puree until smooth. (Be sure to fill the blender only halfway and process with the lid vented.) Return the soup to the pot and gently reheat.

Serve hot, garnished with a drizzle of the olive oil and a sprinkling of the crispy shiitakes, if desired.

Note: Save leek trimmings in an airtight container in the freezer until you have enough vegetable trimmings to make broth (see page 122).

MAKE IT YOURS

Light Pairings: Instead of the shiitakes, sprinkle the soup with chopped Maple Harissa Cashews (page 208) or chopped Rosemary Almonds (page 210).

Hearty Pairings: Top the soup with a pile of Favorite Sautéed Leafy Greens (page 152) or some Roasted Sweet Potato Cubes (page 146).

Simple Swaps: Use broccoli or Romanesco in place of the cauliflower. Or, replace the cauliflower with 4 cups of roasted cauliflower or broccoli (see page 144), adding it to the pot when the zucchini is tender and cooking for just a few minutes before blending.

Butternut Squash Soup
with Rosemary

SERVES 4

2 tablespoons ghee or avocado oil

1 medium white onion, diced

1 fresh rosemary sprig

1 medium butternut squash, peeled, seeded, and cubed (about 4 cups; see Note)

3 to 4 cups Mom's Chicken Broth (page 124) or Vegetable Broth (page 122)

1¼ teaspoons fine sea salt, or more as needed

MAKE IT YOURS

Hearty Pairings: Top with roasted cauliflower (see page 144), chopped Rosemary Almonds (page 210), roasted pumpkin seeds, or Maple Harissa Cashews (page 208).

I very often say, "Keep it simple." It's a mantra of sorts for me. This soup is an expression of that—it's a combination of just six ingredients that make a super-nutritious meal. Butternut squash is one of my favorite vegetables. I especially love it with a little rosemary for its piney flavor. Smooth, sweet, and fragrant—why add anything more?

Warm a Dutch oven over medium heat and when hot, add the ghee. Then add the onion and rosemary sprig, stir, and cook until the onion is soft and translucent, stirring periodically, 7 to 10 minutes.

Stir in the squash. Add 3 cups of the broth and the salt. The squash should be just covered with the broth; add more only if needed (you can always adjust the consistency later). Bring to a simmer over medium-high heat, then cover partially, reduce to medium-low, and simmer until the squash is tender and easily pierced with a knife, 20 to 30 minutes.

Remove the rosemary sprig and discard. Working in batches, transfer the solids and most of the liquid to a blender and puree until smooth. (Be sure to fill the blender only halfway and process with the lid vented.) Return the soup to the pot and gently reheat. If the texture is too thick, add broth, ¼ cup at a time. Taste for seasoning and serve hot.

Note: Save the butternut squash peels in an airtight container in the freezer until you have enough vegetable trimmings to make broth (see page 122).

ADDING INTENTION TO EVERYDAY EATING

Time is our most valuable asset—and we all get a limited amount of it! If you are always distracted, rushing around, or multitasking, it can feel like there is little joy to be found. But eating is always an opportunity for joy and gratitude, if you can bring intention to it. Whether it is planning what to eat, picking vegetables from the garden, cooking the ingredients, sitting down for a meal, or, yes, doing the dishes afterward, by adding intention to these activities you gain so much more from your experience. For example, I pause to bless my food prior to my first bite, acknowledging the origin, look, and smell of what I'm about to eat. Beyond ingesting nutrients, feeling good while eating has a positive impact on my digestion and my happiness, too. This can make an ordinary experience into something so much more meaningful. Why not bring more appreciation and gratitude to something you do three times a day? There is so much beauty in life if you slow down, open your eyes, and take a look.

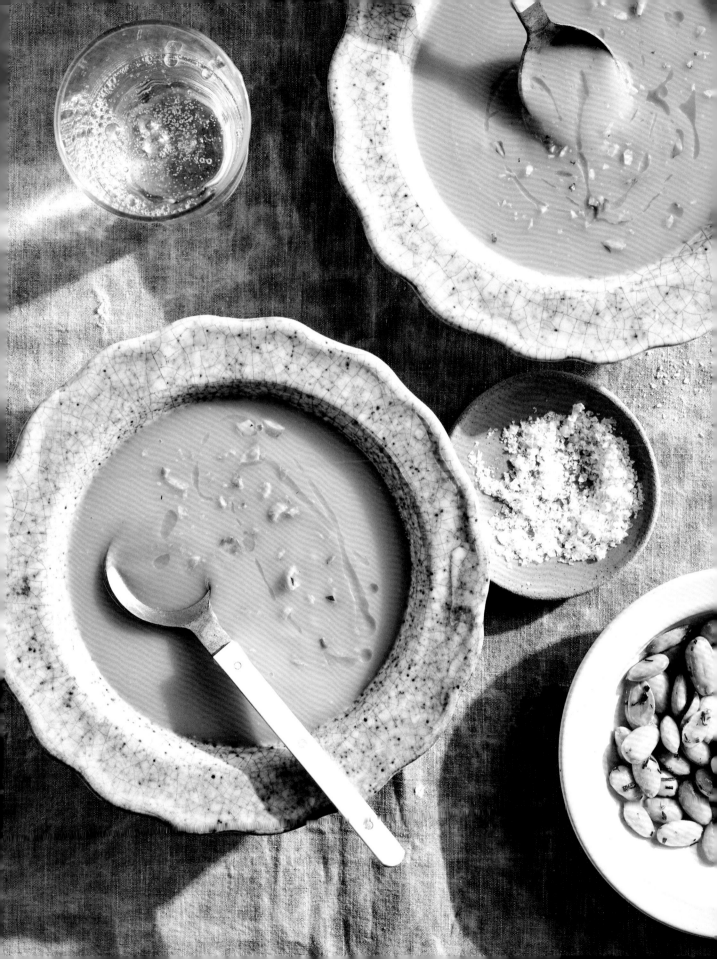

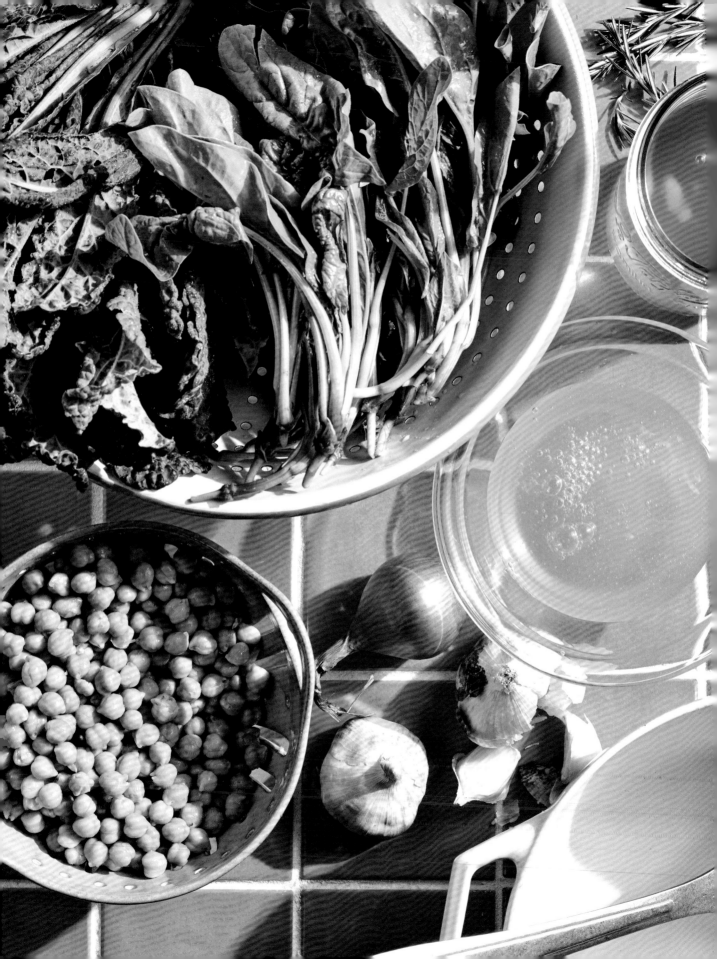

Beans and Greens Soup

SERVES 4 TO 6

3 tablespoons avocado oil
or ghee

2 large shallots or 1 medium
white onion, minced

5 garlic cloves, sliced

4 cups Mom's Chicken Broth
(page 124) or Vegetable Broth
(page 122)

3 cups cooked chickpeas (see
page 179), cannellini beans,
or navy beans, plus about
1 cup cooking liquid (or if using
canned, boxed, or jarred beans,
see Note)

2 teaspoons minced
fresh rosemary leaves

1 pound Tuscan kale, mature
spinach, or combination of
hearty greens, washed, tough
stems removed, and chopped
into bite-sized pieces

Fine sea salt

Big handful of fresh parsley
leaves, coarsely chopped

Extra-virgin olive oil

When working on this book, I couldn't decide which version of beans and greens soup I wanted to highlight, so I decided to include them all! Here is a flexible recipe that uses any type of quick-cooking greens you have around or that are in season—kale, spinach, and so on— and any cooked white beans, like cannellini or navy beans, or even chickpeas (which aren't a bean but are also a legume). With the collagen in the broth, the iron in the greens, and the protein in the beans, this soup offers an entire bowl of health benefits in a tasty format. (Be sure to keep the tough stems from the chard or kale for making broth, so nothing goes to waste.) I flavor this with a little rosemary and garlic, my favorites, but don't hesitate to swap in other herbs or spices if you want to customize it. Take this simple recipe and make it your own!

Place a soup pot or Dutch oven over medium heat, and when hot, drizzle in the avocado oil. Add the shallots and garlic and sauté until softened and translucent, another 5 minutes or so. Stir in the broth, beans and their liquid, and rosemary. Bring the mixture to a boil, then reduce the heat to low, partially cover the pot with a lid, and simmer for 10 to 12 minutes. (For a thicker soup, remove about a cup of cooked beans and broth and blend until smooth in a blender, then mix back into the pot.) Add the greens and continue to cook until wilted and tender, 12 to 15 minutes depending on the type. Season to taste with sea salt.

Just before serving, stir in the chopped parsley. Ladle into bowls and garnish with a drizzle of olive oil.

Note: Use a good-quality brand of canned, boxed, or jarred chickpeas or beans, drained and rinsed, if you don't have home-cooked. Substitute filtered water or additional broth for the cooking liquid.

MAKE IT YOURS

Light Pairings. Top the soup with Crunchy Spiced Chickpeas (page 213). A spoonful of Pesto (page 224) can also be stirred in for extra flavor.

Hearty Pairings: Add shredded cooked chicken or Chicken Meatballs (page 194).

For the Kids: My kids like some chopped Roasted Vegetables (page 144) on top.

Ramen-Style Soup
with Steamed Vegetables

SERVES 4

About 2 pounds assorted fresh vegetables, such as:

• 4 small wedges kabocha, red kuri, or hubbard squash

• 1 small bunch baby turnips, trimmed and halved or quartered

• 2 cups broccoli or cauliflower florets

• 4 small wedges green cabbage, cut from ¼ head

• 4 ounces fresh green beans, trimmed

• 1 cup sugar snap peas

10 ounces brown rice, millet, or quinoa ramen noodles

6 cups Mom's Chicken Broth (page 124) or Vegetable Broth (page 122)

2 tablespoons miso paste (red or white)

3 tablespoons tahini (optional)

3 tablespoons Tamari Dressing (page 228)

Optional Toppings

4 or 5 fresh shiitake or button mushroom caps, thinly sliced

2 scallions, green and white parts, trimmed and thinly sliced

4 squares toasted nori

Finely grated fresh ginger

Toasted sesame seeds

When I lived in Japan as a 14-year-old, I didn't eat much local food—to be honest, it was a lot of burgers and instant soup. I was focused on building my modeling career, so my hours were strange, I had no money, and the language barrier was intense. But Japanese soup culture is serious, and I did go to ramen shops occasionally with some of the other girls I met there. As foreign as I felt, there was something comforting about this type of food when I felt lonely and homesick. This is still true for me, especially in cold weather; I love soup and eat it many nights a week.

This ramen-style soup—made my way, with lots of vegetables and homemade broth—is a special favorite for my kids, who love the salty flavor of the miso and the millet or rice noodles (which are gluten free). It's fun to let everyone assemble their own bowls, just the way they like. When I use vegetable broth instead of chicken broth, I find a drizzle of tahini enriches the soup nicely.

Fill a pot or Dutch oven with 1 to 2 inches of water and fit it with a collapsible steaming basket or stacking steamer insert. Set a sheet pan or platter to the side, for the cooked vegetables.

Bring the water in the pot to a simmer over medium heat. One at a time, add the vegetables to the basket, cover the pot, and steam until just tender (taste to test for doneness): the squash will take 6 to 10 minutes, the baby turnips 5 to 7 minutes, the broccoli or cauliflower 3 to 5 minutes, the cabbage 2 to 4 minutes, the green beans 1 to 2 minutes, and the snap peas 30 to 45 seconds. As you finish cooking each batch, transfer it to the platter, keeping them separate.

Rinse out the pot and return it to the stove. Cook the noodles according to the package instructions, then rinse under cool water and drain well. Place the noodles in a medium bowl.

Pour the broth into the pot and bring to a simmer over medium heat. Place the miso paste in a medium bowl and add the tahini (if using), then add a ladleful or two of the hot broth, whisking vigorously until smooth. Pour the miso mixture back into the pot and stir in the dressing. The broth should be strongly flavored; If not strong enough for you, adjust the

(recipe continues)

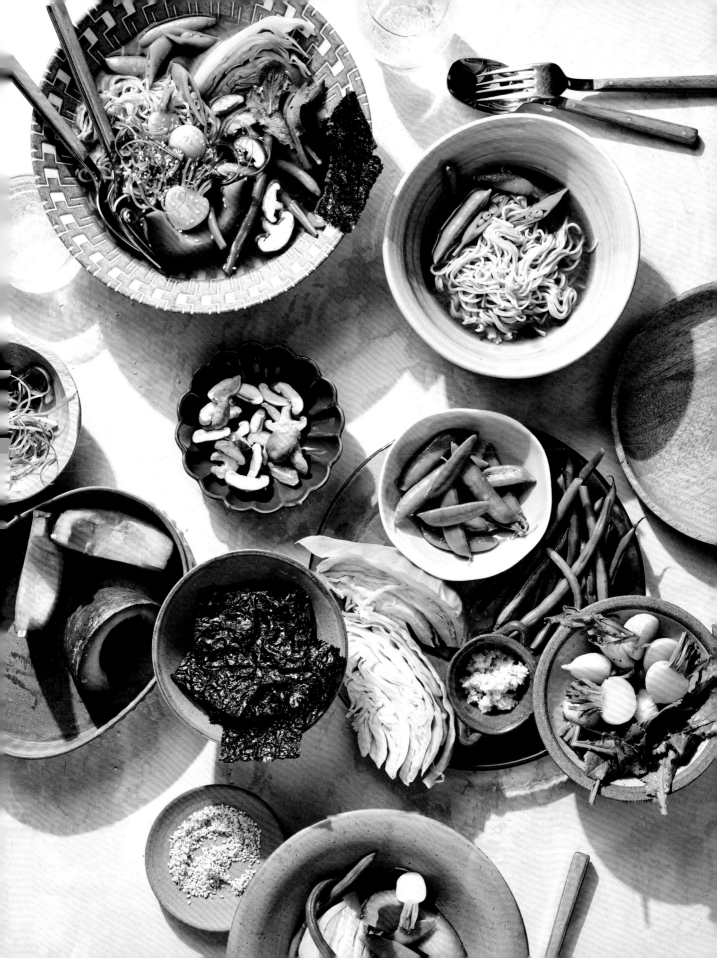

Hearty Pairings: Slices of cooked chicken or even a few Chicken Meatballs (page 194) would be a great addition here. A soft- or hard-boiled egg is traditional and delicious, too.

Simple Swaps: For a speedy version of this soup, use any leftover blanched vegetables in place of the steamed ones; or add fresh leafy greens directly to the broth to wilt. Crispy Roasted Shiitake Mushrooms (page 214) would be delicious instead of the fresh.

seasonings by adding more dressing and miso. Keep the pot covered and warm over low heat.

For the toppings, arrange the mushroom, scallions, and nori on a small platter. Put the ginger and sesame seeds in small bowls.

Bring the pot of broth, the platter of vegetables, the bowl of noodles, and the toppings to the table, so everyone can build their own bowl just as they like it. (Alternatively, you can divide the vegetables and noodles among the bowls, top them with the broth and toppings, and serve.)

GARDENING

When I was growing up, I spent most of my school holidays with my grandmother Vó Maria, who lived in the countryside, where she had an amazing garden. Her family had moved to a German colony in the south of Brazil in the late 1800s, so she spoke mostly German. She knew so much about plants and their healing abilities. Though I didn't speak much German, I would just follow her around, helping her water the garden, feed the animals, and husk the corn. Without a car, she traveled only by cow cart or by foot, so she didn't leave her land very often. Most important, she was born in tough times and so she continued to waste absolutely nothing. (When I say nothing went to waste, I really mean it. I was amazed when I once saw her kill a chicken for dinner and feed the other chickens the corn left

inside its stomach!) Every little thing was so precious to her. This was a philosophy I learned from her without words, just by following her around and working with her.

Gardening is an art *and* a seven-days-a-week job; I have enormous respect for anyone who gardens, especially professional farmers and gardeners who bring so many things to life. I've had some version of a garden in all the places I've ever lived, even if it's just a pot of basil or rosemary on the windowsill. I am lucky to have a nice garden in Costa Rica, where we grow most of the produce we eat. My absolute favorites to grow are the turmeric, ginger, herbs, cucumbers, carrots, and lettuces, while the kids love the cherry tomatoes and red peppers. We had to plant most of the garden

in raised beds so the iguanas wouldn't eat everything.

Working in the garden can be like a meditation. It's amazing to see the tiny seeds grow into the foods that nourish us. I love to witness all the different colors, shapes, and sizes—an assortment that nature provides. The kids—and their friends, during picnic playdates—get to pick cherry tomatoes, cucumbers, and green beans directly from the plants and eat them. I think my grandmother would be proud that I am teaching my children where our food comes from, about the cycles of nature, and the time, patience, and respect gardening requires. I am also lucky that through the years I have had incredible gardeners keep my gardens flourishing when I am not there.

Spiced Lentil Soup

2 tablespoons avocado oil or ghee

2 medium carrots, diced

1 white or yellow medium onion, diced

2 large celery stalks, diced

2 dried bay leaves

1½ teaspoons fine sea salt

5 garlic cloves, minced

2 teaspoons curry powder

1½ teaspoons ground cumin

½ teaspoon ground turmeric

Freshly ground black pepper

1 cup brown lentils

5 cups Mom's Chicken Broth (page 124) or Vegetable Broth (page 122)

Extra-virgin olive oil

I spent many winters in Boston, and I admit it was difficult for me to keep warm. While I never got used to cold weather, sipping on hot broth definitely helped heat me from within. Soups became my wintertime salvation—and so began my deep love for them. Especially lentil soup, which is rich with fiber, potassium, iron, and folate, and is so savory. Flavored with warm spices, onions, carrots, and celery, this is a naturally hearty soup you'll be dreaming about the moment the weather turns chilly.

Place a soup pot or Dutch oven over medium heat, and when hot, swirl in the oil. Then add the carrots, onion, celery, and bay leaves, plus ½ teaspoon of the salt. Cook until the vegetables soften and even begin to caramelize, 8 to 12 minutes, stirring often. Stir in the garlic, curry powder, cumin, turmeric, and a few grinds of black pepper (or skip the spices for a plainer taste), and once it's very fragrant, add the lentils, broth, and remaining 1 teaspoon salt. Bring to a boil, then reduce the heat to medium-low, partially cover, and simmer, stirring every now and then, until the lentils are tender, 20 to 25 minutes. Remove the bay leaves.

Ladle the soup into bowls and garnish with a drizzle of olive oil, if desired.

MAKE IT YOURS

Light Pairings: A few Seed Crackers (page 218) are always good on the side; just before serving, add up to 8 ounces stemmed baby spinach, chard, or Tuscan kale, and cook until just tender.

Coconut-Curry Vegetable Soup

MAKES 4 SERVINGS

3 tablespoons unrefined virgin coconut oil

1 small yellow onion, diced

1 garlic clove, minced

1 tablespoon curry powder

½ teaspoon ground turmeric

¼ teaspoon ground cinnamon

Fine sea salt

Freshly ground black pepper

3 small carrots, thinly sliced

3 cups Mom's Chicken Broth (page 124) or Vegetable Broth (page 122)

4 cups small fresh cauliflower or broccoli florets, or a combination

1½ cups Coconut Milk (page 72) or full-fat coconut milk

1 cup From-Scratch Chickpeas (page 179) or boxed or jarred chickpeas, rinsed

Big handful of fresh spinach, stemmed and chopped

Lime wedges (optional)

Chopped cilantro (optional)

Coconuts are incredibly versatile, as well as nutritious, with essential minerals like manganese, selenium, copper, and iron. In this filling vegetable soup, the rich, naturally sweet coconut milk is mixed with homemade broth and seasoned with aromatics like garlic, curry powder, turmeric, and cinnamon; the result is a surprisingly complex broth.

I like to include a variety of vegetables in this—some hard (carrots), some soft (chickpeas), plus some spinach and cauliflower—so that every bite offers a variety of textures.

In a Dutch oven or soup pot, heat 2 tablespoons of the coconut oil over medium heat. Add the onion and cook for 1 minute. Stir in the garlic and cook 1 more minute, stirring often—don't let it brown. Add the curry powder, turmeric, cinnamon,1 teaspoon salt, and a grind or two of pepper. Toast the spices lightly, stirring, for 1 minute. Add the remaining tablespoon oil and the carrots and cook, stirring often, for 2 to 3 minutes. Turn the heat down to medium-low, stir in ¼ cup of the broth, then scrape the bottom of the pan with a wooden spoon to loosen the browned bits, and cook for another minute.

Add the cauliflower florets, coconut milk, chickpeas, and remaining 2¾ cups broth. Simmer, covered, until the carrots and cauliflower are just tender, about 10 to 15 minutes.

Fold in the spinach and stir until wilted, another minute. Taste and add salt, if needed.

Spoon into individual bowls and serve with lime wedges and cilantro, if you like.

MAKE IT YOURS

Hearty Pairings: This is great served with a seared or pan-fried fillet of fish, like salmon, halibut, or cod. Or, add shredded cooked chicken or Chicken Meatballs (page 194), or serve over cooked rice noodles or wild rice.

Simple Swaps: Add a diced peeled sweet potato to the pot along with the carrots. If you have any blanched vegetables, chop and add 1 cup of them right before you drop in the spinach. If you want a little heat, add ½ teaspoon of cayenne with the spices.

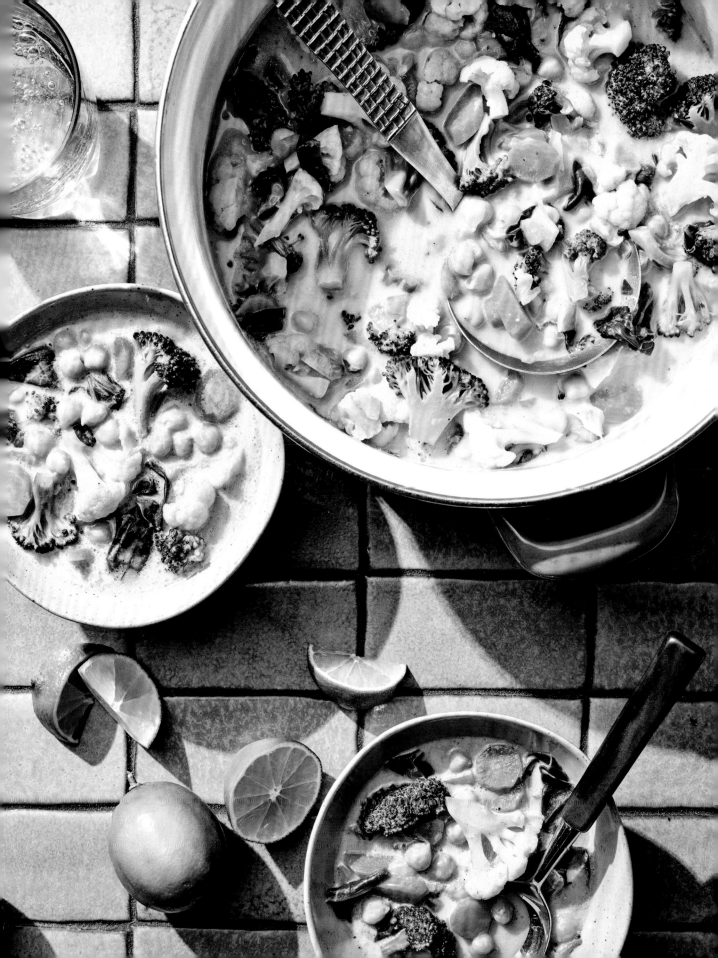

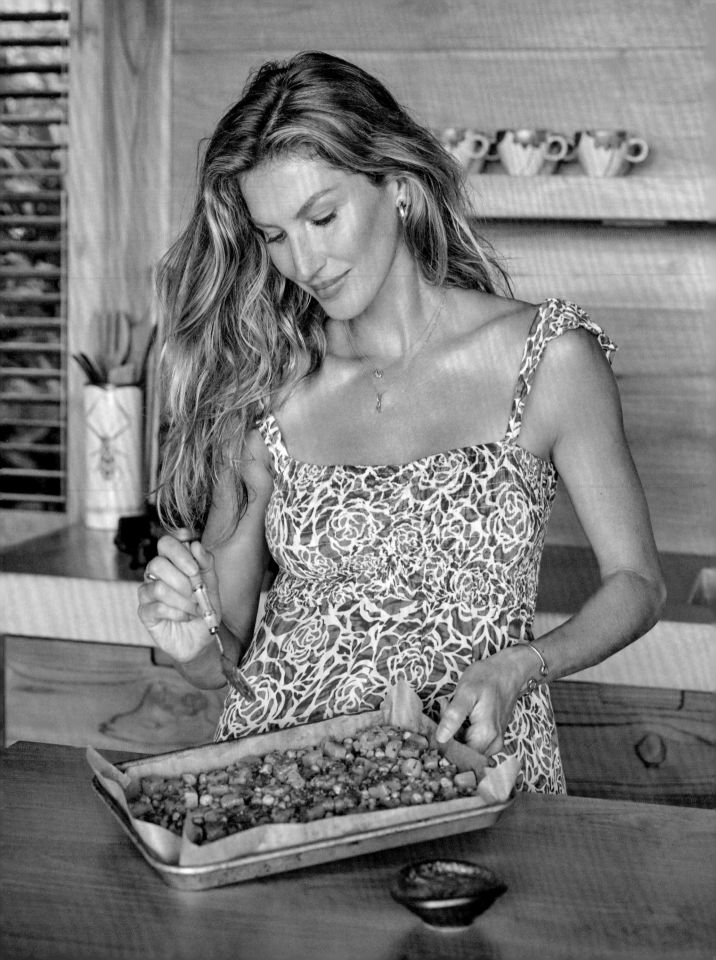

Everyday Vegetables

Vegetables make up the majority of my diet. I love to mix and match them, roast them, blanch them, shred them, stir-fry them, sauté them, puree them, add them to pizza, and roll them up in rice paper. So, pair the recipes that follow with a favorite protein or eat the veggies on their own. Nature provides an amazing rainbow of options—take advantage of the full spectrum, and your body will thank you!

Roasted Vegetables

SERVES 4

3 tablespoons avocado oil, coconut oil, or ghee

1½ to 2 pounds hearty seasonal vegetables, such as:

• 1 large cauliflower, trimmed, cut into florets (see Note)

• 2 or 3 full heads of broccoli or broccoli crowns, trimmed, cut into small florets (see Note)

• Brussels sprouts, trimmed and halved

• 1 to 2 pounds thick or thin carrots, sliced (if thick, in ½-inch coins; if thin, halved lengthwise)

• 1 acorn or butternut squash, peeled, seeded, and cut into wedges or cubes (see Note)

½ teaspoon fine sea salt, or more as needed

MAKE IT YOURS

Light Pairings: Puree some of these roasted vegetables with some homemade broth (pages 122 or 124) for a simple soup. Or add some roasted vegetables to a salad.

Hearty Pairings: Serve with Pan-Fried Falafel (page 177), toss with zucchini noodles (page 166), or include as part of a frittata (see page 87).

For the Kids: On taco night (see page 202), tuck some roasted veggies into your tortillas. Use to top a pizza (see page 173), along with your favorite cheese.

Roasted vegetables are a staple in our household for three reasons: they are easy to make, they are full of nutrients, and the caramelized flavors are delicious. This is why we often make a couple types at a time (each on their own sheet pan), and it's why we eat them so often. Cauliflower and Brussels sprouts are some of my favorites, but try this technique with fennel, broccoli, butternut squash, or anything else that's organic and seasonal. (I love roasted sweet potatoes so much I have a separate set of recipes for them on page 147.) Whether served hot, cold, or at room temperature, these roasted vegetables are some of my favorite things to keep in the fridge for quick meals.

Preheat the oven to 400°F. Line 2 sheet pans with parchment.

Place the oil in a large bowl, then add the vegetables; if using multiple varieties, mix each type separately. Add the salt, tossing well so that every piece is coated with oil. Put the oiled vegetables on the pans, keeping each type separate so you can remove them as they finish cooking. Spread in an even layer.

Place the pans in the oven and roast the vegetables until lightly caramelized and tender, turning them over with a metal spatula midway through. The cauliflower, broccoli, and carrots will take 20 to 30 minutes; the Brussels sprouts will take 25 to 30 minutes; and the squash will take 25 to 40 minutes. As the vegetables are finished, remove them from the oven and season with a few extra pinches of salt, if needed.

Serve the roasted vegetables hot, warm, or at room temperature. Or cool and then pack them in airtight glass containers, and refrigerate for up to 3 days.

Note: When prepping broccoli or cauliflower, trim off the tough outer layer of the stems, cut into thick coins, and roast as well! Other varieties of winter squash—like delicata, kabocha, kuri, and hubbard—have skins that will soften as they roast, so no need to peel them.

SPICE UP YOUR VEG

Change things up by tossing your vegetables with 1 teaspoon of your favorite spice blend, along with the salt, before roasting them. (I love the earthy Moroccan spice blend ras el hanout.) Or, after cooking, sprinkle with crushed pistachios or roasted pumpkin seeds or drizzle with a good balsamic or fresh lemon juice just before serving.

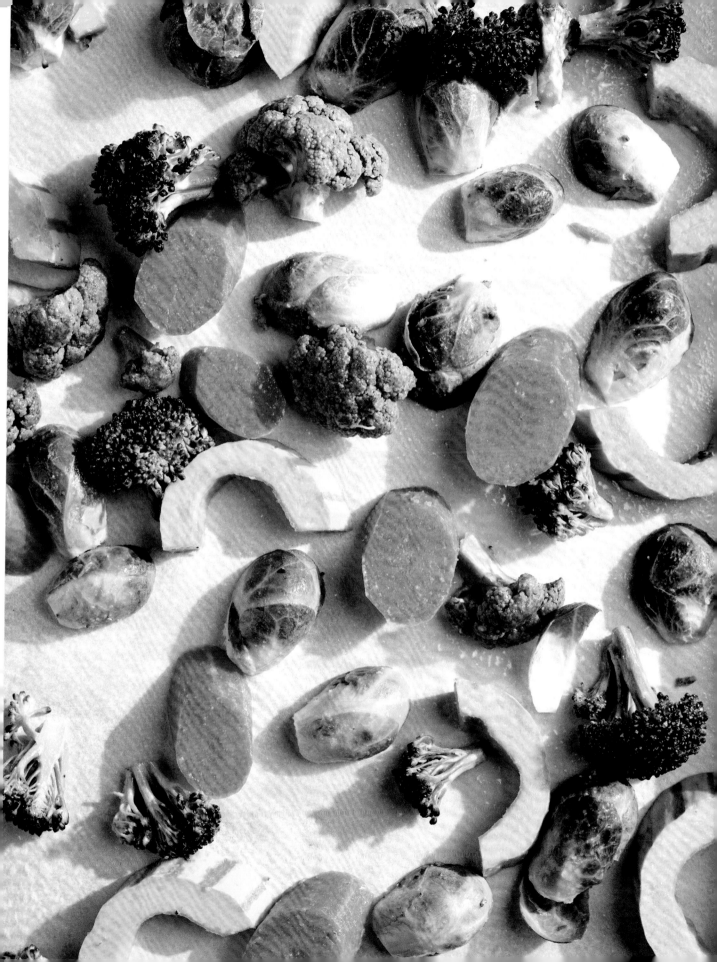

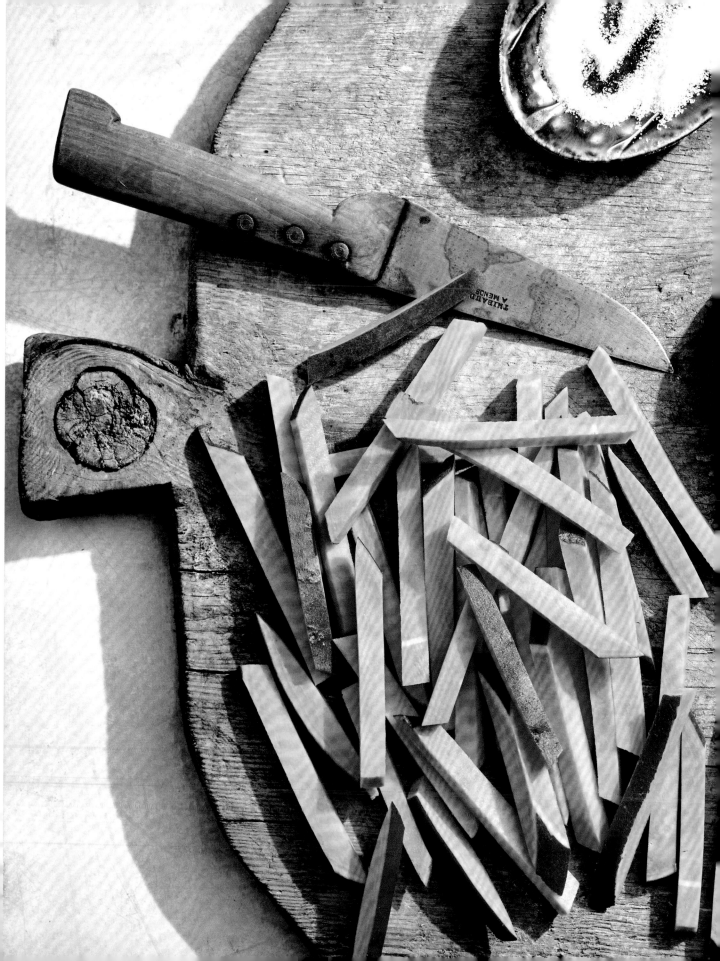

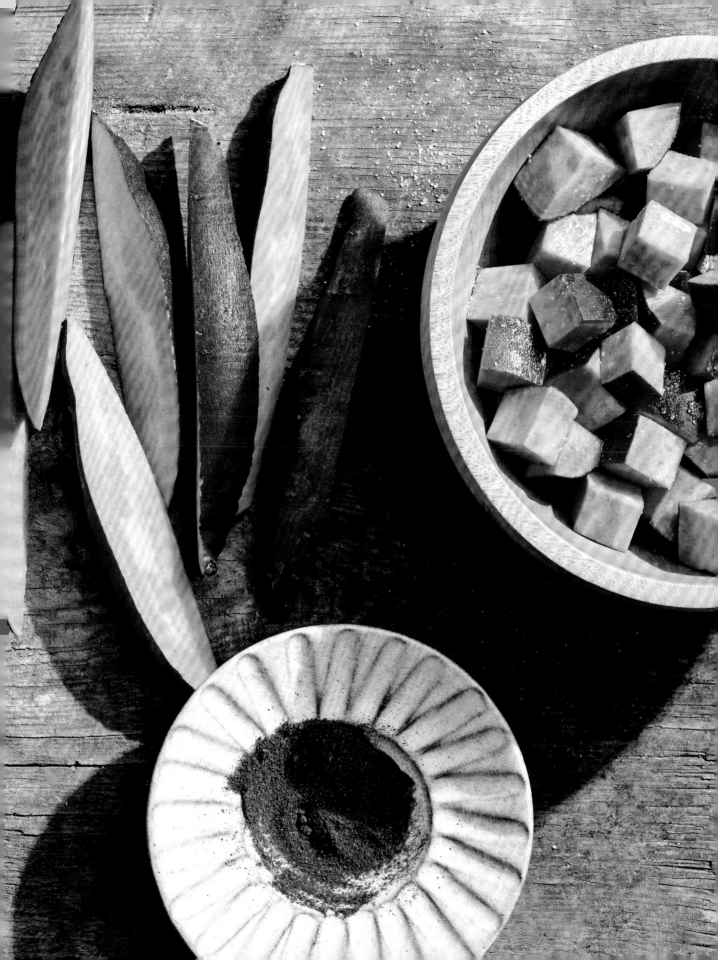

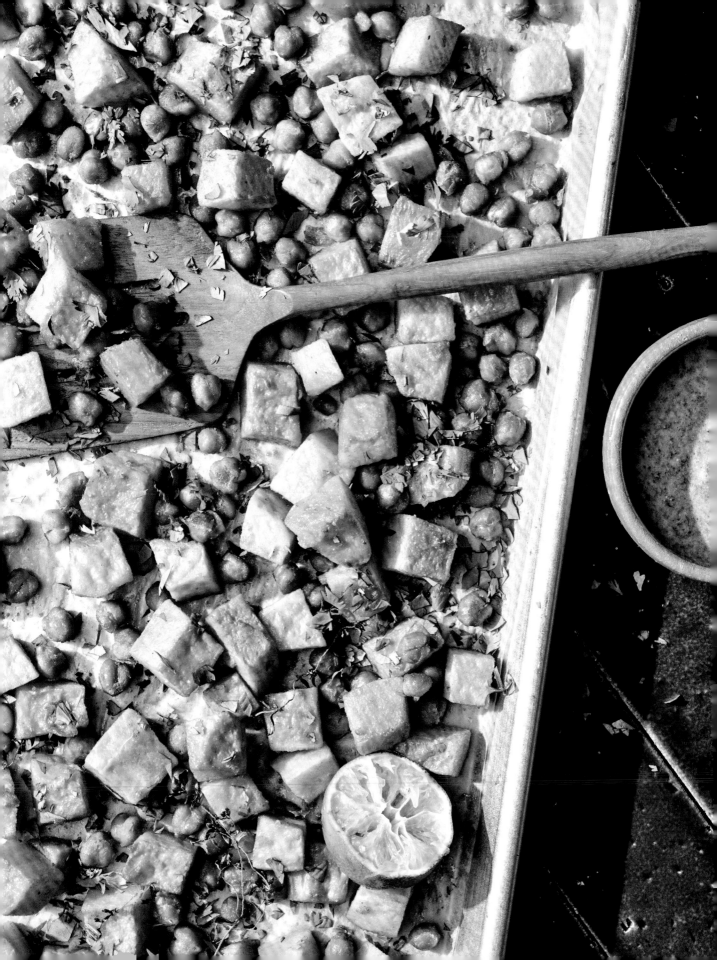

Sheet-Pan Squash
and Chickpeas

SERVES 2 TO 4

2 tablespoons unrefined virgin coconut oil or avocado oil, plus more for the pan

2 small or 1 large butternut squash, peeled, seeded, and cut into ½-inch cubes (3 to 4 cups)

1 teaspoon ground cumin

½ teaspoon fine sea salt, or more as needed

3 to 4 sprigs fresh thyme

1¾ cups From-Scratch Chickpeas (page 179) or jarred or boxed chickpeas, drained and rinsed

1 tablespoon fresh lime juice

2 tablespoons chopped fresh cilantro or flat-leaf parsley

Cilantro-Mint Dressing (page 221), for serving

Assembling the elements of a dinner on a sheet pan is my idea of simple. Here, you toss butternut squash and chickpeas with oil and cumin, and bake them until done—so easy! This vegetable-heavy dish can go in so many directions; serve it as a bowl, as part of a salad, or in a taco. You just might make it every week. I often do!

Preheat the oven to 400°F. Line a sheet pan with parchment and then lightly brush with oil.

In a medium bowl, combine the squash with 1 tablespoon oil, the cumin, and ½ teaspoon salt. Spread evenly on the prepared sheet pan. Place the thyme sprigs on top. Roast for 20 minutes. Meanwhile, put the chickpeas in the same bowl and toss with the remaining 1 tablespoon oil and a pinch of salt.

Remove the squash from the oven and flip with a spatula. Add the seasoned chickpeas and spread out evenly. Continue to roast until the chickpeas are toasted and the squash is tender, another 15 to 20 minutes.

Taste for salt, adding more as needed. Drizzle the squash mixture with the lime juice and top with the cilantro. Serve with the dressing, if you like.

MAKE IT YOURS

Light Pairings: Add a scoop of shredded fresh greens for a quick lunch or dinner.

Hearty Pairings: This is delicious with Miso-Mustard Roasted Whole Cauliflower (page 170) or with a fried egg on top.

For the Kids: This combo makes an amazing taco filling (see page 202).

Simple Swap: Instead of cumin, season with ½ teaspoon ground coriander, ground fennel, or smoked paprika.

Favorite Sautéed Leafy Greens

SERVES 4

2 tablespoons avocado oil
or ghee

2 garlic cloves, minced
or finely grated

1 pound fresh spinach or Swiss
chard, tough stems removed
and leaves chopped (see Note)

Fine sea salt

In my early twenties I ate a ton of green vegetables to try to calm my body, as it was one of the only foods my doctor approved during this reset time. Before that, I was more into pizza and french fries, with the occasional piece of fruit. But once I started eating sautéed leafy greens on a regular basis, I began to crave them all the time. Their pure, clean greenness filled me with such satisfaction; they felt like a gift to my body. It helps, too, that they are so easy to prepare. Get the best-quality greens you can (ideally from a farmer's market or your own garden, but anything organic is great), sauté them with garlic, oil, and salt until wilted and tender, then enjoy!

Place a Dutch oven or wide skillet over medium heat and when hot, add the oil. Add the garlic and cook until just golden and fragrant, stirring constantly, about 1 minute. Pile in the greens and sprinkle with a big pinch of salt. Toss the greens, using tongs, until wilted, about 2 minutes for spinach or 5 minutes for chard.

Taste for seasoning, then transfer to a serving plate and serve. If stored in an airtight glass container in the refrigerator, the greens will keep for about 3 days.

Note: Save the chard stems for making broth (see page 122). If you have only just washed your greens, don't worry about spinning them dry. The steam from a little water on the leaves helps them cook.

MAKE IT YOURS

Hearty Pairings: Add some sautéed greens to Creamy Cauliflower Soup (page 131). Or, serve with Garlicky Clams with Rice Noodles (page 187) or Baked Risotto with Asparagus (page 169). Or, serve with Warm Wild Rice Salad (page 116) and top with a fried egg.

For the Kids: My kids love these sautéed greens tucked into Egg and Cheese Quesadillas (page 84) for a nutrient-packed breakfast.

Simple Swaps: Try with curly kale, adding ½ cup of broth with the greens and cooking until tender, about 8 to 10 minutes.

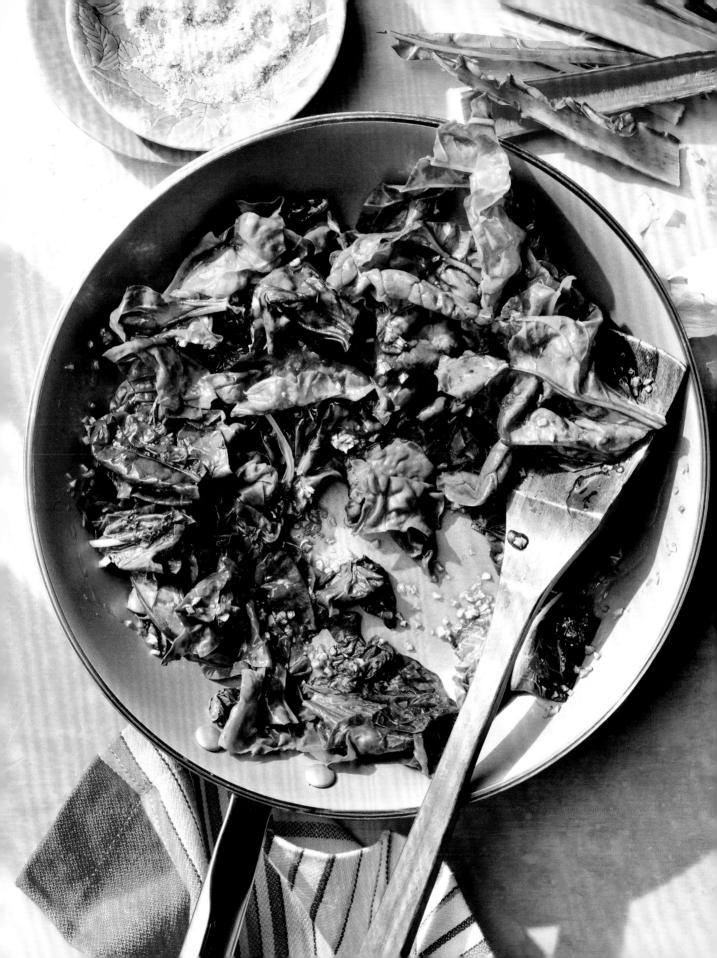

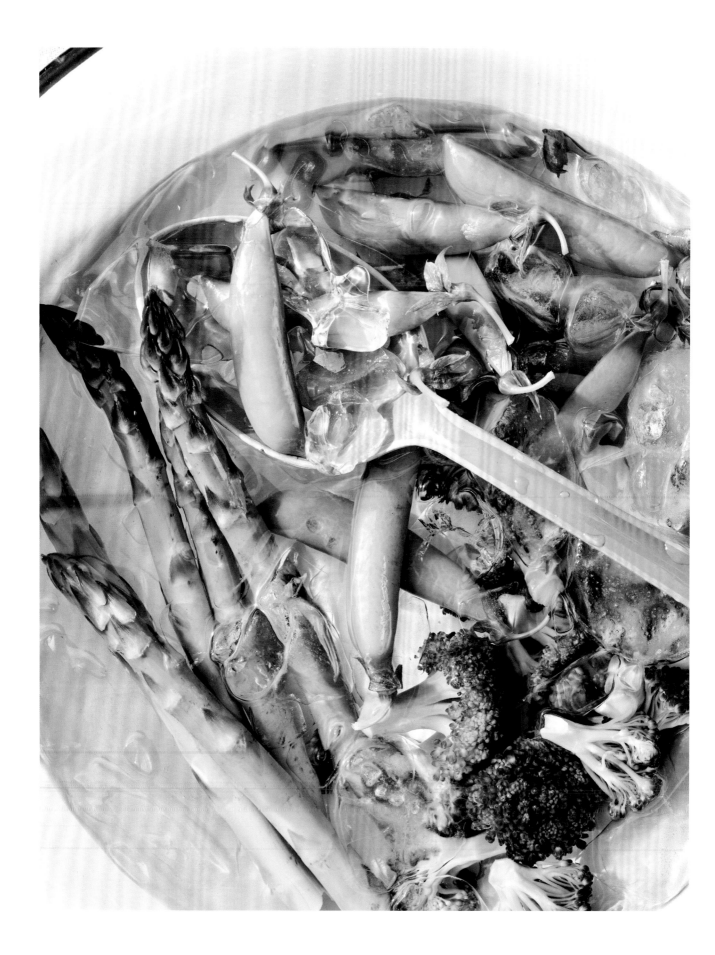

Best Blanched Vegetables

SERVES 4

2 tablespoons fine sea salt, or more as needed

1 pound fresh seasonal vegetables, such as:

• 2 or 3 broccoli heads, cut into small florets

• Broccolini, tough ends trimmed

• Sugar snap peas, trimmed and any strings removed

• Green beans, trimmed

• Asparagus spears, tough ends trimmed, spears left whole or sliced

• Carrots, quartered or halved lengthwise if thick, or left whole if thin

When I was on a raw-food diet, I discovered that while I love cucumbers and celery in their natural state, many other vegetables, like green beans, broccoli, and broccolini, I prefer slightly cooked. To blanch, simply place veggies into a big pot of boiling water and cook just until the color brightens; the texture should be barely tender and still quite crisp. An ice bath stops the cooking.

Cooking to al dente makes nutrients like calcium easier for the body to absorb and limits loss of water-soluble vitamins, so you get maximum nutritional value with easier digestion.

I like to make a big batch of these at one time and refrigerate them to later add to a salad or broth for a heathy meal. I also—big surprise!—love to eat them simply drizzled with a little olive oil and seasoned with salt.

Make an ice bath by filling a large bowl with ice cubes and water.

Fill a large pot with filtered water and bring to a boil over high heat. Add the salt, then add the vegetables, one type at a time if doing a few, and cook briefly, until just slightly tender, about 1 minute for the broccoli and sugar snap peas; 2 minutes for the asparagus, broccolini, and green beans; and 3 to 4 minutes for the carrots. Taste a piece to see if it's done.

Using a spider or slotted spoon, transfer the vegetables to the ice bath to shock them and stop the cooking. Drain the vegetables, and dry on a dishtowel, if you like. Stored in a glass container in the fridge, the blanched vegetables will keep up to 3 days.

MAKE IT YOURS

Light Pairings: Tuck some of these blanched veggies into Extra-Crunchy Summer Rolls (page 156) or Pesto Chicken Lettuce Wraps (page 193). Or, add them to any bowl or salad, especially Benny's Shaved Salad (page 102).

Hearty Pairings: Add some blanched vegetables to Mom's Chicken Broth (page 124) along with some cooked chicken for a fast soup. Or, include blanched veggies in your ramen (see page 136) or a frittata (see page 87).

For the Kids: Blanch a whole rainbow of vegetables, then serve them with Hummus (page 180), Tahini Dressing (page 220), or Cashew Ranch (page 227).

Simple Swaps: Use blanched vegetables instead of raw in a stir-fry (see page 162) or in Coconut-Curry Vegetable Soup (page 140) for a faster prep.

Extra-Crunchy Summer Rolls

MAKES 8 ROLLS

8 rice paper wrappers, preferably from brown rice

¼ medium green cabbage, cored and shredded

2 medium carrots, julienned or coarsely shredded

1 seedless cucumber, peeled and julienned

1 firm apple, cored and thinly sliced

1 avocado, peeled, pitted, and sliced

Ginger-Cashew Sauce (page 223), for serving

TIP: I usually use a mandoline to quickly prep the cabbage, carrots, and cucumber.

This is one of my favorite recipes in this book. Unlike fried spring rolls, these rolls are soft, made from softened rice paper filled with fresh vegetables and fruit. I love the different textures of this extra-crunchy version: cabbage, carrot, and cucumber, with juicy apple and creamy avocado, wrapped up in a chewy wrapper. Vivi loves the simpler version with just cucumber and avocado. But like many other recipes in this book, this one is flexible: use whatever produce you have, and serve with any sauces you like. The Ginger-Cashew (page 223) is my absolute favorite, creamy and salty; Vivi loves the Almond Butter–Sesame (page 223), which is a little sweet. These rolls are great for company, too; you can even have your guests roll up their own versions—all you need do is set out the fillings and wrappers.

Fill a wide, flat bowl with 1 to 2 inches of very warm water. Place one rice paper wrapper in the water for a few seconds, until just softened and pliable (do not let the wrapper sit too long or it will get too soft).

Place the wrapper on a cutting board. On the bottom third, leaving 1 inch on each side bare, neatly stack a thin bundle of cabbage, a few carrot and cucumber slices, a couple apple slices, and a couple avocado slices. Carefully fold the bottom edge of the wrapper up and over the fillings, fold in the sides, and roll up like a burrito. Repeat with the remaining wrappers and filling ingredients.

Serve immediately, with the sauce on the side for dipping.

VIVI'S CUCUMBER-AVOCADO ROLLS

In a medium bowl, gently toss the cucumber, avocado, the juice of 1 lime, and about 2 tablespoons chopped fresh cilantro. Fill wrappers and roll them up. Serve with Almond Butter–Sesame Sauce (page 223).

MAKE IT YOURS

Light Pairings: Serve the rolls with some raw or blanched vegetables (page 155) to dip in the sauce.

Hearty Pairings: Add a little cooked steak (see page 199) or chicken (like shredded Rosemary-Lemon Chicken Paillards on page 197) to the filling if you want some extra protein.

Simple Swap: Use shredded romaine Napa cabbage instead of green cabbage.

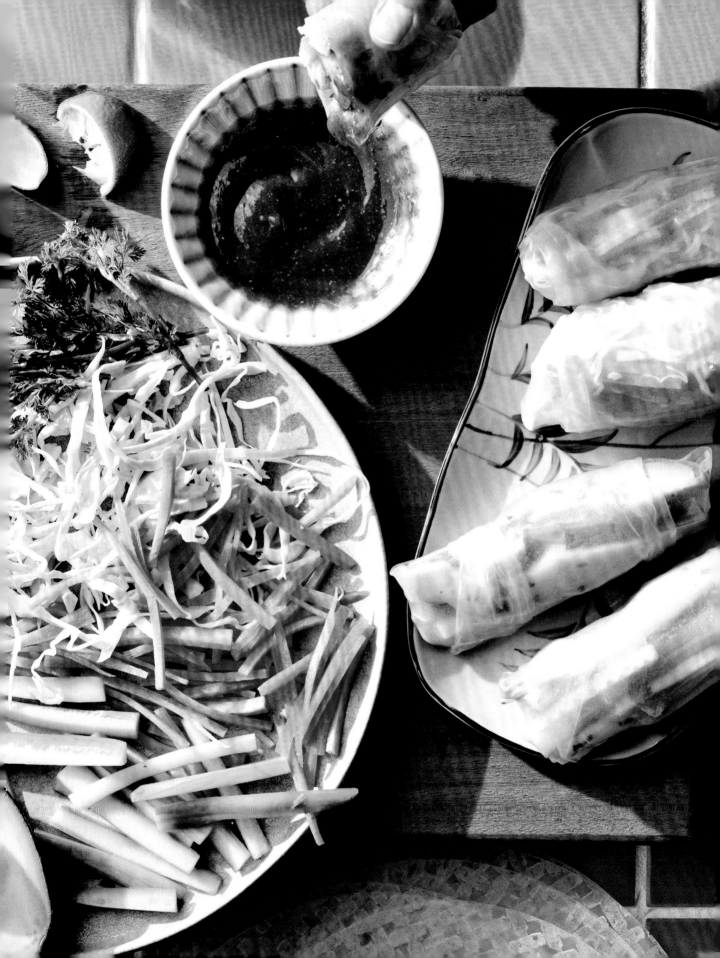

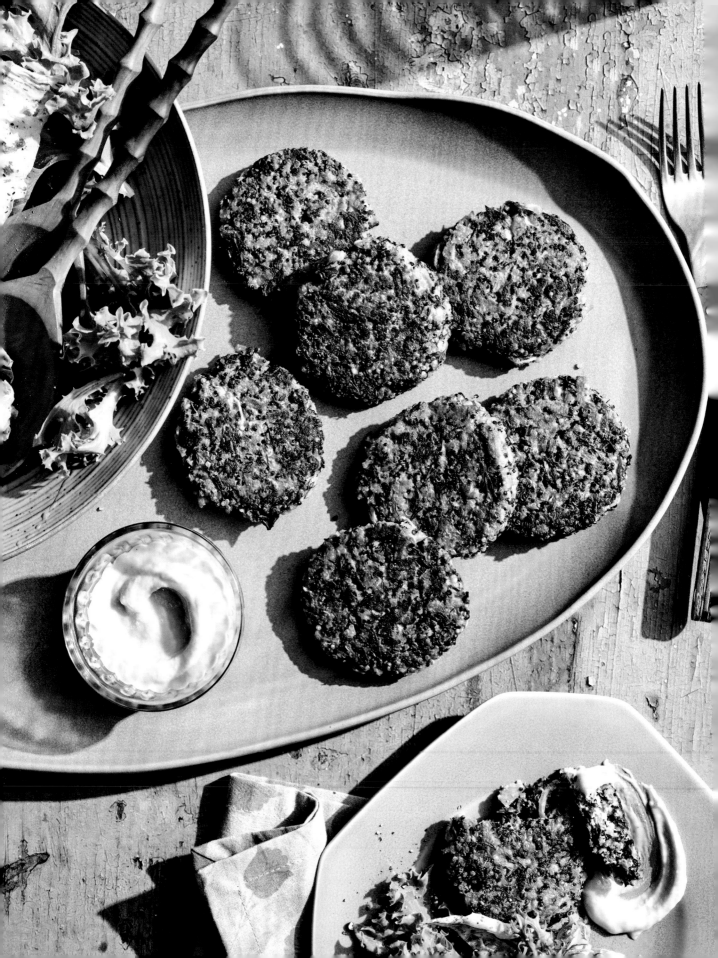

Vegetable-Quinoa Cakes

MAKES 8 CAKES

3 tablespoons avocado oil, plus more for pan-frying

1 medium shallot or ½ small white onion, minced

1 garlic clove, minced or finely grated

½ cup tricolor quinoa, rinsed

¾ cup filtered water

1 teaspoon fine sea salt

5 cups (5 ounces) packed fresh spinach leaves

2 large eggs

½ cup coarsely grated carrot

½ cup coarsely grated zucchini or yellow squash

¼ cup coarsely chopped fresh dill or parsley

3 tablespoons almond flour

Tahini Dressing (page 220), Cashew Ranch (page 227), Ginger-Cashew Sauce (page 223), or any of the Tamari Dressing variations (see page 228), for serving

These delicious pan-fried cakes are a nutritional powerhouse—a combination of protein-rich quinoa and almond flour, iron-packed spinach, antioxidant-loaded zucchini, and more. Plus, the tricolor quinoa, the abundance of herbs, and a rainbow of produce make for a fun spectrum of color. A couple of these cakes are great topping any salad or bowl, but they are also fun on their own when having friends over or with kids—just add any sauce you like for dipping (see suggestions). Also, try making a double batch and freezing half; the frozen cakes heat up quickly for a fast meal. If you can't find tricolor quinoa, any other kind of quinoa will do.

Place a medium saucepan over medium heat and when hot, add about ½ tablespoon of the oil, followed by the shallot. Cook, stirring often, until softened and translucent, 2 to 3 minutes. Stir in the garlic and then the quinoa. Pour in the water and ½ teaspoon of salt and bring to a boil, reduce the heat to low, cover the pan, and cook until the quinoa is tender and the water is absorbed, about 15 minutes. Allow to cool, uncovered. (You can speed this up by spreading the quinoa on a sheet pan.)

Warm a large sauté pan over medium heat and when hot, add about ½ tablespoon oil. Pile in the spinach and cook, tossing with tongs, until wilted, about 1 minute. Transfer to a plate to cool, then gently squeeze out the liquid and coarsely chop the greens.

In a medium bowl, whisk the eggs. Stir in the cooled quinoa and spinach, and add the carrot, zucchini, dill, almond flour, and the remaining ½ teaspoon salt. (The mixture will be a bit wet and loose, but it'll firm up when cooked.) Use a ¼ cup measuring cup to divide the mixture into 8 portions, shaping them into little cakes and arranging them on a cutting board or in a sheet pan.

(recipe continues)

MAKE IT YOURS

Light Pairings: Eat these cakes with a simple salad topped with Tahini Dressing (page 220) or Cashew Ranch (page 227).

Hearty Pairings: Serve the cakes with a scoop of Benny's Shaved Salad (page 102) or tuck them into a bowl or wrap in lettuce leaves along with some roasted vegetables or greens, with a sauce for dipping.

Simple Swap: About ¼ cup of Favorite Sautéed Leafy Greens (page 152) can replace the freshly sautéed spinach.

Rinse out the sauté pan, then return it to the stove and place over medium-low heat. When hot, add 1 tablespoon of the oil, swirling the pan to coat it evenly. Arrange 4 cakes in the pan and use a spatula to gently flatten them into patties about ½ inch thick. Cook without disturbing until golden brown on the bottom, about 5 minutes. Slide the spatula under the cakes and quickly flip. Brown the other sides, another 4 to 5 minutes. Transfer the cooked patties to a clean plate or sheet pan and repeat to cook the remaining cakes, adding another tablespoon of oil to the pan.

Serve immediately with desired sauce. (The cooked cakes can be stored in an airtight container in the refrigerator for up to 3 days, or layered between sheets of parchment in a airtight container in the freezer for up to 1 month. Reheat the frozen patties in a 350°F oven until warmed through and crisped, 8 to 15 minutes, flipping them halfway through.)

AVOIDING FOOD WASTE

In the United States, food waste accounts for 30 to 40 percent of the country's food supply. I hate to imagine all that food being thrown away, especially when so much work, resources, time, and money went into growing, transporting, and selling it. More important, there are so many hungry people who could be benefiting from that food. Take responsibility for not creating more waste by buying only the groceries you will use, cooking and eating what you have, and using up any leftovers.

Sometimes I buy a lot of produce and then my or the kids' schedule changes, and I don't have a plan to use it all. That's when I turn to one of these flexible recipes that will work with a variety of fruits or vegetables:

Smoothies (pages 55–57)

Ice Pops (page 62)

Veggie Frittata (page 87)

Benny's Shaved Salad (page 102)

Mom's Chicken Broth (page 124)

Vegetable Broth (page 122)

Ramen-Style Soup with Steamed Vegetables (page 136)

Coconut-Curry Vegetable Soup (page 140)

Roasted Vegetables (page 144)

Favorite Sautéed Leafy Greens (page 152)

Best Blanched Vegetables (page 155)

Easy Sautéed Veggies with Garlic (page 165)

Zucchini Noodles with Pesto-Cashew Cream (page 166)

Baked Risotto with Asparagus (page 169)

Veggie Stir-Fry (page 162)

Extra-Crunchy Summer Rolls (page 156)

Taco Night! (page 202)

You can be part of the solution to eliminate food waste—it feels good and it helps our planet.

COMPOSTING

Organic fresh produce is so precious that I aim to get as much use out of it as possible. Finding a use for the plant-based waste from the kitchen is satisfying. Vegetable ends, stems, and cores are bonus ingredients in Vegetable Broth (page 122) or Mom's Chicken Broth (page 124), which extract plenty of nutrients and flavors from these less usable parts. Any other kitchen scraps, like most seeds, peels, and skins—including those from fruit, nuts, plus the spent remnants from making broth—end up in the compost. There, this produce has a second life, as it breaks down into rich soil that then makes our garden flourish. I get a lot of joy knowing that the waste we create can be put to good use, and that this cycle is beneficial to the next season of produce.

Cauliflower Puree

1 medium cauliflower, cut into florets, core peeled and sliced

¾ to 1 cup Vegetable Broth (page 122) or Mom's Chicken Broth (page 124)

2 tablespoons extra-virgin olive oil

Fine sea salt

Similar to mashed potatoes but thinner and smoother, cauliflower puree is a perfect neutral side dish with grilled meat or fish. But instead of using cream, as one would for mashed potatoes, I use homemade broth and olive oil, so the puree is full of nutrition and flavor. I like mashed cauliflower smooth and rich, so I blend it longer than you might think necessary, then emulsify the olive oil into the puree at the last second for a velvety finish.

This recipe uses fresh cauliflower, but don't miss the variations that follow in the Simple Swap, which use roasted cauliflower and roasted garlic.

Place the cauliflower florets and core in a medium saucepan and add ¾ cup broth. Bring to a low boil over medium-high heat, then cover the pan, reduce the heat to low, and simmer until the cauliflower is very tender and easily pierced with a knife, 7 to 10 minutes.

Transfer the mixture to a blender and puree until very smooth (don't fill the blender too much or the hot puree could cause the blender to erupt). Add up to ¼ cup more broth if you'd like the consistency to be thinner. With the blender motor running, pour in the olive oil and blend until emulsified. Taste for salt and serve hot.

MAKE IT YOURS

Light Pairing: Add extra broth to turn the cauliflower puree into a smooth and delicious soup.

Hearty Pairings: Serve as a side dish with Grilled Rib Eye with Chimichurri (page 199) or Crispy Salmon (page 184). Or, spread the puree on a plate and top with Miso-Mustard Roasted Whole Cauliflower (page 170) for a double cauliflower meal!

For the Kids: Blend the cauliflower puree into a pasta sauce for extra nutrition, or use as a pasta sauce by itself, or spread it on a pizza crust along with other toppings and bake.

Simple Swap: Use cooked cauliflower: In a saucepan, warm 3½ cups of roasted, steamed, or blanched cauliflower with ¾ cup broth, then transfer to a blender and proceed with the recipe.

ROASTED GARLIC

I often roast garlic alongside other veggies—I love it blended into hummus (page 180) or added it to the blender with the cauliflower when making this puree.

To make it, cut off the top ¼ inch of the pointy end of a head of garlic, exposing each clove. Drizzle with a little avocado oil, sprinkle with salt, and place cut side up on a piece of parchment paper. Brush the edge of the paper with a little oil and fold it over the garlic head, crimping the edges to fully seal (or use twine to tie it closed). Roast on a baking sheet at 400°F until the cloves are tender and golden, 45 to 55 minutes. Cool completely, then squeeze the soft garlic out of its skin. Roasted garlic keeps in an airtight container in the fridge for up to a week—and don't discard the roasted skins— you can save them to add flavor to your next broth (page 122).

Veggie Stir-Fry

SERVES 4

For the Sauce

½ cup Mom's Chicken Broth (page 124) or Vegetable Broth (page 122)

3 tablespoons tamari

1 teaspoon apple cider vinegar

1 teaspoon toasted sesame oil

1 teaspoon arrowroot powder

2 garlic cloves, minced

½ teaspoon fine sea salt

For the Veggies

2 tablespoons unrefined virgin coconut oil, ghee, or avocado oil

4 ounces fresh mushrooms, tough stems removed, caps sliced

2 medium carrots, thinly sliced

1 celery stalk, thinly sliced

½ small white onion, sliced

About 3 cups chopped assorted veggies, such as:

• Broccoli or cauliflower florets

• Asparagus, tough ends trimmed

• Sugar snap peas, trimmed

• Green beans, trimmed

• Small zucchini or yellow squash

1 tablespoon toasted sesame seeds

Almost any vegetable pairs well with this super-savory, umami-loaded sauce of tamari, vinegar, and sesame oil. Broccoli, green beans, carrots, and celery are almost always in my fridge, but you could use whatever your CSA, farmer's market, or fridge has in abundance. The vegetables in the stir-fry should remain vibrant and full of crunch, which retains more of their nutrients.

Make the sauce: In a small bowl, whisk together the broth, tamari, vinegar, sesame oil, arrowroot, garlic, and salt.

Make the stir-fry: Place a wok or large sauté pan over medium-high heat and when hot, pour in 1 tablespoon of the oil. Add the mushrooms and a pinch of salt, and cook, tossing and stirring frequently, just until glistening and softened but not completely limp, 2 to 3 minutes. Transfer to a plate.

Add the remaining tablespoon oil to the wok, then add the carrots, celery, onion, and a pinch of salt, and cook, tossing frequently, until the onion is just starting to soften, 2 to 3 minutes. Add the other vegetables and continue stirring and tossing until they're almost tender, another 2 to 3 minutes. Return the mushrooms to the wok, then pour in the sauce. Toss the vegetables to coat and cook until the sauce is bubbling and thickened, and the vegetables are glazed and just tender, about 3 minutes.

Transfer the stir-fry to a serving bowl or a large platter. Garnish with the sesame seeds, if desired, and serve immediately.

VEGGIE STIR-FRIED NOODLES

Soak 8 ounces of rice noodles in warm water, until softened (check the package instructions for guidelines). Drain and rinse. Make a double batch of the sauce. Add the noodles to the stir-fry with the sauce, tossing well, until warmed through, about 3 minutes.

CHICKEN OR BEEF STIR-FRY

Make a double batch of the sauce. Marinate 8 ounces of boneless beef strips or cubed chicken breast in one batch of sauce for 15 to 20 minutes. Add 1 tablespoon oil to the wok and heat over medium-high heat. Remove the meat from the marinade and sear in the hot oil until just cooked through, 3 to 5 minutes. Transfer to a plate and continue with the recipe. Add the meat to the stir-fry with the fresh sauce, tossing well, until warmed through, 2 to 3 minutes.

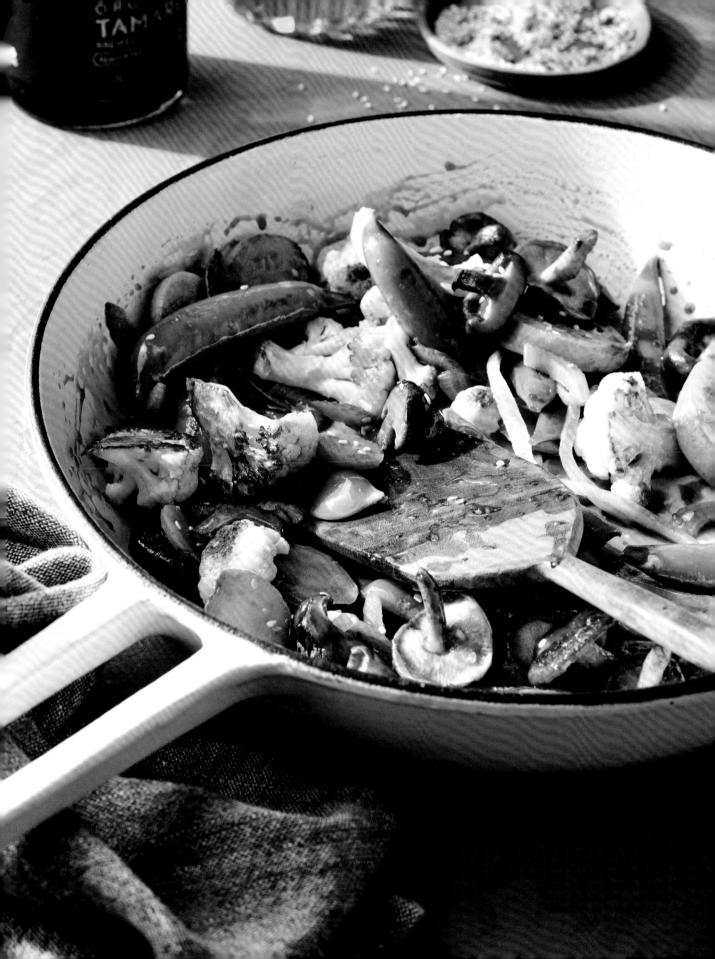

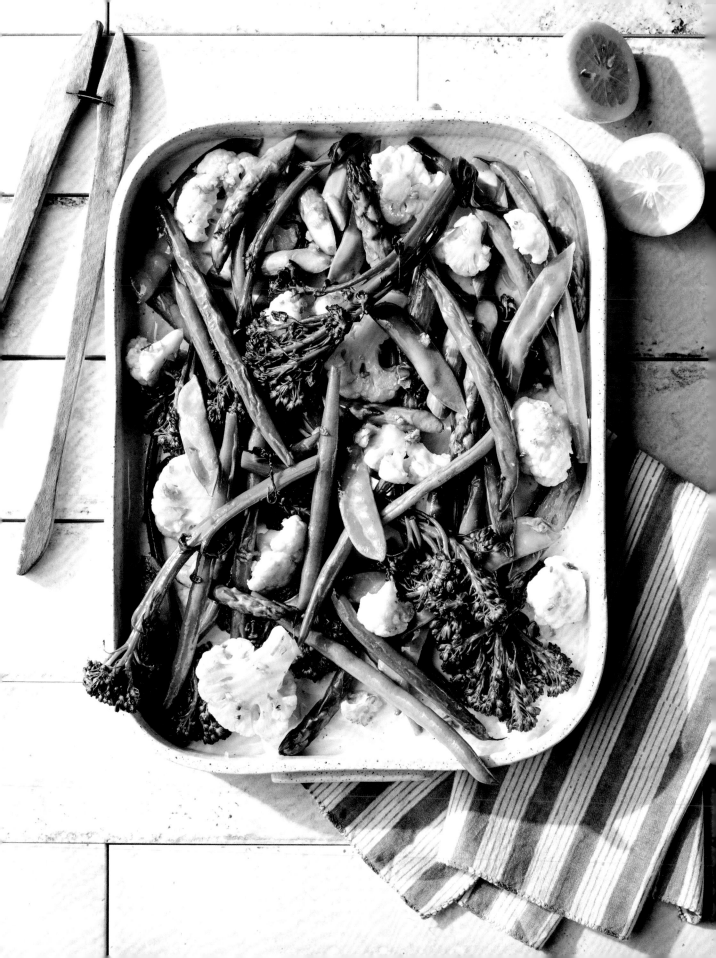

Easy Sautéed Veggies
with Garlic

SERVES 4

2 tablespoons avocado oil
or ghee

4 garlic cloves, minced
or finely grated

1 pound fresh seasonal
vegetables, such as:

• 1 head of broccoli
or cauliflower, cut into
bite-sized florets (see Note,
page 144)

• Broccolini, tough ends
trimmed

• Sugar snap peas, trimmed
and any strings removed

• Green beans, trimmed

• Asparagus spears, tough ends
trimmed, cut into bite-sized
pieces

½ teaspoon fine sea salt

½ cup Mom's Chicken Broth
(page 124) or Vegetable Broth
(page 122)

Usually I love simple meals most: a beautiful piece of steamed fish, some blanched veggies with olive oil and sea salt, a simple salad, fresh juice, and homemade broth. But on days when I want something a little different, this is what I make. Just adding some garlic and broth to my favorite green veggies (here, I suggest broccoli, sugar snap peas, green beans, or asparagus) adds a bit of extra flavor without overshadowing the essence of the veggies.

Heat the oil in a large sauté pan set over medium heat. Add the garlic and sauté until golden brown and fragrant, about 1 minute. Add the vegetables and salt, staggering them so the longest-cooking ones are first and get a head start: cook broccoli or cauliflower for 4 minutes; broccolini, asparagus, or green beans for 2 minutes; and snap peas for 1 minute.

Add the broth to the pan and cook until the vegetables are just tender, only another minute or so, taking care to avoid overcooking. Taste and season with more salt, if desired.

Transfer the veggies to a platter and serve.

MAKE IT YOURS

Hearty Pairings: Pile the sautéed vegetables on top of a bed of Hummus (page 180), then top with a scattering of Crunchy Spiced Chickpeas (page 213). Or, spread the veggies on plates and top with French Lentil and Mushroom Ragout (page 183). Or, serve as a side dish with Fish Baked in Parchment (page 188).

For the Kids: Serve on the side of Rosemary-Lemon Chicken Paillards (page 197).

Zucchini Noodles
with Pesto-Cashew Cream

SERVES 4

1 tablespoon avocado oil
or ghee

1 small shallot, finely diced,
or 2 tablespoons finely diced
white onion

1 garlic clove, minced
or finely grated

2 cups bite-sized broccoli
florets (see Note, page 144)

1 cup sliced green beans,
in ½-inch pieces

1 medium yellow squash,
finely diced

½ teaspoon fine sea salt,
or more as needed

Cashew Cream (page 221)

¼ cup Pesto (page 224)
or good-quality store-bought

3 medium zucchini, spiralized,
or 8 cups store-bought
spiralized zucchini

You better believe I will order pasta if I'm in Italy and a croissant when in Paris—and will *really* enjoy them. But most of the time I am gluten free because wheat just doesn't do any good for my body. So, it makes sense that zucchini noodles—zucchini cut into ribbons using a spiralizer or specialized peeler (also known as zoodles)—are very popular in our house. And nothing makes them more delicious than a creamy Alfredo-style sauce made of quick-soaked cashews instead of heavy cream. This dish is so nourishing, especially with the broccoli, green beans, and yellow squash added—good for me, delicious, and comforting!

Heat the oil in a Dutch oven over medium heat. Add the shallot and garlic and sauté until lightly golden-brown and fragrant, about 2 minutes. Stir in the broccoli and green beans, along with 3 tablespoons of filtered water. Cover the pan and cook for 1 minute to soften the vegetables. Stir in the yellow squash and ½ teaspoon salt, cover, and cook until all the vegetables are just tender, about 1 minute more.

Fold the cashew cream and pesto into the vegetables until everything is evenly coated. Reduce the heat to low and add the zucchini, tossing well to just wilt and soften the zucchini, 4 to 6 minutes. Taste for salt, adjusting as needed, then serve immediately.

MAKE IT YOURS

Light Pairings: Sprinkle the zoodles with Crispy Roasted Shiitake Mushrooms (page 214) or grate Midnight Moon over the dish.

Hearty Pairings: Add shredded cooked chicken or Roasted Vegetables (page 144) to the sauce.

For the Kids: Serve the zoodles with Chicken Meatballs (page 194).

Simple Swaps: Omit the pesto for a simpler Alfredo-style sauce. Or, leave out the cashew cream and pesto entirely, and instead toss with Tamari Dressing (page 228). You could also, to save time, substitute some Best Blanched Veggies (page 155) for the broccoli and green beans, and cook just until warmed through.

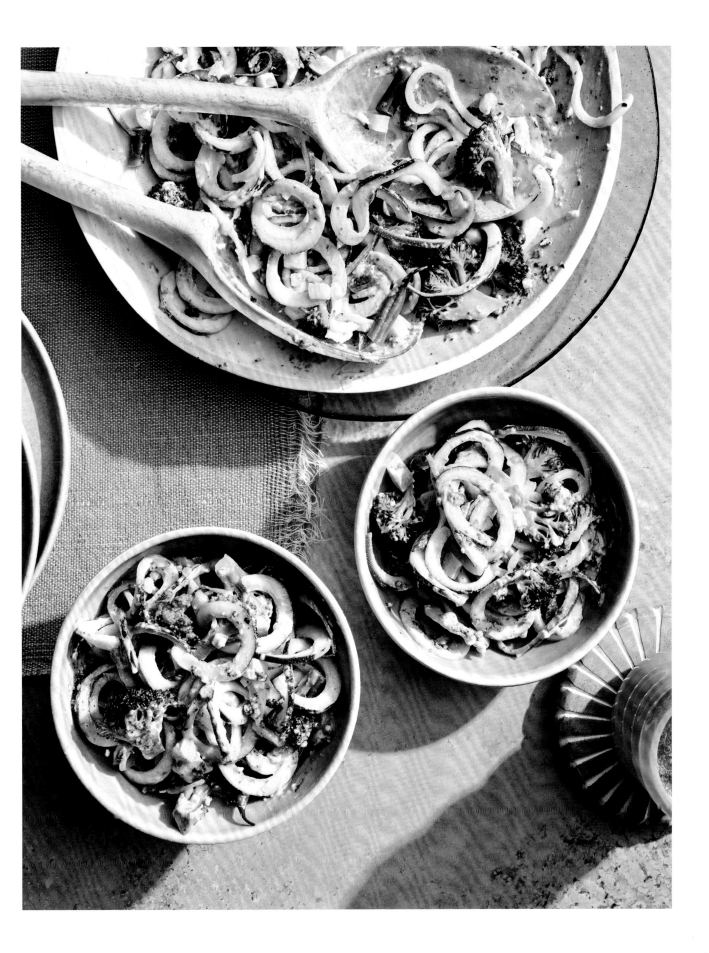

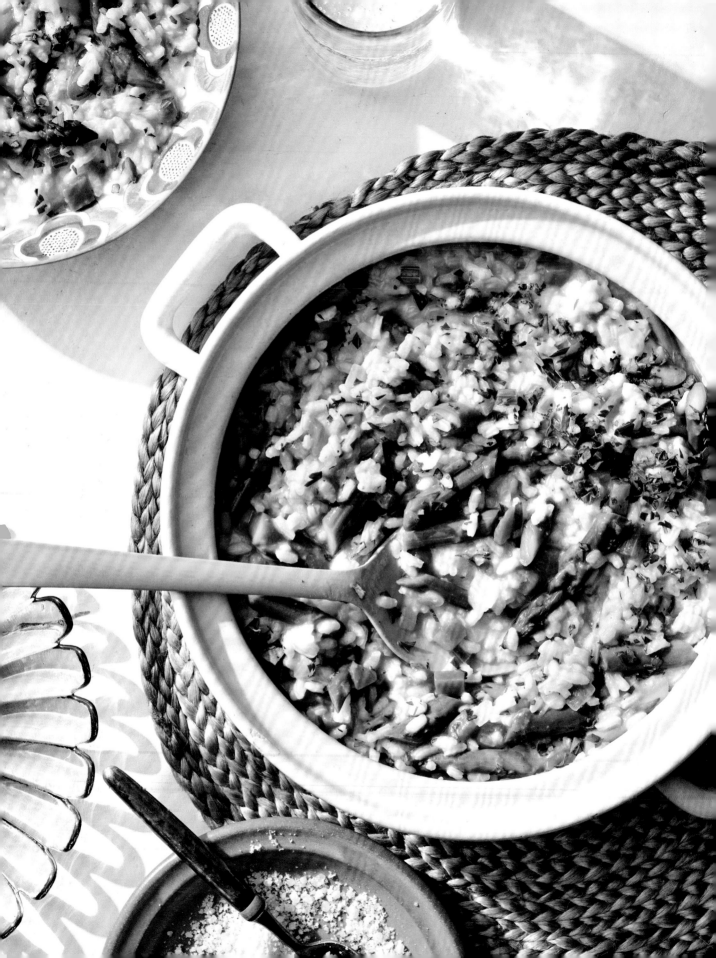

Baked Risotto
with Asparagus

SERVES 4

3½ cups Mom's Chicken Broth (page 124) or Vegetable Broth (page 122)

3 tablespoons unsalted butter

2 medium shallots or 1 small white onion, minced

1 medium carrot, diced

1 celery stalk, diced

¼ teaspoon fine sea salt, or more as needed

1½ cups arborio rice

1 garlic clove, minced

1 pound fresh asparagus, tough ends trimmed, cut into bite-sized pieces

¼ cup finely grated Parmesan cheese, plus more for serving (optional)

¼ cup coarsely chopped flat-leaf parsley leaves

Extra-virgin olive oil

Risotto is the perfect meal to make when a friend is coming over—a little sophisticated, a little indulgent, and most of all delicious. Who can resist? But I don't love standing by the stove stirring for a half hour. Luckily, this version cooks in a covered pot in the oven, so it requires minimal hands-on time. The asparagus is added toward the end of cooking, so it steams lightly on top of the rice. The final step is vital: finishing the risotto with butter, cheese, and additional broth, and stirring for a full minute or two. This is the key to the super-creamy result, so use your muscles! A drizzle of olive oil at the end puts it over the top.

Preheat the oven to 350°F. Place the broth in a medium saucepan and gently heat over medium-low, covered.

Place a Dutch oven over medium heat and when hot, add 1½ tablespoons of the butter. Add the shallots, carrot, celery, and a pinch of salt, and cook, stirring occasionally, until the vegetables are glistening and beginning to soften, 4 to 5 minutes. Add the rice and garlic and toast it in the pan, stirring often, until fragrant and slightly translucent, 2 to 3 minutes.

Stir in 3 cups of the warm broth and the ¼ teaspoon salt. Bring the liquid to a simmer, then cover and transfer to the oven.

Bake the rice for 15 minutes. Remove the pot from the oven, uncover, and carefully arrange the asparagus in a single layer on top of the rice, without stirring. Cover and return the pot to the oven for 3 to 4 minutes more, until the asparagus is tender. Remove from the oven.

Add the remaining 1½ tablespoons butter, the cheese (if using), and ¼ cup of the remaining warm broth. Stir with a sturdy spatula or wooden spoon for 1 to 2 minutes, until the rice is *very* creamy. Taste for salt and stir in additional warm broth to make a looser risotto, if you prefer. Lastly, stir in the parsley. Serve immediately with a drizzle of olive oil and additional cheese, if you like.

MAKE IT YOURS

Simple Swaps: Instead of asparagus, use other vegetables, like fava beans, fresh peas, snow peas, bite-sized broccoli florets, or diced baby zucchini. Add to the top of the rice and steam until tender.

Miso-Mustard Roasted Whole Cauliflower

SERVES 4

1 medium to large cauliflower (about 2 pounds)

¼ cup avocado oil

¼ cup Mom's Chicken Broth (page 124) or Vegetable Broth (page 122), or filtered water

2 garlic cloves, grated or finely minced

1 tablespoon miso paste (red or white)

1 tablespoon grainy Dijon mustard

1 teaspoon rice wine vinegar (or white wine vinegar)

½ teaspoon fine sea salt

A roasted whole cauliflower is impressive in the best way: it's beautiful, simple, and pure. This is a great main dish for a vegetable-focused dinner, especially when served with the French Lentil and Mushroom Ragout (page 183), which adds a sauciness and depth of flavor, plus protein. The rub applied to the cauliflower—miso, mustard, and garlic—comes together in about 30 seconds and can be used on other vegetables, or even on fish or chicken, before grilling or roasting. It's easy, vegan, and just so good!

Preheat the oven to 400°F. Line a baking sheet with parchment.

Wash the cauliflower and drain. Remove most of the leaves and dig out some of the core, being careful not to cut away parts connecting the florets (you want it to remain intact).

In a large bowl, whisk together the oil, broth, garlic, miso, mustard, vinegar, and salt. Place the cauliflower in the bowl and use your hands to turn it over in the marinade and massage it into the little nooks and crannies on top.

Place the cauliflower upright on the baking sheet; retain the remaining marinade. Roast, brushing the cauliflower with the remaining marinade halfway through cooking, until tender but not mushy (a wooden skewer should easily slip in), 50 to 60 minutes depending on size. For a more charred finish, run the cauliflower under the broiler for a couple minutes. Let cool slightly, then cut the cauliflower into quarters.

MAKE IT YOURS

Light Pairings: Sprinkle the cauliflower with microgreens or chives. Or, serve with Cashew Cream (page 221). A simple puree of blanched sugar snap peas or asparagus (see page 155) would make a delicious and beautiful base.

Hearty Pairings: This is so good on top of Sheet-Pan Squash and Chickpeas (page 151). Or, serve it on top of Hummus (page 180), with some blanched asparagus or other green vegetable (see page 155), Crispy Roasted Shiitake Mushrooms (page 214), and Tahini Dressing (page 220).

Simple Swaps: This marinade works great with broccoli florets or whole carrots that are to be roasted, or massaged on raw chicken or fish before grilling. Or use the same technique but marinate with Tamari Dressing (page 228) or Almond Butter–Sesame Sauce (page 223).

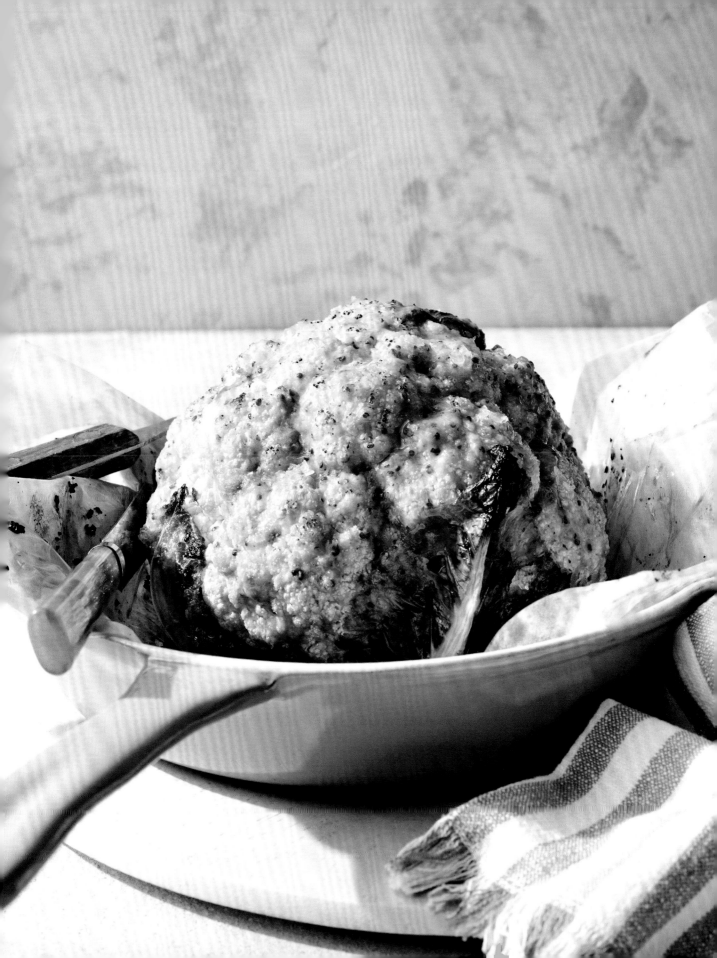

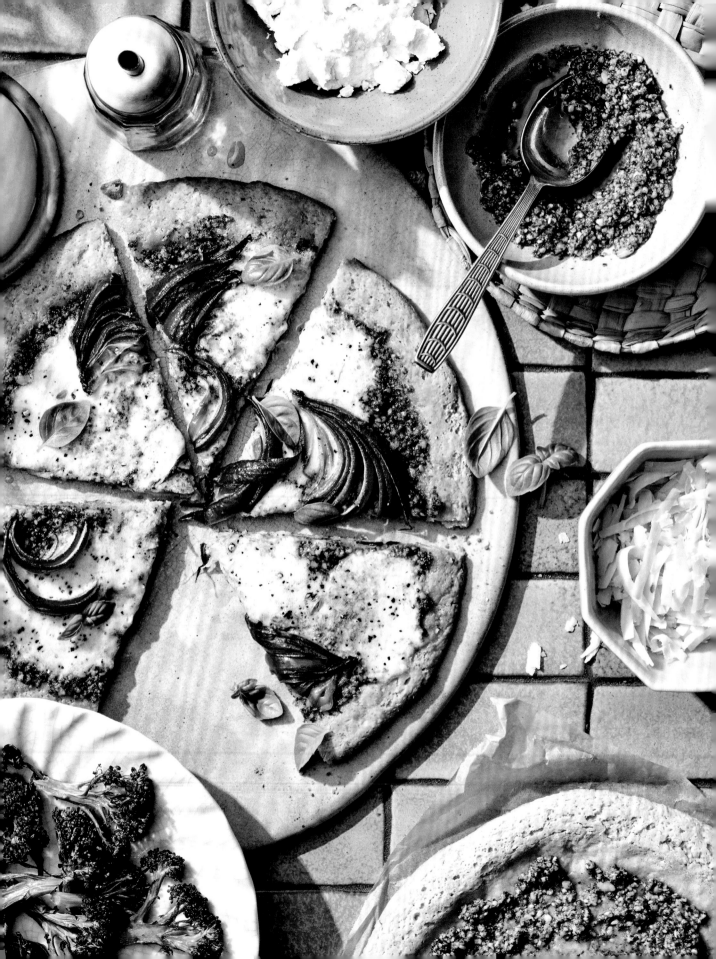

Pizza Night!

MAKES 2 (12-INCH)
PIZZAS

3 cups gluten-free flour
(such as Bob's Red Mill)

1 package (2¼ teaspoons)
instant yeast

2 teaspoons psyllium husk
powder

1 teaspoon fine sea salt

2 large eggs

1 cup warm filtered water

1 tablespoon honey

Avocado oil

Suggested Toppings

Pesto (page 224) and
crumbled goat cheese

Slices of queijo minas and a
sprinkling of dried oregano,
with olive oil drizzled over
after baking

Fresh buffalo mozzarella
and fresh basil

Roasted Vegetables (page
144) and grated manchego
cheese

Crispy Roasted Shiitake
Mushrooms (page 214) and
grated Midnight Moon cheese

We all love pizza night! It's one of those meals everyone looks forward to and can make just the way they like. Pizza is great for guests, and equally fun when it's just family. Using gluten-free flour, yeast, and psyllium husk powder (which creates a gel that helps increase the airiness of the yeast), this simple dough yields two crusts, so I suggest making both but topping and serving just one, while freezing the other to keep for another time. In fact, having a crust in the freezer ready to go is so helpful when time is crunched—dinner can be on the table in no time. Everyone is happy!

In a stand mixer fitted with the paddle attachment, combine the flour, yeast, psyllium husk powder, and salt.

In a large measuring glass, whisk together the eggs, warm water, and honey.

With the mixer running on low speed, slowly add the egg mixture to the dry ingredients and mix until the dough is thoroughly combined, thick, and slightly sticky, 2 to 3 minutes. Cover the bowl with a clean kitchen towel and set aside at room temperature for 30 minutes to let the dough rest. (If you don't have a stand mixer, you can also mix the dough by hand, but it requires some strength; use a sturdy spoon or spatula and stir until the dough is thick and slightly sticky, 3 to 4 minutes.)

Preheat the oven to 450°F. Line 2 baking sheets with parchment and drizzle a bit of oil in the center of each.

Divide the dough in half. Scrape each half onto the center of each pan, then use well-oiled hands to press into a round with slightly raised edges about 12 inches in diameter. Drizzle the surface of each crust with a little more oil and use your fingers to gently smear it all over the surface. Let the dough rest for another 30 minutes, until puffed slightly and soft.

Place the pans in the oven and bake until the crusts are lightly browned and crisp, but soft inside, 12 minutes, rotating the pans halfway through baking. Remove the crusts from the oven but keep the oven turned on. (If desired, cool one crust, then wrap it tightly and place in a freezer ziptop bag and freeze for use later; it will last in the freezer for up to 2 months.)

Arrange whatever toppings you like on the crust(s), then return to the oven to bake for another 10 minutes, until the cheese is blistering and a bit crusty at the edges. Slice and serve immediately.

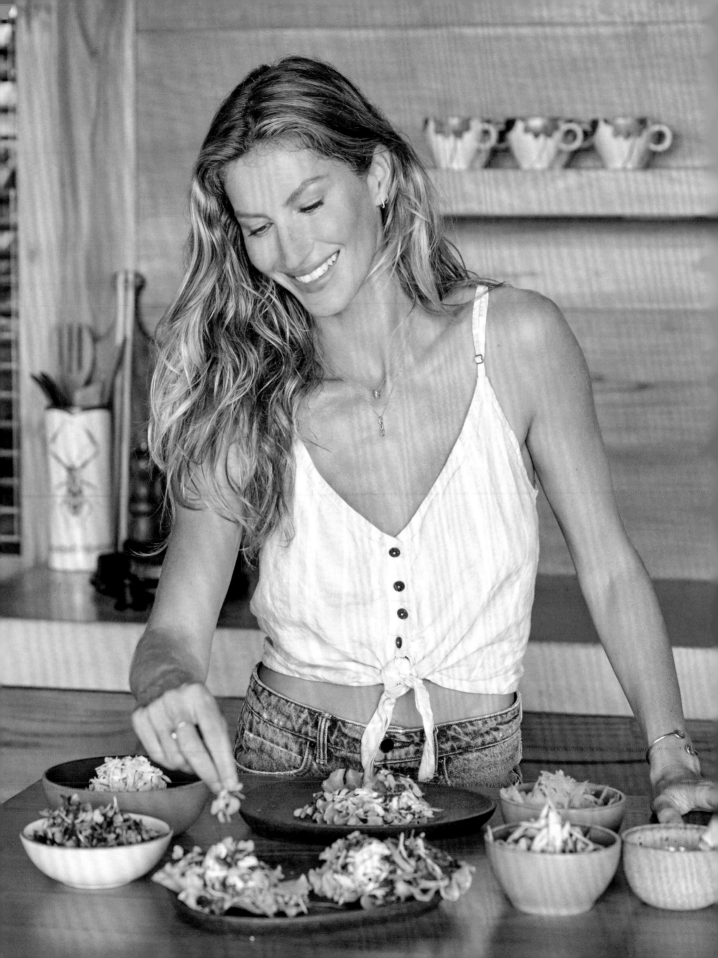

Favorite Proteins

Protein is super important for a healthy body, as it helps build
and rebuild muscle, as well as provides tons of important nutrients,
like iron. Whether the protein is humanely raised meat or fish,
or is plant-derived beans or chickpeas, I am very intentional
about eating protein a few times a week.

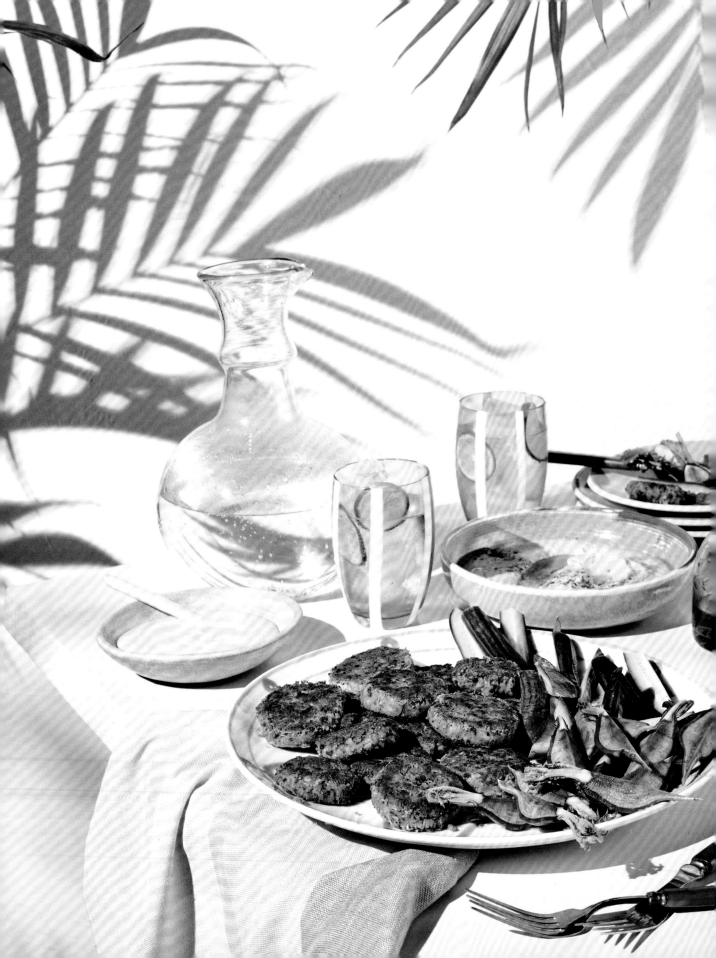

Pan-Fried Falafel

2 cups From-Scratch
Chickpeas (page 179) or boxed
or jarred chickpeas, drained
and rinsed

1 small white onion,
finely diced (see Note)

1 cup packed fresh flat-leaf
parsley leaves

1 tablespoon ground cumin

1 teaspoon fine sea salt,
or more as needed

3 tablespoons chickpea flour,
plus more as needed

Freshly ground black pepper

Avocado oil

Tahini Dressing (page 220),
for serving

I love chickpeas, as they have tons of protein and fiber, as well
as vitamins and minerals like iron, potassium, and folate. These
simple patties are one of my favorite ways of eating them; a rich
tahini dressing is always served on the side, to drizzle over. While
traditional falafel is made with soaked raw chickpeas that are ground
with herbs and spices, and then deep-fried, here I use home-cooked
chickpeas that get pulsed in the food processor with fresh parsley
and earthy cumin. (If you aren't able to cook your own chickpeas,
use a box or jar of organic chickpeas rather than those in a can; the
quality is usually better and they will certainly be BPA free.)

A few tips: If I have the time, I like to peel the chickpeas first to
get rid of any rough texture, and then grind and shape them. I've also
discovered that refrigerating the patties for an hour ensures they
don't fall apart during their quick pan-sear. Lastly, I freeze any extra
patties to pull out anytime for a quick lunch or dinner.

Follow the instructions on page 179 to remove the peels of the chickpeas,
if you like. Dry them on a clean kitchen towel.

Place the chickpeas, onion, parsley, cumin, and 1 teaspoon salt in a food
processor. Pulse in 15 to 20 1-second bursts, scraping down the sides
once or twice, until evenly chopped and thoroughly combined. Do not
grind the mixture into a paste.

Add the chickpea flour to the processor 1 tablespoon at a time and pulse
to form a coarse dough that is lightly moist and malleable but doesn't
stick to your fingers; pulse in more chickpea flour, 1 tablespoon at a time,
if necessary to achieve that consistency. Taste and add additional salt and
some pepper as needed.

(recipe continues)

MAKE IT YOURS

Light Pairings: I love falafel atop mixed greens, with some chopped cucumber
alongside and dressed with the Cilantro-Mint Dressing (page 221). Or, place the
falafel in a gluten-free wrap with some shredded carrots.

For the Kids: Have a falafel party! Arrange the falafel on a large platter, with a
rainbow of blanched and raw veggies that your kids love, and place the Tahini
Dressing or Hummus (page 180) in the middle for dipping

Line a baking sheet with parchment. Tip the chickpea mixture onto a cutting board and shape into a 16-inch-long log, then cut the log into 16 1-inch-thick slices. Shape each slice into a ¾- to 1-inch-thick patty. Arrange the patties on the prepared baking sheet. Cover lightly with a clean kitchen towel and refrigerate for at least 1 hour, or, even better, up to 1 day ahead. (If chilling the dough for more than 1 hour, arrange the patties between sheets of parchment and store in an airtight glass container.)

Heat a medium sauté pan over medium heat. Add 1 to 2 tablespoons of avocado oil (enough to coat the bottom of the pan), then add as many falafel as will fit in a single layer without crowding. Cook, flipping once, until crispy and browned, 2 to 3 minutes per side. Transfer the cooked falafel to a covered plate to keep warm, then wipe out the sauté pan and heat more oil to cook the remaining patties.

Serve the falafel hot, warm, or at room temperature with the dressing. Store extra falafel in an airtight glass container in the refrigerator for up to 2 days, or in the freezer for up to 1 month. Reheat the patties (even if still frozen) in a 350°F oven until warmed through and crisped, 6 to 12 minutes.

Note: Be sure to very finely chop the onion before adding it to the food processor, so the texture of the cooked falafel isn't too chunky or wet.

THE IMPORTANCE OF GOOD FAT

Fat is important for your health. I like to use a variety of oils and healthy fats in my cooking, and most recipes in this book offer options, based on preferences or availability.

I prefer the taste of unrefined virgin coconut oil in anything involving sweet potatoes, popcorn, or sweets. When I want to give a dish a richer flavor, I use ghee, which is clarified butter. Avocado oil is a convenient, neutral-tasting oil that can be used raw or for cooking. Olive oil is my favorite fat, but I don't usually use it for cooking, as heat kills some of its nutritional benefits. I love olive oil drizzled on cooked vegetables, in salads, and as a finishing oil for cooked fish. I also blend it into Cauliflower Puree (page 161) and Hummus (page 180) for richness.

And most important, I keep a bottle of the best olive oil on my table for drizzling over whatever needs a little extra love.

These healthy fats, especially the olive oil, help to lubricate the digestive system and provide excellent health benefits—and they make everything taste extra delicious.

From-Scratch Chickpeas

**MAKES 3 CUPS COOKED
CHICKPEAS**

1 cup dried chickpeas

Filtered water, cold

1 teaspoon baking soda

1 teaspoon salt

Cooking chickpeas from scratch is worthwhile, especially if you use really high-quality dried chickpeas that haven't been sitting on a supermarket shelf for years; not only do they taste better, but they don't include preservatives or excess salt. Removing the skins can be a little tedious, but the reward is a super-creamy texture—if you don't have the time or energy, don't worry about it.

Use these home-cooked chickpeas for making Pan-Fried Falafel (page 177) or the Beans and Greens Soup (page 135), and especially Hummus (page 180). Note that the chickpeas do need to soak overnight so that they cook evenly the next day.

Place the chickpeas in a large bowl and cover with at least 3 inches of cold water. Soak overnight, or up to 24 hours.

Rinse and drain the chickpeas, then place in a large pot. Add enough filtered water to cover the chickpeas by 4 inches. Bring to a boil over high heat, add the baking soda and salt, then reduce the heat to low and simmer for 35 to 40 minutes, skimming off any foam that rises to the surface. Use the back of a spoon to smash a chickpea against the side of the pot to check if they are done and soft. (Note: Older chickpeas will take longer to become tender.) Allow the chickpeas to cool in their cooking liquid before storing. Refrigerate cooked chickpeas in their cooking liquid for up to 5 days or freeze for up to 3 months.

To remove the skins from the chickpeas, drain the chickpeas and run under cold water to cool. Place in a large bowl and cover with water. Lightly rub the chickpeas together to loosen their skins, which will rise to the surface. Use a slotted spoon or strainer to collect and remove the skins. Drain and repeat as needed until all chickpeas are peeled.

Hummus

3 cups From-Scratch Chickpeas (page 179) or boxed or jarred chickpeas, drained, plus ¾ cup cooking liquid or filtered water

1 cup good-quality stirred tahini

¼ cup fresh lemon juice

4 scallions, white parts only, chopped

2 to 4 garlic cloves

Handful of fresh flat-leaf parsley leaves (optional)

1 teaspoon fine sea salt

1 teaspoon ground cumin or 1 teaspoon ras al hanout, harissa, or other North African spice blend (optional)

2 tablespoons extra-virgin olive oil, plus more for drizzling

Everyone in my house loves hummus, especially the recipe our chef James Kelly taught me how to make. It is extra-smooth and creamy, with lots of garlic, meaning it's extra-delicious! Plus, it's dense with nutrition: the chickpeas alone are full of protein, fiber, and many vitamins and minerals, like folate, iron, and magnesium.

If you are trying to incorporate more vegetables into your life, start here. You'll be amazed how enthusiastic you'll become about raw celery, carrots, cucumbers, fennel, and radishes, as well as anything else you can find to dip into it. Vivi especially loves this hummus with raw green beans—they magically disappear when she is around!

Follow the instructions on page 179 to remove the peels of the chickpeas, if you like.

Add the chickpeas, tahini, lemon juice, scallion whites, garlic, parsley (if using), salt, and cumin to a food processor, and process for a full minute. Scrape down the sides with a silicone spatula, then blend for another minute, until completely smooth.

With the processor running, drizzle in the 2 tablespoons olive oil, followed by ½ cup of the cooking water, and process until the hummus is the consistency you like. I usually add a bit more liquid, since we like our hummus a little loose (and the hummus will thicken up in the refrigerator).

To serve, spoon some hummus onto a small plate, use the back of a spoon to create a small well in the center, and drizzle with some olive oil. Stored in an airtight glass container, hummus will keep in the fridge for up to 5 days. If it's a little dried out from being in the fridge, drizzle a little olive oil on top and mix it in before serving.

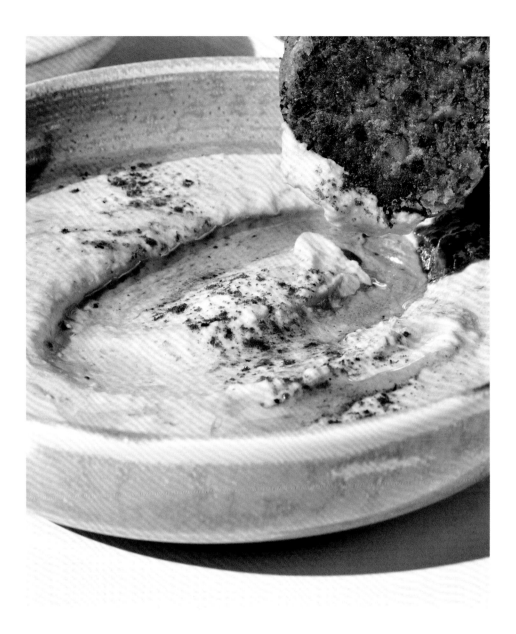

Hearty Pairings: Crunchy Spiced Chickpeas (page 213) are yummy sprinkled on top. Or make a nutrient-packed lunch bowl or wrap with hummus, some Roasted Vegetables (page 144), shredded kale, a couple Pan-Fried Falafel (page 177), or shredded cooked chicken, and Tahini Dressing (page 228).

For the Kids: My kids love carrots, cucumbers, celery, green beans, and red peppers (or any raw or blanched vegetables) or Seed Crackers (page 218) for dipping.

Simple Swaps: Try other cooked beans, like cannellini, in place of the chickpeas. Or add 1 or 2 small roasted beets (see page 144) when pureeing, but start with only ¼ cup of the cooking water so the texture isn't too loose.

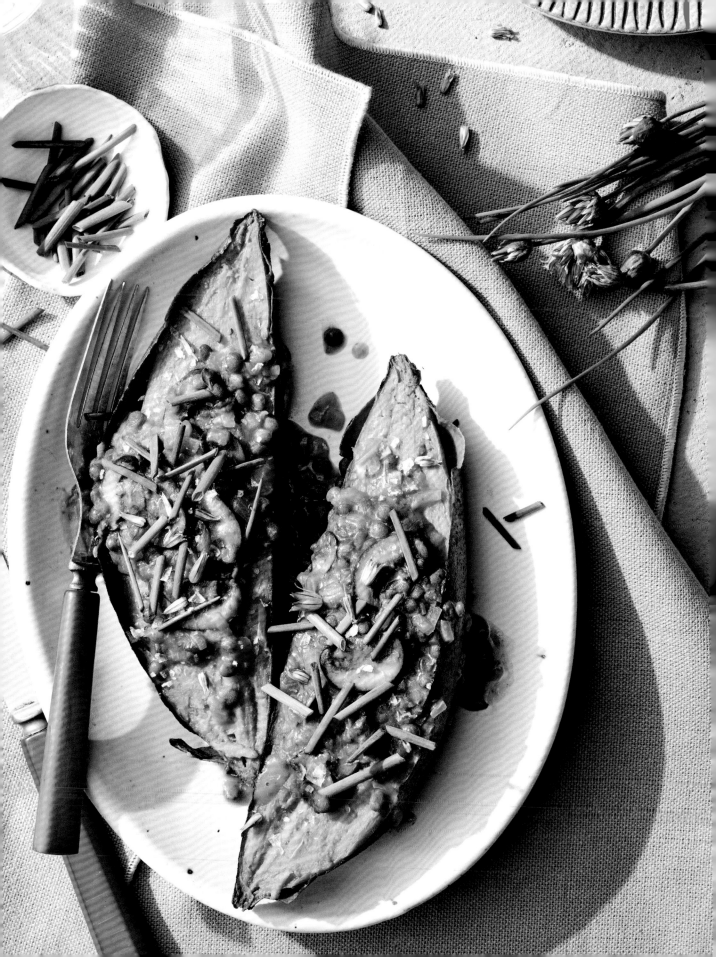

French Lentil and Mushroom Ragout
over Baked Sweet Potatoes

SERVES 2 TO 4

4 cups Vegetable Broth
(page 122) or water

½ teaspoon fine sea salt

½ cup French lentils
(or brown, if unavailable)

1 tablespoon avocado oil
or ghee

1 small white or yellow onion,
finely diced

1 garlic clove, minced

8 to 12 shiitake or cremini
mushrooms, stemmed, caps
thinly sliced

Leaves from 1 fresh thyme
sprig

1 teaspoon Dijon mustard

1 teaspoon tamari

1 tablespoon arrowroot
powder or tapioca starch

Chopped fresh chives
or tarragon leaves

2 Whole Roasted Sweet
Potatoes (page 147), halved

This saucy, mustard-flavored ragout features sautéed mushrooms and French lentils—a protein-rich small green legume—which keep their shape especially well after long cooking, providing both firm texture and heartiness. Somewhere between a sauce and a stew, this is a perfectly balanced, substantial vegan dish on its own, but there is so much flexibility in how you serve it. Scoop over roasted sweet potato halves for a family-friendly meal; or serve it under a whole roasted cauliflower (see page 170) and you have something worthy of guests.

In a medium saucepan, bring 3 cups of the broth to a boil over medium-high heat. Add the salt. Stir in the lentils, return to a boil, and reduce the heat to low and simmer until just tender, about 20 minutes. Drain, if needed, and place lentils in a bowl. (If you like a creamier texture, puree half the lentils and combine with the remaining lentils.) Wipe out the saucepan.

Place the saucepan over medium-high heat. Add the oil and onion and sauté, stirring constantly, until starting to soften, about 2 minutes. Add the garlic and cook, stirring, for 1 more minute. Add the mushrooms and thyme leaves and cook until slightly browned and tender, about 3 minutes, stirring occasionally.

Add 1 more cup of broth to the saucepan along with the mustard and tamari; bring to a boil. Add the cooked lentils, stir well, reduce the heat to medium, and return to a low simmer.

In a small bowl, mix the arrowroot with the remaining ⅓ cup broth. Stir the arrowroot slurry into the lentils, bring back to a simmer, and gently cook until slightly thickened, 2 to 3 minutes. Add the fresh herbs. Serve over the sweet potato halves.

Crispy Salmon

SERVES 2

2 (6-ounce) wild-caught,
skin-on salmon fillets

Fine sea salt

1 tablespoon fresh lemon juice

1 tablespoon extra-virgin
olive oil

1 to 2 tablespoons avocado oil,
plus more as needed

2 tablespoons chopped
fresh mixed herbs

One of the many benefits of eating animal protein only once or twice a week is that it is easier to justify buying the best quality. Sustainably fished, seasonal wild-caught salmon (fresh in late spring and early summer, frozen the rest of the year) is such a treat. Searing it, undisturbed, on top of the stove makes the skin get super crispy while the inside stays soft and rare. Served very simply, with just lemon, olive oil, and fresh herbs (I like a mix of parsley, dill, or tarragon), this is my favorite way to enjoy this gift from nature.

Pat the salmon dry. Season both sides generously with salt.

In a small bowl, whisk together the lemon juice, olive oil, and a pinch of salt until emulsified.

Place a large nonstick pan over medium-high heat and when hot, drizzle in enough of the avocado oil to cover the bottom of the pan, 1 to 2 tablespoons. Carefully add the fillets, placing them skin side down in the pan. Sear until the skin is crispy and browned and the fish easily releases from the pan, about 3 minutes. Try your best not to disturb the fish as it cooks; you can gently tuck a thin spatula under a corner and lift it an inch or so to check its progress. Flip the fillets and cook on the second side until the fish begins to flake when gently pressed, about 3 minutes more for rare, 5 minutes for well done.

Transfer the salmon skin side up to individual plates and sprinkle with the fresh herbs. Drizzle the lemon-oil mixture around the fish (but not on the skin, as it will get soggy). Serve immediately.

MAKE IT YOURS

Light Pairings: I love this salmon with a simple arugula salad or any blanched veggies (see page 155).

Hearty Pairings: Salmon is delicious served on a bed of French Lentil and Mushroom Ragout (page 183), or with the Veggie Stir-Fry (page 162), or the Baked Risotto with Asparagus (page 109). Or, serve it with Cauliflower Puree (page 161) and sautéed asparagus (see page 165).

For the Kids: My kids love this salmon with wild rice, drizzled with a little Tamari Dressing (page 228) or with Benny's Shaved Salad (page 102).

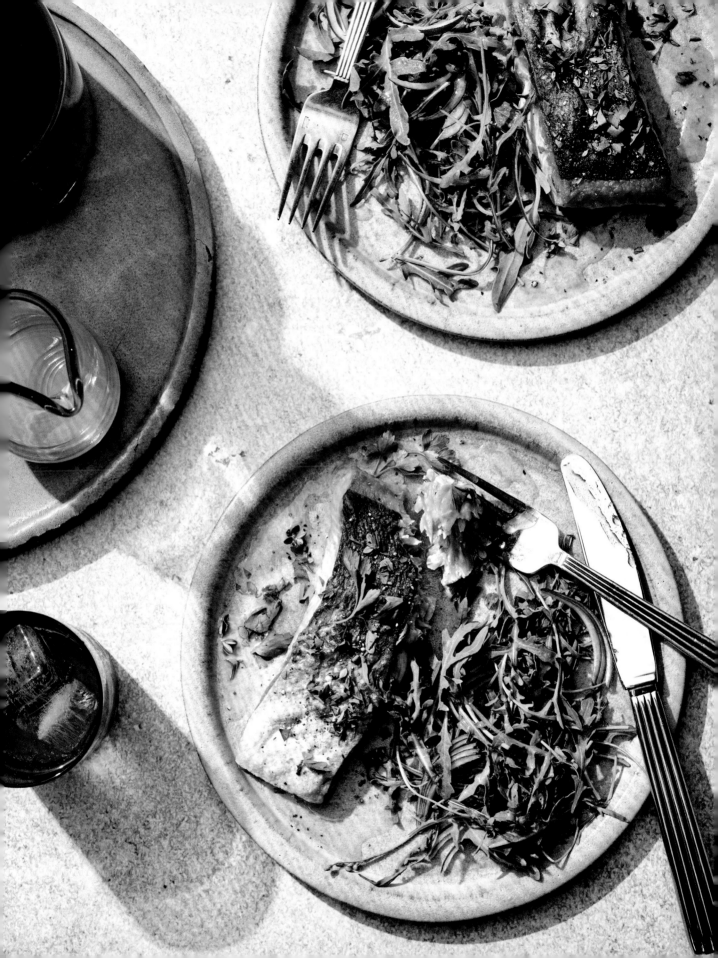

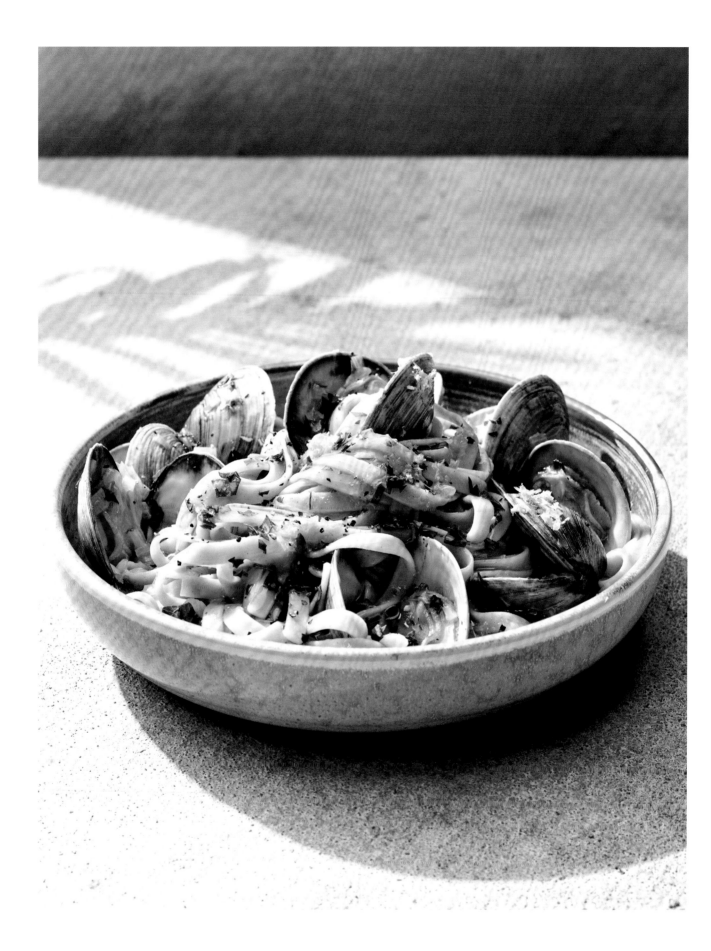

Garlicky Clams with Rice Noodles

SERVES 4

12 ounces rice linguini
or rice spaghetti

2 pounds littleneck clams
(about 24)

2 tablespoons unsalted butter

5 garlic cloves, thinly sliced

1 medium shallot, diced

½ teaspoon fine sea salt,
or more as needed

1½ cups Mom's Chicken Broth
(page 124), Vegetable Broth
(page 122), or fish stock

Zest and juice of 1 lemon

¼ cup coarsely chopped
fresh flat-leaf parsley

Freshly ground black pepper

Extra-virgin olive oil

MAKE IT YOURS

Light Pairings: Easy Sautéed
Veggies with Garlic (page 165) is a
nice accompaniment; I especially
like it with asparagus or broccolini.
Or, serve this with the Favorite
Sautéed Leafy Greens (page 152),
either on the side or tossed in
with the cooked noodles.

Hearty Pairing: Serve this with a
Beet and Arugula Salad (page 105).

Simple Swaps: Use another
gluten-free pasta instead, or
serve the cooked clams and sauce
over cooked wild rice. Or, omit the
fresh herbs and lemon juice and
stir in 2 to 3 tablespoons of Pesto
(page 224).

I try to eat in harmony with the planet—in this case, by choosing only high-quality, sustainable shellfish. Clams are one of the best choices you can make when it comes to cooking sustainable seafood (check out the Monterey Bay Aquarium's *Seafood Watch* website for more info), as clams are harvested responsibly and the method is not destructive to any other species.

This succulent pasta dish brings me right to Italy, where I always like to indulge in pasta alla vongole, one of my all-time favorite dishes. At home, I make it gluten free by using rice noodles. The pasta is dressed with sweet, briny clams and a combination of herbs, lemon, and butter. It tastes yummy and comes together quickly!

Place the rice linguini in a wide, shallow bowl and cover with hot water. Soak the pasta until softened, 20 to 30 minutes, then drain and rinse under cool water.

Put the clams in a large bowl and cover with cold water. Soak for at least 20 minutes, or up to 1 hour, so they release any sand trapped inside their shells. Rinse each clam, inspecting for any grit on the surface and scrubbing, if necessary. Discard any with cracked or broken shells.

Set a large wide skillet or a Dutch oven over medium heat. Add the butter, swirling to melt, and when the foaming subsides, stir in the garlic, shallot, and ½ teaspoon salt. Cook, stirring often, until fragrant, about 2 minutes, then add the broth. Bring to a simmer and add the clams, cover the pan, and cook until the clams open, 4 to 6 minutes.

Use tongs to transfer the clams to a bowl, discarding any unopened ones, then add the noodles to the skillet. Toss in the sauce until they're well coated and tender, about 2 minutes. Add the lemon zest and half the lemon juice, and sprinkle with the parsley and some pepper. Taste for seasoning, adding additional lemon juice and more salt as needed.

Divide the noodles among 4 pasta bowls and top with the clams. Serve immediately, drizzling the top with the olive oil at the table.

Fish Baked in Parchment

SERVES 2

1 small lemon, thinly sliced

2 (6-ounce) fresh fish fillets (like sole, cod, halibut, grouper, sea bass, or salmon)

Fine sea salt and freshly ground black pepper

4 teaspoons avocado oil

4 fresh thyme sprigs

There are many wonderful things about spending time in Costa Rica, where I've had a home since I was in my early twenties. I love being surrounded by nature—the lush landscape, the mountains, and the sea nourish my soul. And being a girl from Brazil, I am happiest in the sunshine. Fresh fish is usually the protein of choice there, because the local options are all so delicious. Though it sounds fancy, wrapping fish in banana leaves (which we have so many of in Costa Rica) or parchment and baking it is a surprisingly quick and easy method.

At its most basic, I season the fish with lemon slices, fresh thyme, olive oil, and salt; the fish gently steams in about 15 minutes. Or pick one of the variations. Either way, its natural flavor is trapped in the package and the end result is a tender, juicy fillet that tastes pure and delicious. If you are serving more than two people, just double or triple the recipe to make more packages.

Preheat the oven to 400°F. Fold a 12-inch square of parchment in half diagonally, then open and lay it flat on a work surface.

Place half the lemon slices in the center of the square, and set the fish fillet on top. Season with salt and pepper, drizzle half the avocado oil over the fish, and top with half the thyme sprigs. Close the package by crimping around the fish in a half-moon shape, sealing the fish inside. Repeat with another 12-inch square of parchment and the remaining fish fillet.

Place the 2 packages on a sheet pan and place in the oven. Bake until the fish just flakes when gently pressed with a spatula or butter knife, 10 to 12 minutes for thin fillets and up to 16 minutes for thicker ones (the packages may also puff up!). You can carefully unwrap a package to check if it's done, then seal it back up and return it to the oven if more baking is necessary.

Place each package on a serving plate and cut open, being careful of escaping steam. Remove the thyme sprigs and serve immediately.

MAKE IT YOURS

Light Pairings: I love to serve this with the Hearts of Palm, Avocado, and Cucumber Salad (page 98). Or, drizzle the fish after baking with Chimichurri (page 224).

Hearty Pairings: The baked fish goes well with a warm Green Bean Salad (page 119) or any Roasted Vegetables (page 144).

GRILLED FISH IN BANANA LEAVES

Prepare an outdoor grill for indirect cooking: heat one side of the grill on medium-high heat and do not heat the other side, which will be used for indirect heat.

Place each prepared fish fillet on a banana leaf (thawed, if frozen) and tuck or fold the excess leaf under the fish. Place the wrapped packages directly on the grill grates on the side with indirect heat and close the grill. Cook and serve as instructed in the recipe.

FIVE EASY VARIATIONS FOR FISH IN PARCHMENT

To mix things up a bit, include some other ingredients in the fish package before cooking:

- Add ½ small seeded and julienned zucchini to each fillet before wrapping.

- Skip the thyme and spread a teaspoon of Pesto (page 224) on top of each fillet before wrapping.

- Skip the olive oil, thyme, and lemon, and add a small handful of baby bok choy leaves and/or blanched broccolini (see page 155), then drizzle the fish with 1 tablespoon Tamari Dressing (page 228) before wrapping.

- Add a few spears of fresh asparagus, split lengthwise, on top of the fillet before wrapping.

- Place 5 pitted Kalamata olives and 1 teaspoon capers on each fillet before wrapping.

PORTION SIZE

You might notice that the serving sizes of most of these protein recipes are small. This is because what makes up most of my plate is vegetables, with the fish or meat as an accent. A great way to turn a small piece of protein into a full meal is to combine it with salads, steamed vegetables, sautéed greens, or any leftover vegetable-based dishes in your fridge. Having a variety of vegetables on the plate keeps things dynamic while allowing you to consume less animal protein.

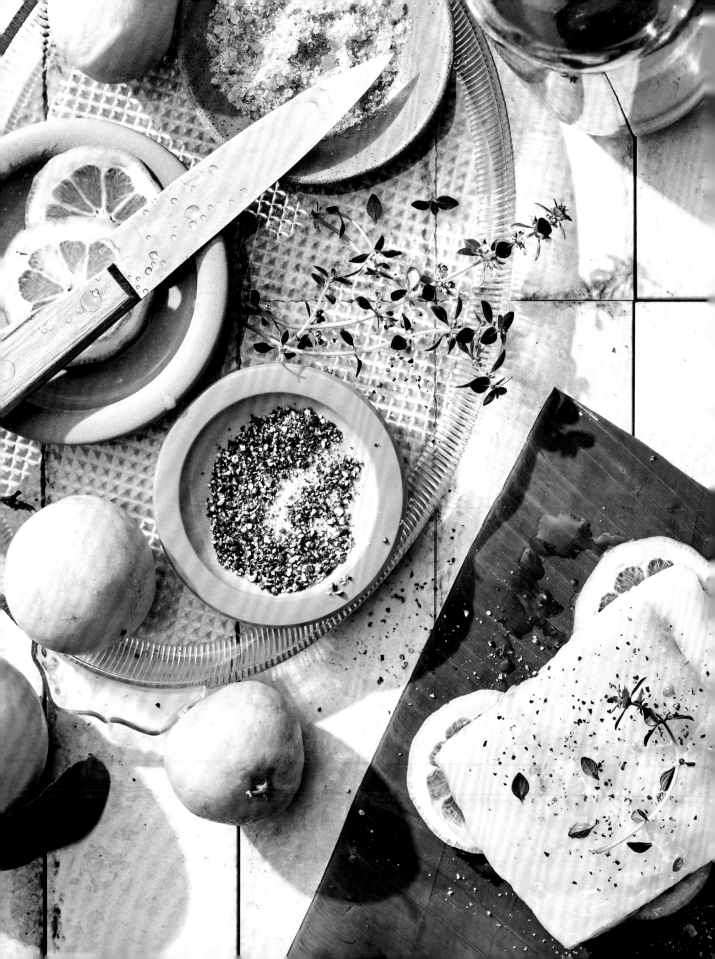

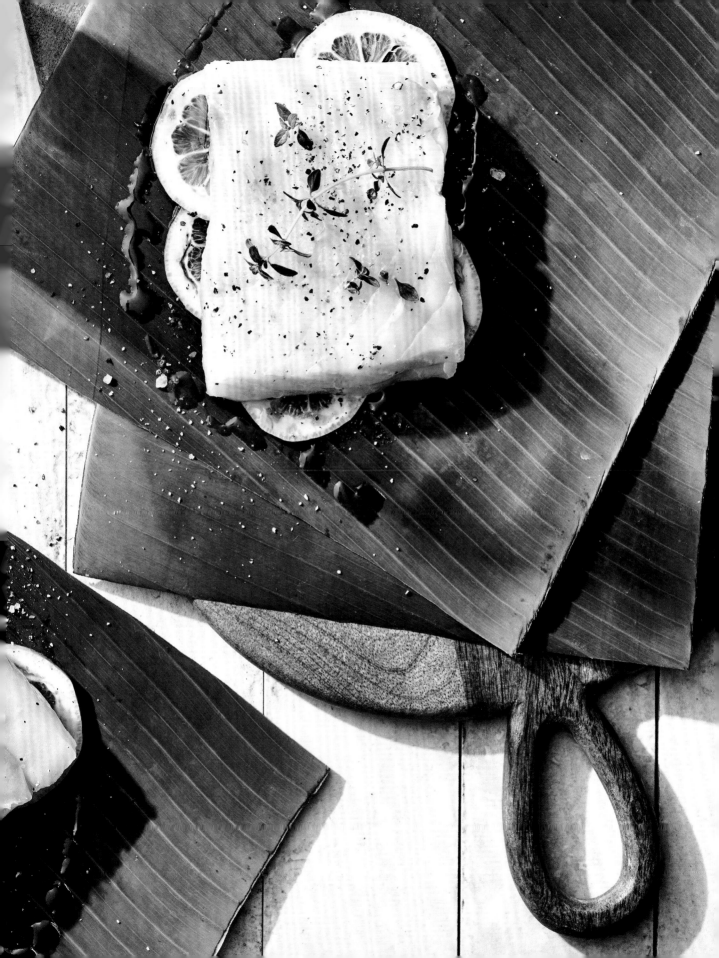

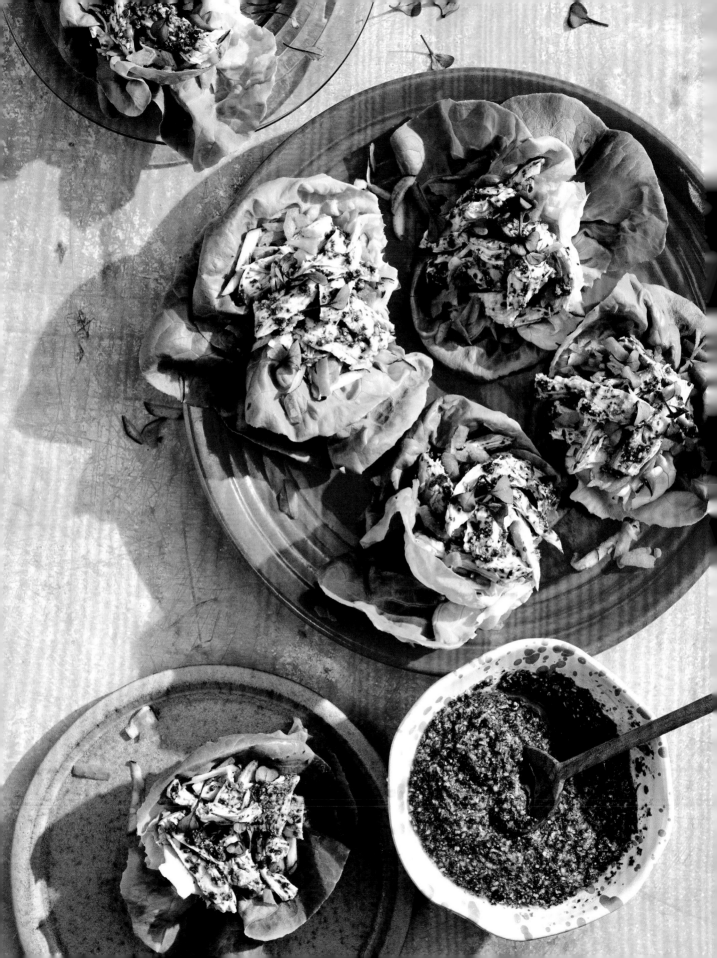

Pesto Chicken Lettuce Wraps

SERVES 2

2 cups thinly sliced
or shredded cooked chicken

3 tablespoons Pesto (page
224) or store-bought pesto

Extra-virgin olive oil

12 large Bibb lettuce leaves
(from about 2 heads)

1 medium carrot, coarsely
shredded

1 medium zucchini, coarsely
shredded

1½ teaspoons apple cider
vinegar

Fine sea salt and freshly
ground black pepper

½ cup microgreens (optional)

My kids eat very well, but Benny, my firstborn, had the benefit of my exclusive attention when it came to his early meals—I made them as nutrient dense and clean as possible. As our family grew (and grew up), I realized my idealized meals weren't always practical or popular across the household. Even if I had wanted to eat mostly simply prepared vegetables, sometimes my kids didn't want that. Behold the power of a lettuce wrap! For children, there's something exciting about being told to eat with your hands; and as a mom, I'm just thrilled that they enjoy lettuce leaves stuffed with shredded carrots and zucchini, lean chicken, and other good-for-them ingredients. Super-nutritious and kid-friendly, these are a win-win.

In a medium bowl, combine the chicken and 2 tablespoons of the pesto, stirring to coat. In a small bowl, thin out the remaining tablespoon pesto with 1 to 2 tablespoons olive oil—just enough to be sauce-like.

Divide the lettuce leaves into 6 piles of 2 leaves stacked on top of each other. Arrange little piles of the carrot and zucchini on top of each 2-leaf stack, then sprinkle each stack with a bit of vinegar and a couple small pinches of salt and pepper.

Divide scoops of the dressed chicken over the vegetables, and then drizzle each stack with a bit of the pesto sauce. Garnish with a few microgreens, if using, then serve.

MAKE IT YOURS

Hearty Pairing: Placing a few slices of avocado on each wrap adds delicious creaminess.

Simple Swap: Substitute Ginger-Cashew Sauce (page 223) or Tahini Dressing (page 220) for the pesto.

Chicken Meatballs

MAKES 12 MEATBALLS

Avocado oil

1 pound ground chicken,
not lean

½ cup chopped fresh flat-leaf
parsley

¼ cup Mom's Chicken Broth
(page 124) or Vegetable Broth
(page 122)

¼ cup almond flour or
gluten-free breadcrumbs

1 large egg, lightly beaten

1½ teaspoons onion powder

1½ teaspoons garlic powder

1 teaspoon dried oregano

1 teaspoon fine sea salt

Why do children love meatballs so much? I have no idea, but let's be honest, I love them, too! These juicy chicken meatballs are flavored with garlic and oregano, and are bound with protein-rich, gluten-free almond flour, rendering them a secret weapon for making an otherwise standard, healthy meal irresistible to kids. Served atop noodles or a salad, dropped into a soup, or stuffed into a wrap, these baked meatballs are so delicious. I like to make a double batch and store them in chicken broth in the fridge, which keeps them moist.

Preheat the oven to 375°F. Line a sheet pan with parchment and brush lightly with a little avocado oil.

In a large bowl, combine the chicken, parsley, broth, almond flour, egg, onion powder, garlic powder, oregano, and salt, then use your hands to mix well. Put the mixture in the refrigerator for 20 to 30 minutes to chill.

Divide the mixture into approximately 12 equal portions (about the size of a golf ball); I often use a small spring-loaded scoop. Then, using wet hands, roll them into smooth balls and place on the sheet pan.

Bake for 12 minutes, then turn the meatballs over and continue baking until fully cooked, another 12 minutes. The cooked meatballs can be refrigerated up to 3 days (preferably in chicken broth to keep them moist), or frozen in an airtight container for up to 1 month.

MAKE IT YOURS

Light Pairings: Simmer some veggies and meatballs in chicken broth (see page 124) for a simple soup.

Hearty Pairings: Slice or crumble the meatballs into the Beans and Greens Soup (page 135). Or, place the meatballs in an almond or cauliflower tortilla (or lettuce leaf) along with some Roasted Vegetables (page 144), salad greens, and grated manchego cheese. Or, crumble or slice a few meatballs for a pizza topping (see page 173).

For the Kids: Make meatball sliders by topping the meatballs with melted cheese on gluten-free buns. Add the meatballs to Zucchini Noodles with Pesto-Cashew Cream (page 166), or make rice noodles with tomato sauce for a nourishing spaghetti and meatballs.

Simple Swaps: Replace the parsley with fresh cilantro or dill; or substitute ground cumin or coriander for the oregano.

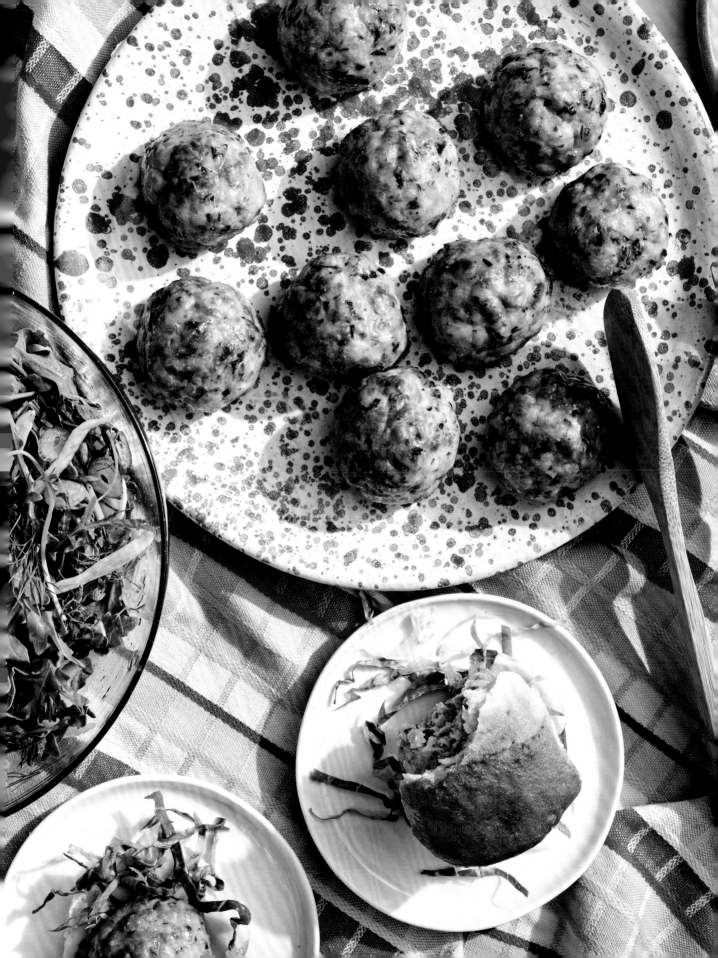

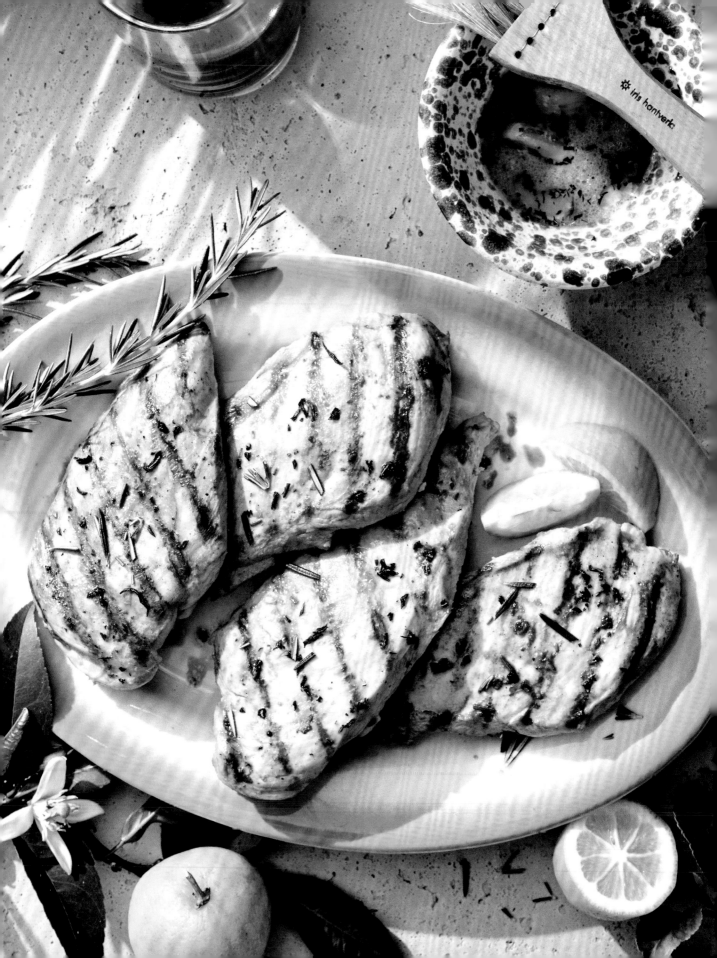

Rosemary-Lemon Chicken Paillards

SERVES 4

2 pounds boneless, skinless chicken breasts (about 4)

½ cup extra-virgin olive oil, plus more as needed

¼ cup red wine vinegar

2 lemons, 1 juiced and 1 sliced

3 garlic cloves, smashed

2 tablespoons chopped fresh rosemary

1 tablespoon Dijon mustard

Fine sea salt

Avocado oil

Indoor-outdoor living is a real benefit of life in Florida, where the mild, sunny weather suits this Brazilian girl very well. I am always looking for more ways to spend time outdoors, so grilling is one of my favorite ways to cook. (Though an indoor grill pan gives very delicious results, too.) This lemony, mustardy marinade makes boneless and skinless chicken breasts—here pounded into weeknight-friendly, quick-cooking paillards—tender, juicy, and full of flavor. This is one of our favorite recipes from Susan Ryan, a wonderful chef who cooked for our family for years. My kids absolutely love these.

In case you prefer dark-meat chicken, the marinade works just as well on bone-in pieces or even on a whole bird (see the variation below). In any event, the leftovers can be sliced or shredded, then added to soups, salads, and more—so be sure to make plenty!

Lay out the chicken pieces on a cutting board and cover with a sheet of parchment. Using the smooth side of a meat-tenderizing mallet, pound the chicken breasts to an even thickness, between ¼ and ½ inch.

In a medium bowl, whisk together the ½ cup olive oil, the vinegar, lemon juice, garlic, rosemary, and mustard. Add the chicken and the sliced lemon and toss to coat. Cover and marinate the chicken at room temperature for 30 minutes, or place in the refrigerator for up to 2 hours.

Preheat a stovetop grill pan over high heat, or heat an outdoor grill to medium-high, leaving space on the grate to cook indirectly (see page 189 for more detail).

(recipe continues)

MAKE IT YOURS

Light Pairings: Serve with Roasted Vegetables (page 144) or Favorite Sautéed Leafy Greens (page 152). Any leftovers can be shredded or sliced and added to a salad, especially the Arugula and Chicken Salad (page 115), or added to a soup, or included as part of the Pesto Chicken Lettuce Wraps (page 193) or the Extra-Crunchy Summer Rolls (page 156).

For the Kids. Shred the cooked chicken and add to the Ramen-Style Soup (page 136). Or, slice the chicken into strips for tacos (see page 202). Or, serve with oven-roasted Sweet Potato Fries (page 146) and blanched green beans (see page 155) on the side.

Simple Swaps: Replace the rosemary with fresh thyme or 1 tablespoon herbes de Provence.

Remove the chicken from the marinade and pat dry with paper towels. Sprinkle the chicken with some salt.

If cooking on the stovetop, lower the heat under the grill pan to medium, brush the pan lightly with a little avocado oil, then carefully arrange the chicken to fit in a single layer; you may have to cook in 2 batches.

If grilling outdoors, brush the grates with oil, arrange the chicken on the grates over indirect heat, and close the lid.

In either case, cook without disturbing for 3 to 4 minutes, then gently use a spatula to check if the chicken lifts away easily from the grill and has nice grill marks. (If the chicken sticks, it is not ready to be flipped—be patient.) Flip the chicken and continue cooking until grill marks appear on the bottom and the chicken is cooked through, about 3 more minutes.

Transfer the cooked chicken to a cutting board or plate. Let rest for at least 5 minutes, then serve. Chicken can be refrigerated, covered, in an airtight glass container for up to 2 days.

ROASTED WHOLE CHICKEN

Use a 3½- to 4-pound chicken. Place the marinade in a large bowl, add the chicken, cover, and marinate at room temperature for 30 minutes and up to 2 hours in the refrigerator. When ready to cook, preheat the oven to 400°F. Pat the chicken dry, sprinkle all over with salt, and arrange breast side up in a large baking dish. Stuff the cavity with a halved lemon and a bunch of fresh rosemary, then roast until the skin is browned and crispy and an instant-read thermometer reads 165°F when inserted into the thickest part of a thigh (juices at the thigh joint should run clear), 60 to 80 minutes. Let rest for at least 10 minutes before carving.

ROASTED BONE-IN CHICKEN BREASTS, THIGHS, OR DRUMSTICKS

Use 3 to 4 pounds of bone-in chicken thighs, drumsticks, or breasts. Place the marinade in a large bowl, add the chicken pieces, cover, and marinate at room temperature for 30 minutes and up to 2 hours in the refrigerator. When ready to cook, preheat the oven to 400°F. Pat the chicken dry, sprinkle all over with salt, and arrange the pieces on a sheet pan lined with parchment. Roast until the skin is browned and crispy and an instant-read thermometer reads 165°F when inserted into the thickest part of the thigh (the juices should run clear), 30 to 45 minutes. Let rest for at least 10 minutes before serving.

Grilled Rib Eye
with Chimichurri

SERVES 4 TO 6

1 large (2 to 2½ pounds)
bone-in rib eye steak
(1½ inches thick),
at room temperature

1½ teaspoons coarse salt,
or more as needed

Avocado oil

2 tablespoons unsalted butter
Chimichurri (page 224)

If you're from the south of Brazil, like me, you know that eating steak is part of the culture. My father grilled steak on a stick—churrasco—pretty much every Sunday. We all loved it. I truly missed it when I was vegetarian or vegan. Plus the iron in red meat is especially helpful for my health, which is why I went back to eating meat. These days, I source really high-quality options, ideally from a small ranch or farm, but I eat it less frequently.

This is a treat to serve when the weather is nice, especially if you are able to grill outside, but there is also a variation for cooking on the stovetop. The chimichurri is delicious on the side, or serve the steak with just salt—if you buy good-quality meat, you don't really need much else!

Set the steak in a baking dish and pat dry with paper towels. Sprinkle salt all over and massage it into the meat with your fingers. (This is the secret to a flavorful and juicy steak!) Allow the meat to marinate for at least 30 minutes (or if you have time, put it in a covered glass container in the refrigerator overnight). When ready to cook, remove the steak from the fridge and let it come to room temperature.

Preheat your outdoor grill to high heat, leaving areas for both direct and indirect cooking. Brush the steak with some oil, then set it over direct heat. Cover the grill and cook until the steak starts to develop a dark brown crust, about 3 minutes. Use tongs to flip it over and cook for another 3 minutes, until you have a dark brown crust on the second side.

(recipe continues)

MAKE IT YOURS

Light Pairings: Sautéed spinach (see page 159) and grilled asparagus are classics for a reason.

Hearty Pairings: Cauliflower Puree (page 161) is a delicious accompaniment.

Simple Swaps: Pesto (page 224), thinned out a bit with some extra-virgin olive oil, or Cilantro-Mint Dressing (page 221), is delicious drizzled on top instead of the chimichurri.

Move the steak to indirect heat. Cover the grill again, and continue cooking for another 3 to 6 minutes—3 minutes for more rare and up to 6 minutes for well done. To check, make a small cut with a paring knife into the thickest part of the steak.

Transfer the steak to a carving board or serving platter, top with thin slices of the butter, and let rest for 10 minutes. Remove the meat from the bone in one large piece, then slice thinly against the grain. Serve warm, with any collected juices spooned over the steak and the chimichurri on the side.

STOVETOP BUTTER-BASTED RIB EYE

Season and marinate the steak as instructed. Set a large cast-iron skillet over medium-high heat and preheat for 5 to 10 minutes. Add about 3 tablespoons oil to generously coat the bottom, then add the steak. Cook, using tongs to rotate (not flip) the steak periodically so it browns evenly on the bottom, developing a brown crust, 4 to 6 minutes. Then flip and repeat on the other side.

Add 2 tablespoons of unsalted butter to the pan, along with 2 smashed garlic cloves and a few thyme or rosemary sprigs, if you like. Tilt the pan toward you so that the butter pools in one part of the pan, then use a spoon to collect it and pour over the top of the steak to baste it. Continue cooking this way, flipping, rotating, and basting until the steak is well browned all over, another 3 to 6 minutes, depending on how you like it. To check, make a small cut with a paring knife into the thickest part of the steak. Let rest for 10 minutes, then slice against the grain.

MAKE TIME TO MARINATE

I always say, "Don't put off to tomorrow what you can do today." And that is one reason I love marinating meats. Marinating is such a simple thing, and the taste difference is huge—steaks and chicken are juicier and more flavorful. Plus, when I marinate ahead of time, the decision about what's for dinner is already made and the work is begun; all I have to do later is put the meat on the grill or in a pan and cook some veggies on the side.

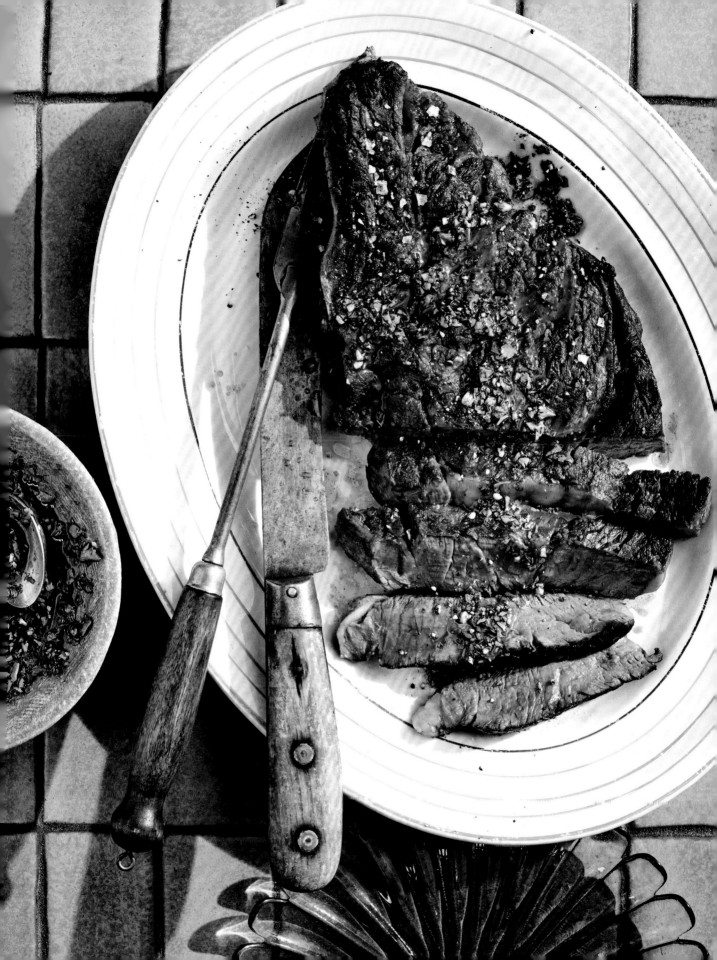

Taco Night!

In our house, Taco Night is an event we all look forward to. It's a fun (and smart!) meal to have when friends come over, as you never know what everyone's preferences, portion sizes, or allergies might be. Here, the recipes are for grilled chicken and flank steak—you can make both, just one, or neither, as you can also fill your tortillas with any combination of other toppings (see list on opposite page for our favorites). Whatever way you like tacos, these have wholesome ingredients and all the fun— something we all can celebrate!

Chicken Tacos with Corn

SERVES 4 TO 6

¼ cup avocado oil

Juice of 1 lime

1 teaspoon fresh thyme leaves

1 teaspoon coarse salt

1½ pounds boneless, skinless chicken thighs (4 to 6 pieces)

2 ears corn, husked and silk removed

8 to 12 tortillas (almond flour, chickpea flour, or Hero brand)

MAKE IT YOURS

Simple Swaps: Substitute Rosemary-Lemon Chicken Paillards (page 197) for the grilled chicken. Or try grilled fish instead of chicken.

Whisk together the oil, lime juice, thyme, and salt in a large bowl, then add the chicken, stirring to coat. Cover and marinate for 20 to 30 minutes at room temperature, or refrigerate up to 2 hours.

While the chicken marinates, cook the corn. Bring a large pot of filtered water to a boil over high heat. Add the corn and blanch just for 3 to 4 minutes, until tender. Remove from the pot and let cool.

Hold an ear of corn vertically, with the broad end down, on your cutting board and use a sharp knife to cut down along the side to trim off a strip of kernels. Rotate the cob, and continue to slice off strips, rotating as you go. Repeat with the other ear of corn. Break up the strips so you have separate kernels and transfer to a serving bowl.

Prepare an outdoor grill for direct cooking over medium-high heat, or set a large nonstick sauté pan or grill pan over medium-high heat. When hot, use tongs to arrange the chicken on the grates over direct heat or in a single layer in the sauté pan; you may need to cook in 2 batches. In either case, cook without disturbing for 6 to 8 minutes, then gently use a spatula to check if the chicken lifts easily from the grill or pan and has nice grill marks. (If the chicken sticks, it is not ready to be flipped—be patient.) Flip and continue cooking until the outside is caramelized and the juices run clear, or an instant-read thermometer reads 165°F, about 8 minutes more.

Transfer the chicken to a plate or cutting board to rest for 10 minutes, then slice, chop, or shred.

Warm the tortillas and wrap them in a clean kitchen towel. Set out all the toppings you'll be offering (see possible toppings, opposite). Encourage everyone to make their own tacos, just the way they like!

Flank Steak Tacos

SERVES 4 TO 6

1½ pounds boneless
flank steak

Coarse salt

Fresh rosemary sprig, leaves
only (optional)

Avocado oil

8 to 12 tortillas (almond flour,
chickpea flour, or Hero brand)

Possible toppings

Simple Cabbage Slaw
(page 101)

Roasted cauliflower florets
(see page 144)

Roasted Sweet Potato Cubes
(page 147)

Sheet-Pan Squash and
Chickpeas (page 151)

1 cup coarsely shredded
manchego or Midnight Moon
cheese

1 cup roasted corn nuts

Sliced avocados

Sour cream or plain cultured
coconut yogurt

½ cup Crispy Roasted Shiitake
Mushrooms (page 214)

The steak is marinated, then grilled or broiled as you like.

Lay the steak on a cutting board and blot it dry with paper towels. Sprinkle with 1 teaspoon of coarse salt. If desired, sprinkle the steak with the rosemary leaves. Massage the seasonings into the meat with your fingers. Cover and marinate for 20 to 30 minutes at room temperature, or up to 8 hours in the refrigerator; bring to room temperature before cooking.

If using an outdoor grill: Prepare your grill for direct and indirect cooking, heating one side over high heat. Lightly brush the grate with avocado oil and, when hot, place the steak over direct heat and cook without disturbing for 2 to 4 minutes, until charred on the edges and grill marks have developed. Use tongs to flip and repeat on the second side, cooking for another 2 to 4 minutes, depending on preference: 2 minutes for rare, 4 minutes for medium to well done. To check, make a small cut with a paring knife into the thickest part of the steak. (If the steaks have grill marks but is undercooked, move it to indirect heat for a few more minutes.)

If using the broiler: Arrange an oven rack in the top position and preheat the broiler to high. Line a broiler pan with the pan's insert or an oven-safe rack. Set the steak on the rack and place under the broiler. Cook without disturbing for 3 minutes, until dark and crispy around the edges, then flip and cook the opposite side for another 2 to 4 minutes, until cooked to your preference; medium-rare is about 6 minutes total. To check, make a small cut with a paring knife into the thickest part of the steak. If needed, cook a few minutes more.

Move the steak to a platter and let rest for 10 minutes. Slice as thin as you can against the grain. Dress with any juices that collect on the platter.

Warm the tortillas and wrap them in a clean kitchen towel. Set out all the toppings you'll be offering. Encourage everyone to make their own tacos, just the way they like!

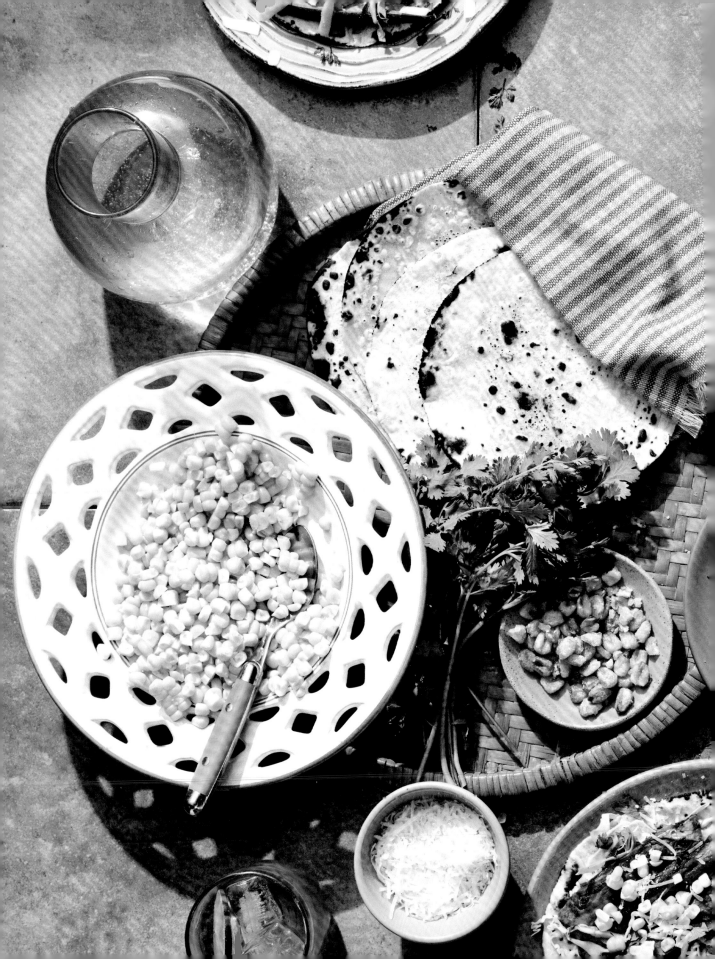

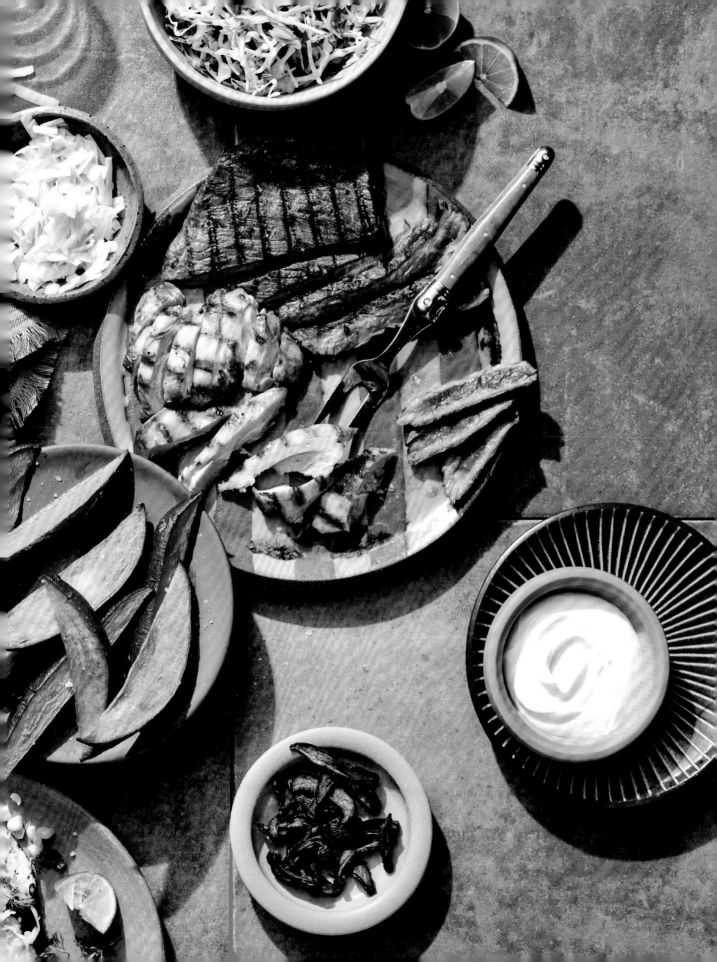

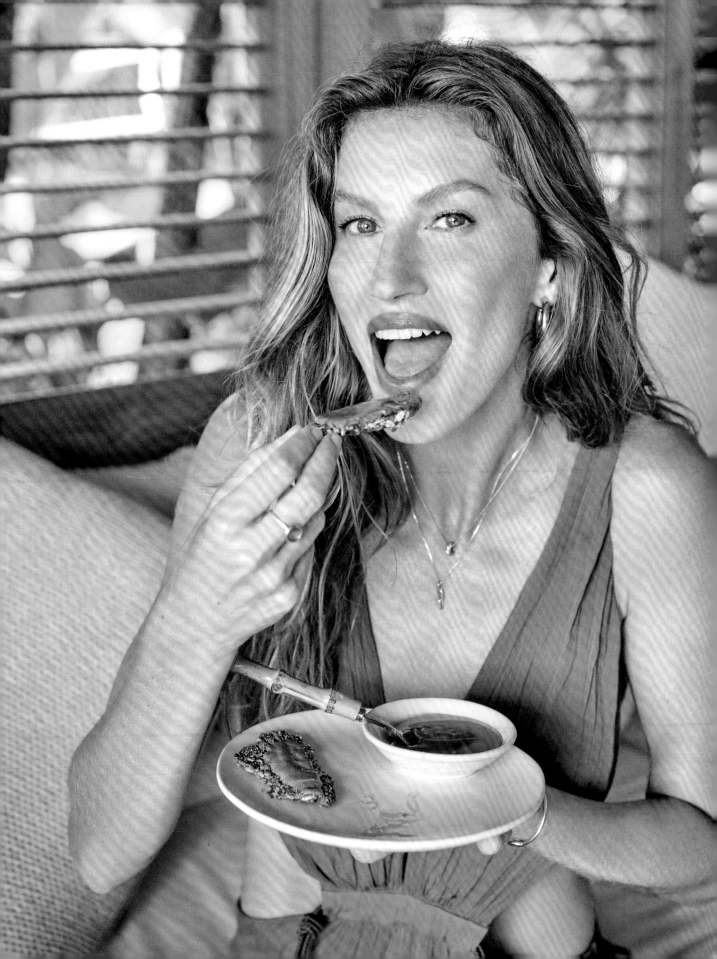

Crunchies & Condiments

I love simple foods, so having some extra textures and a variety of dressings is so helpful to change up a basic meal. Here are my go-to recipes for crunchy sprinkles and delicious, bright, and high-flavor sauces that add so much personality and fun to a dish.
Mix and match and see what you like!

Maple Harissa Cashews

MAKES 4 CUPS

4 cups raw cashews

2 to 3 tablespoons harissa paste (see Note)

3 tablespoons pure maple syrup

1½ tablespoons avocado oil

½ teaspoon fine sea salt, or more as needed

I'm a wimp when it comes to spicy food, but these harissa cashews are an exception. Harissa can be purchased as a paste or as a spice blend. Here, I use the North African spice paste that usually includes dried chiles, garlic, cumin, and caraway—it adds a pleasant warmth that is balanced by maple syrup's sweetness. I find the combination irresistible. I often sprinkle these nuts on salads.

As in other recipes where soaked nuts and seeds get roasted, be patient in allowing them to crisp. While they may not seem completely crisp right out of the oven, as they cool they'll develop an appealing snap. You can make a half batch, if you prefer.

Place the cashews in a large bowl, cover with room-temperature water, and soak at room temperature for 2 to 24 hours (or see page 244 for a quick-soak method).

Preheat the oven to 350°F. Line a baking sheet with parchment.

Rinse the cashews in a colander or fine-mesh sieve, and drain. Spread the nuts out on the baking sheet in an even layer and roast until the nuts are dry to the touch and start to lightly brown, 15 to 20 minutes.

Meanwhile, in a small bowl, stir together the harissa, maple syrup, oil, and ½ teaspoon salt.

Remove the cashews from the oven and use a silicone spatula to scrape the harissa mixture onto them and stir to evenly coat. Return the cashews to the oven and continue roasting until the nuts are golden brown (test by breaking one in half and looking inside) and dry, another 30 to 40 minutes.

Remove the cashews from the oven and immediately sprinkle with a few extra pinches of salt. The cashews will continue to crisp as they cool. (If the nuts aren't as crisp as you'd like after cooling, return them to the oven and roast for 5 to 10 minutes more.) Stored in an airtight glass jar or container, they'll keep up to 7 days.

Note: If you would prefer to use a dried harissa spice blend, use only 1 tablespoon and add 1 tablespoon filtered water with the remaining ingredients.

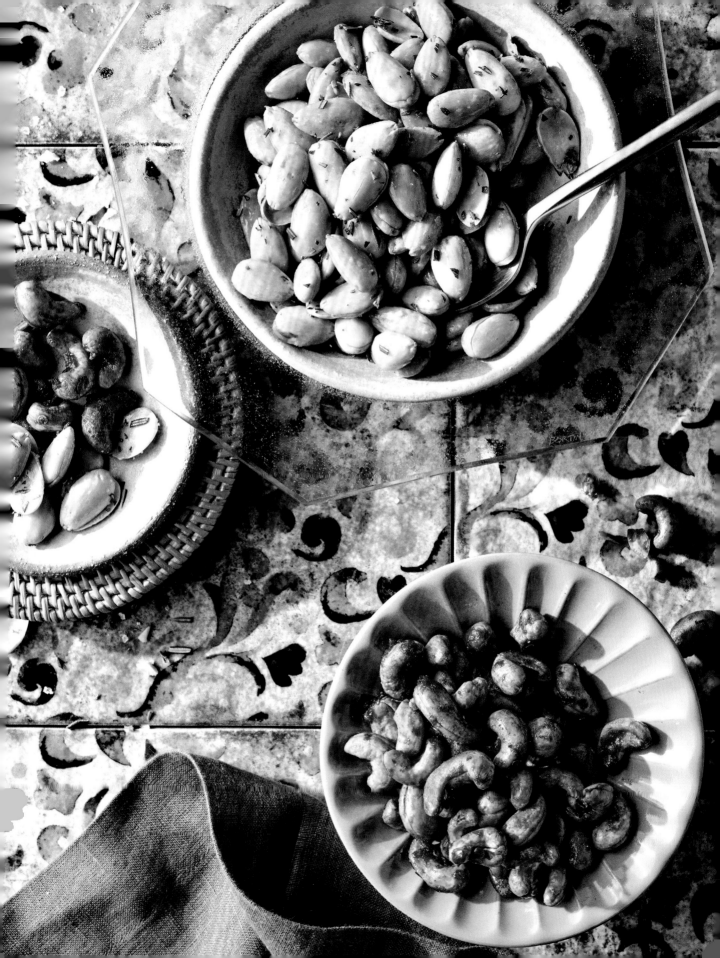

Rosemary Almonds

MAKES 4 CUPS

4 cups raw almonds
(about 1 pound)

2 tablespoons avocado oil

2 to 3 tablespoons coarsely
chopped fresh rosemary or
2 to 3 teaspoons dried

¾ teaspoon fine sea salt,
or more as needed

I used to be a huge snacker, especially on things that were super crunchy, like crackers, nuts, crispy spiced chickpeas—I love them all! But in the last couple of years, I've learned that it is important to give your digestive system a break of four to five hours between meals, so that your body has a chance to properly digest—even if those between-meal snacks are healthy ones. I try my best to do that.

So now, instead of snacking on these herby roasted almonds (you can also use walnuts or pumpkin seeds), I use them to boost the texture and protein of a meal—such as topping a salad or roasted vegetables. I soak the almonds ahead to remove their skins, and while this is great for digestibility, it does take longer for them to roast in the oven, so be patient. Feel free to halve this recipe, if you prefer (though I'm warning you—you'll go through them quickly!).

Place the almonds in a large bowl, cover with room-temperature water, and soak for at least 8 hours or overnight. (If you don't have time to soak, see Note.)

Preheat the oven to 325°F. Line two baking sheets with parchment.

Rinse the nuts in a colander or fine-mesh sieve. Gently pinch each almond to loosen its skin, and then slip it off. (I compost the skins.)

Spread the nuts on the baking sheets in an even layer and roast until dry to the touch and starting to lightly brown, 15 to 20 minutes.

Remove the nuts from the oven (leave oven turned on). In a mixing bowl, stir together the nuts, oil, rosemary, and ¾ teaspoon salt, coating the nuts evenly. Return to the oven and roast until fully golden brown and the rosemary is crisp, 20 to 30 minutes more, stirring every 10 minutes (see Note). Taste and add an extra pinch or two of salt, if you like.

Transfer the nuts to a plate and let cool completely. Once cool, if the nuts aren't as crisp as you'd like, return them to the oven and cook for 5 to 10 minutes more. Stored in an airtight glass jar or container, the nuts will keep up to 7 days.

Note: Soaked nuts take longer to get crunchy in the oven. Be patient and remember that they will continue to crisp up after you remove them from the oven, as they cool. If you don't have time to soak the nuts, blanched almonds can be used, but they take less time to roast. Skip the step to dry them out in the oven, and instead start roasting them with the spice mixture as detailed in the directions above.

MAKE IT YOURS

Light Pairings: These are a delicious crunchy topping for any soup or salad, or even for roasted or sautéed vegetables (see pages 144 or 165).

Simple Swaps: Try other herbs in place of the rosemary, like thyme or herbes de Provence.

ROSEMARY PEPITAS

When I have seeds left from carving pumpkins, I like to roast them. To do so, first place the seeds in a large bowl and cover with water. Using your fingers, remove and discard the pulp from the seeds; drain the cleaned seeds. Bring a large saucepan of salted water to a boil, add the seeds, and cook for 10 minutes, then drain in a sieve. Transfer the seeds to a towel-lined plate to dry further. Then, measure the seeds: for every 1 cup, you'll need about 2 tablespoons avocado oil and 1 tablespoon chopped fresh rosemary leaves (or 1 teaspoon dried).

Preheat the oven to 350°F. Line a baking sheet with parchment. Add the seeds, toss with the oil, and spread them out evenly on the baking sheet. Roast for 10 minutes, then stir in the rosemary and continue roasting for another 5 to 10 minutes, until lightly browned and crisp. Taste and add an extra pinch or two of salt, if you like.

FOOD ON THE GO

I like to plan my meals ahead so even if I'm traveling or running errands, I still have something nutritious to look forward to (and this way, I never find myself starving and without options!). Here are some of my favorite options for bringing on flights, in cars, or any other time I am on the go.

Baru Nut Bars (page 233)—one of these and a cup of tea will definitely satisfy me.

Coconut–Chia Seed Pudding (page 80)—I often make this in small mason jars so I can grab one from the fridge and walk right out the door (don't forget the spoon!).

Seed Crackers (page 218) with smashed avocado.

Crunchy Spiced Chickpeas (page 213) or **Rosemary Almonds** (page 210).

Extra-Crunchy Summer Rolls (page 156) with a container of Ginger-Cashew Sauce (page 223) for dipping.

Benny's Shaved Salad (page 102), often with some chicken.

Best Blanched Vegetables (page 155) or raw carrots and celery do not need to be refrigerated and are delicious at room temperature; a little bit of **Hummus** (page 180) alongside is always nice!

A mason-jar salad. I put dressing on the bottom, then layer in some blanched veggies, followed by salad greens, and top it off with chopped Rosemary Almonds (page 210) or Crunchy Spiced Chickpeas (page 213)—shake and enjoy! Or add the same ingredients to a wrap.

When I don't have any homemade options, I look for simple whole foods or foods with as few ingredients as possible, like **organic fruit**. Real food is always going to be the best.

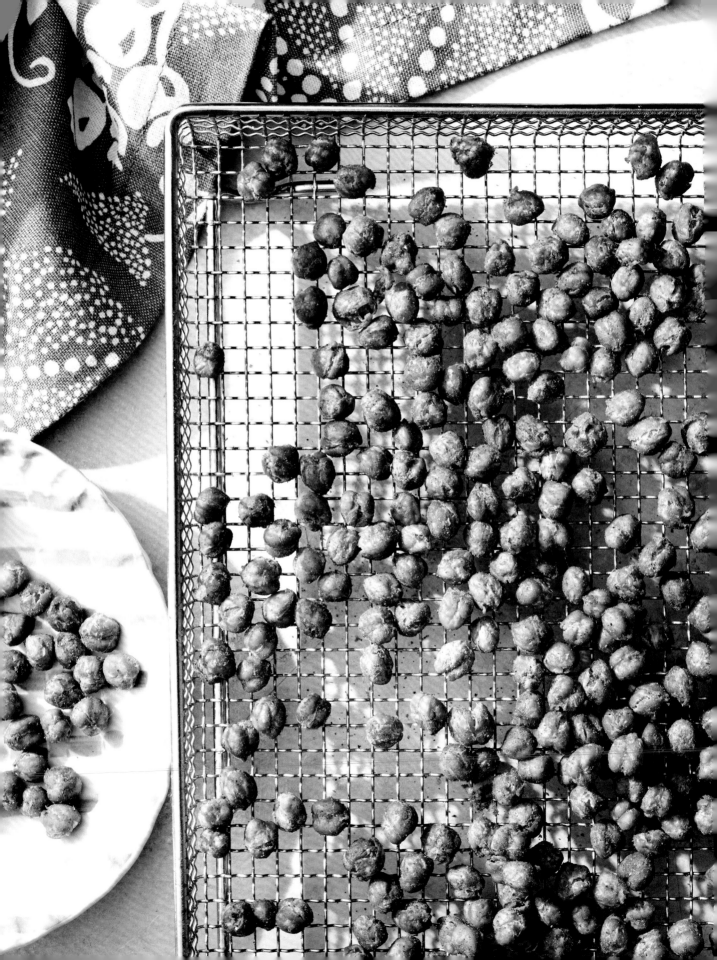

Crunchy Spiced Chickpeas

MAKES ABOUT 3 CUPS

3 cups From-Scratch Chickpeas (page 179) or boxed or jarred chickpeas, rinsed and drained (no need to remove skins)

2 tablespoons avocado oil

1½ teaspoons ras el hanout

1 teaspoon fine sea salt, or more as needed

Roasted and spiced chickpeas are one of my favorite crunchies, but many homemade versions can quickly lose their crisp texture. To achieve maximum crispness, I dry the chickpeas with a kitchen towel and then roast prior to seasoning. This allows even more moisture to evaporate. Once they are fully dried, *then* I toss them with oil and one of my favorite spice blends from Morocco called ras el hanout—a mix of warming spices like coriander, cumin, black pepper, ginger, and cinnamon—and continue roasting. Once they are brown and crisp, I dust them with salt. You can also easily make these in an air-fryer (see variation that follows)!

Preheat the oven to 425°F. Line a sheet pan with parchment.

Spread the chickpeas on a large kitchen towel. Gently roll them around and blot so as to absorb as much moisture as possible. It's important to get the chickpeas as dry as you can for maximum crispiness!

Spread the chickpeas in the sheet pan and roast for about 15 minutes, until further dried out and slightly shriveled. Remove the sheet pan from the oven and add the oil and spice mix, stirring with a spatula to coat evenly. Return the chickpeas to the oven and continue roasting until very crisp, another 30 to 35 minutes, stirring or gently shaking the pan every 10 minutes.

Take the chickpeas out of the oven and immediately sprinkle with ½ teaspoon salt, stirring to coat evenly. Taste and add extra salt or seasoning, if you like.

Let cool completely on the sheet tray, then transfer to an airtight glass jar or container. The chickpeas will keep for up to 3 days.

MAKE IT YOURS

Light Pairings: Sprinkle these on top of a salad or soup instead of croutons.

Simple Swaps: Use any spice blend (another Moroccan blend, an Italian blend, Chinese five spice powder, or Indian curry powder or garam masala) in place of the ras el hanout.

AIR-FRYER CRUNCHY SPICED CHICKPEAS

Following the manufacturer's instructions, preheat the air-fryer to 400°F. Place the chickpeas, the spice mixture, and oil in a medium bowl and toss to coat. Add half the chickpeas to the fryer basket, gently shaking them into an even layer, and cook for 10 to 15 minutes, shaking the basket every 5 minutes, until they're well crisped and evenly browned. Transfer to a bowl or plate and sprinkle with half of the salt. Repeat, cooking and then seasoning the remaining chickpeas.

Crispy Roasted Shiitake Mushrooms

MAKES ABOUT 1 CUP

10 ounces fresh shiitake mushrooms

2 tablespoons avocado oil

½ teaspoon tamari

½ teaspoon fine sea salt

These rich and flavorful roasted mushroom slices are thin and crispy like potato chips. Sprinkle them over any soup, salad, or other dish that could use some texture and savoriness. Just a few can make an impact, as they are so concentrated.

Preheat the oven to 350°F. Line a baking sheet with parchment.

Trim off the mushroom stems (save them for chicken or vegetable broth, pages 124 or 122) and slice the caps into ⅛-inch-thick strips. Add them to a medium bowl and toss with the oil, tamari, and salt to coat thoroughly. Spread in an even layer on the baking sheet.

Place in the oven and bake for 35 to 45 minutes, stirring every 10 minutes, until darkened in color and most have turned crispy. (Watch carefully toward the end—they go from crisp to burnt quickly.) They'll continue to get a bit crispier as they cool.

When completely cooled, store in an airtight glass jar or container at room temperature for up to 3 days (they will soften a bit). To re-crisp, place on a baking sheet in a 350°F oven for 5 to 7 minutes.

MAKE IT YOURS

Light Pairings: These are delicious sprinkled on Benny's Shaved Salad (page 102) or on soups, like the Creamy Cauliflower (page 131).

Hearty Pairings: Add to the Pesto Chicken Lettuce Wraps (page 193) or use in tacos (see page 202).

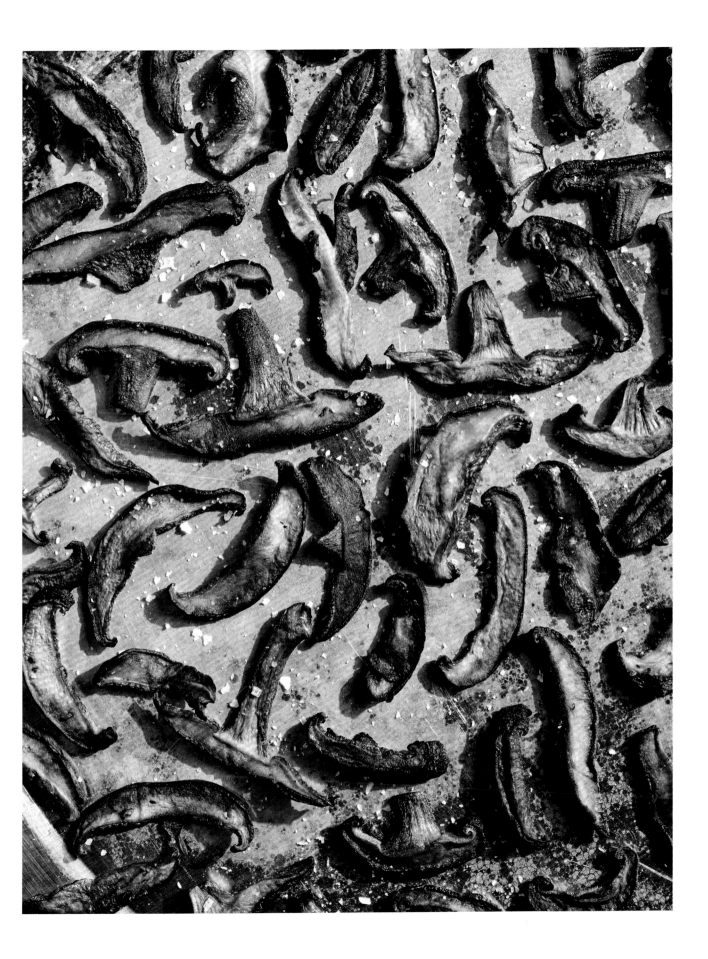

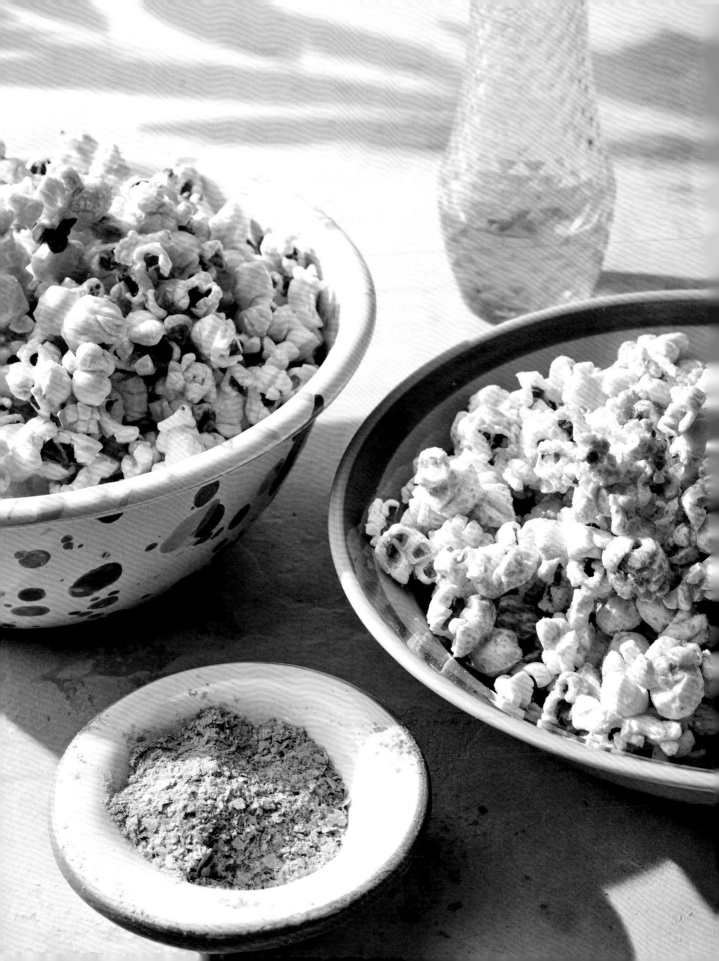

Buttered Popcorn

MAKES 15 CUPS

4 tablespoons unsalted butter, divided

½ cup popcorn kernels

Fine sea salt

Popcorn has a bad reputation. It's true that store-bought or pre-popped popcorn can be very unhealthy—for example, movie theater popcorn "butter" is not actually butter at all; it contains artificial colors, flavors, and hydrogenated GMO soybean oil! But if you make popcorn at home, you can add high-quality toppings, like additional butter (my favorite—I like to melt it and pour into a spray bottle for even coverage), and enjoy a whole-grain snack that can be flavored in a hundred different ways. The variations include a sweet version made with honey and a quick "cheesy" version with nutritional yeast, but also feel free to swap in any dried herbs, spices, or other flavorings you like.

Place a large Dutch oven or other heavy-bottomed large pot over high heat. Add 2 tablespoons of the butter and the popcorn kernels, stirring constantly with a wooden spoon until the butter is melted and the popcorn is lighter in color. Add the remaining 2 tablespoons of butter and continue stirring until the first kernel pops, about 3 to 5 minutes. Immediately cover the pot with a lid (glass is ideal) and turn the heat to medium-high. As the pot begins to fill with popcorn, use mitted hands to occasionally swirl and shake the lidded pot over the heat to redistribute the unpopped kernels inside. Continue cooking until the popping subsides. Turn off the heat.

Toss the popcorn with salt, to taste, and enjoy.

"CHEESY" BUTTERED POPCORN

Sprinkle the finished popcorn with 3 to 4 tablespoons of nutritional yeast for a cheesy flavor with the added benefit of providing protein, B vitamins, folate, and essential amino acids.

SWEET BUTTERED POPCORN

For a kettle corn–caramel corn sweetness, skip the salt and replace the butter with coconut oil, then drizzle 3 to 4 tablespoons warmed honey over the popped corn and toss.

Seed Crackers

MAKES 2 LARGE SHEETS
OF CRACKERS

1⅓ cups raw sunflower seeds

1 cup raw pumpkin seeds

½ cup flax seeds

½ cup raw sesame seeds

2 tablespoons psyllium husk
powder

2 tablespoons almond flour

1 teaspoon fine sea salt

2 cups filtered water, at room
temperature

2 tablespoons poppy seeds

Coarse or flaky salt, such as
Maldon

My five sisters all live in Brazil, so I don't get to see them nearly as much as I want to. But we do make sure we all meet up at least once a year, and since moving to Miami, I sometimes get lucky with a visit from some of them. I often make a cheese plate for us to nibble on before dinner while we are sitting around in comfy clothes, catching up in person. It's a treat for me in every way.

These naturally gluten-free crackers, made of nutritious seeds with a bit of almond flour to hold everything together, are always on that cheese plate as well. They are super crunchy and especially delicious spread with Midnight Moon, my favorite goat cheese. They are also great alongside any soup or salad—we always have a batch on hand.

Preheat the oven to 325°F. Line 2 (18 by 13-inch) baking sheets with parchment.

In a large bowl, mix the sunflower seeds, pumpkin seeds, flax seeds, sesame seeds, psyllium husk powder, almond flour, and sea salt, making sure to distribute the psyllium powder evenly. Stir in the water. The batter that forms will be thin at first, and will then thicken considerably.

Divide the batter between the 2 baking sheets. Using an offset spatula or lightly moistened hands, spread or press the batter into a thin sheet, covering as much of the parchment as possible. Sprinkle with the poppy seeds and several pinches of the coarse or flaky salt. Allow to rest for 5 minutes.

Bake until lightly browned, dry to the touch, and crisp, 60 to 70 minutes, rotating the pans halfway through. Let the cracker sheets cool on the sheet pans, then loosen them carefully from the parchment.

When sheets are cool, break into large pieces. Store the crackers in an airtight glass container at room temperature for up to 1 week.

MAKE IT YOURS

Light Pairings: Dip the crackers in Hummus (page 180) or spread with avocado.

Hearty Pairings: On a serving plate, platter, or wooden board, arrange a few types of cheese. (I eat mostly goat- and sheep-milk cheeses; some of my favorites are Midnight Moon and manchego.) Add some olives, Maple Harissa Cashews (page 208), Rosemary Almonds (page 210), or Crunchy Spiced Chickpeas (page 213).

For the Kids: Serve the crackers with almond butter, drizzled with honey.

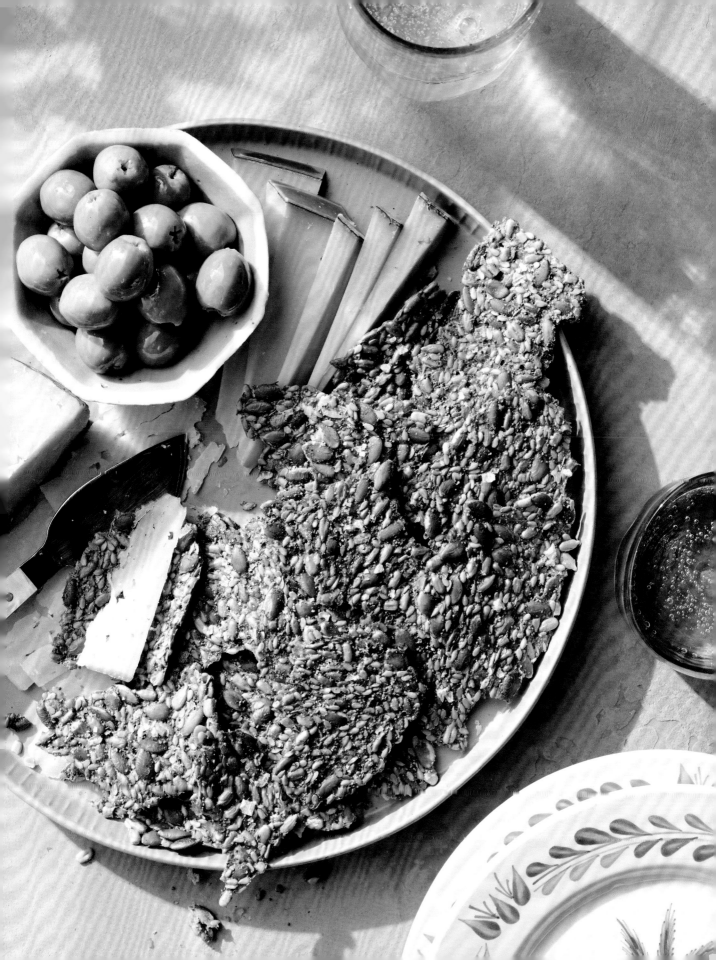

Dad's Honey-Mustard Dressing

MAKES ABOUT ⅔ **CUP**

6 tablespoons extra-virgin olive oil

2 tablespoons apple cider vinegar

1 tablespoon honey

1 tablespoon mustard

½ teaspoon fine sea salt

Freshly ground black pepper

While my mom was in charge of most of what we ate growing up, my dad was the resident griller. This is a big role in Brazil, with our weekly Sunday churrasco—a big mixed grill—which was a time to get together with family and friends. The one exception to this was that he also made the salad dressing—and this simple honey mustard is his recipe. My dad likes assertive flavors, and this is a bit tangy and sweet—and because of that, my kids love it, too.

If I want a salad dressing that has a bit more personality than a light lemon vinaigrette or the olive oil and salt that go with everything, this is what I make. I use Primal Kitchen mustard, as it includes no additives or preservatives, and is organic; my favorite is the Dijon, but all types work great here.

Add the olive oil, vinegar, honey, mustard, salt, and pepper to a lidded jar and shake until emulsified. (Or whisk the ingredients in a small bowl.) Refrigerate, covered, in an airtight glass jar or container for up to 2 weeks (though I prefer to eat most things within 3 days as they will taste much fresher).

Tahini Dressing

MAKES 1 CUP

½ cup stirred tahini

½ cup filtered water, or more as needed

3 tablespoons fresh lemon juice

¼ teaspoon fine sea salt, or more as needed

Nutty and rich, this simple dressing is a must for my kids when eating Pan-Fried Falafel (page 177).

In a medium bowl, whisk together the tahini, water, lemon juice, and salt. The tahini will thicken as you whisk, but continue whisking until the dressing smooths out, adding additional water as needed, 1 tablespoon at a time, until the dressing is creamy and pourable.

Taste and add additional salt as needed. Refrigerate, covered, in an airtight glass container or jar for up to 5 days; stir before using.

Cilantro-Mint Dressing

MAKES ABOUT ⅔ CUP

¼ cup plus 1 tablespoon
Coconut Milk (page 72)
or store-bought full-fat
coconut milk

½ to 1 serrano chile
or jalapeño, stemmed and
seeded (optional)

1 garlic clove, chopped

1 (1-inch) piece fresh ginger,
peeled and roughly chopped

2 tablespoons fresh lime juice

1 teaspoon ground coriander

½ teaspoon fine sea salt

1 cup packed fresh cilantro
leaves

½ cup packed fresh mint
leaves

This dressing is my new favorite: I put it on everything! It has a little bit of heat from the serrano, a little creaminess from the coconut, and tons of flavor from the ginger and garlic. The cilantro and mint (and lime juice) are fresh and bright, so the sauce will wake up anything you pair it with. Try it alongside a grilled steak or fish fillet, or drizzled on Miso-Mustard Roasted Whole Cauliflower (page 170) or Sheet-Pan Squash and Chickpeas (page 151). Or, use it to toss any salad (especially the Green Bean Salad on page 119), or smeared in a wrap. Make this, and you just might eat it with every meal.

In a blender, combine the coconut milk, chile (if using), garlic, ginger, lime juice, ground coriander, and salt and blend until smooth. Add the cilantro and mint and blend until everything is thoroughly combined, scraping the sides down as needed. Refrigerate in a covered container for up to 3 days.

Cashew Cream

MAKES 1 CUP

1¾ cups filtered water, room
temperature, or more as
needed

1 cup raw cashews

1 garlic clove

1 teaspoon fresh lemon juice

1 teaspoon nutritional yeast

½ teaspoon fine sea salt

This creamy, rich sauce is raw and totally delicious—excellent on zucchini noodles (page 166).

In a small saucepan, bring 1 cup of the filtered water to boil, then remove from the heat. Add the cashews and allow to soak for 15 minutes. Drain and rinse, then drain again.

Place the cashews in a blender along with the garlic, lemon juice, nutritional yeast, salt, and remaining ¾ cup water. Blend until smooth and creamy, 45 to 90 seconds, scraping down the sides of the blender once or twice. The sauce should be the consistency of creamy salad dressing. Add more water, a tablespoon at a time, to thin out, if needed. Refrigerate, covered, in an airtight container for up to 5 days.

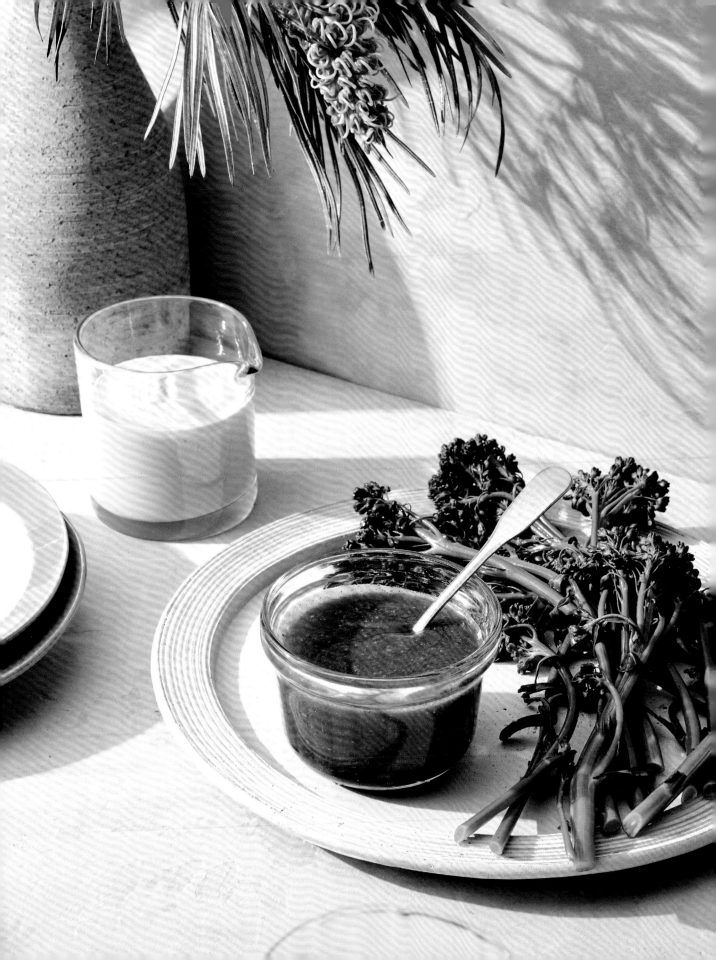

Ginger-Cashew Sauce

MAKES ABOUT 1½ CUPS

1½ cups raw cashews

1 garlic clove

1 (2-inch) piece fresh ginger, peeled and roughly chopped

Juice of ½ lime

2 tablespoons tamari

2 teaspoons yuzu juice (or fresh lemon or lime juice)

¾ cup filtered water

Fine sea salt

I could happily drink this sauce—it's a rich, velvety combination of cashews, yuzu (a sweet-sour Japanese citrus fruit whose juice I buy bottled; fresh lemon juice is a fine substitute), and tamari mixed up in a blender. But usually I have it on the side with my Extra-Crunchy Summer Rolls (page 156). This is an especially easy recipe as you don't have to presoak the cashews, but feel free to, because it will increase digestability.

To a blender, add the cashews, garlic, ginger, lime juice, tamari, yuzu juice, and water and puree until very creamy. The sauce should be the consistency of a creamy dressing; add another tablespoon or so of water to thin out, as necessary. Taste and add salt if you like. The dressing can be stored in a glass container, covered and refrigerated, for up to 3 days.

Almond Butter–Sesame Sauce

MAKES ABOUT 1 CUP

5 tablespoons almond butter

¼ cup tamari

¼ cup avocado oil

¼ cup toasted sesame oil

3 tablespoons pure maple syrup

This is Vivi's favorite sauce to have with Extra-Crunchy Summer Rolls (page 156), especially the avocado-cucumber variation. It's a little savory and a little sweet and is easy to whip up with just a whisk and a bowl.

Place the almond butter, tamari, avocado oil, sesame oil, and maple syrup in a small bowl and whisk until smooth. Refrigerate, covered, in an airtight glass container for up to 5 days.

Pesto

MAKES ABOUT ½ CUP

¼ cup freshly grated
Parmesan cheese (optional)

2 tablespoons toasted pine
nuts or toasted walnuts

1 garlic clove, coarsely
chopped

Fine sea salt

1 cup packed fresh basil leaves

⅓ cup extra-virgin olive oil,
plus more for storage

Fresh, vibrant pesto is a summertime staple in our house; we use it on rice noodles for a quick dinner, drizzled on chicken wraps, and as a sauce for pizza. The cheese is optional, if you want to keep it vegan. Feel free to double the recipe to use for a couple of applications.

In a blender or a food processor, combine the cheese (if using), nuts, garlic, and a pinch of salt, pulsing until the mixture is ground. Add the basil and process, pushing the mixture with the tamper or scraping down the sides a couple of times, until the basil is evenly chopped. With the motor running, slowly pour in the olive oil, processing until the pesto is as smooth as you like.

Taste, adding additional salt, if needed. Store, covered, in an airtight glass container in the refrigerator, topped with a thin layer of olive oil to prevent it from turning brown, for up to 4 days.

Chimichurri

MAKES ABOUT 1 CUP

2 to 3 garlic cloves, roughly
chopped

2 tablespoons red wine vinegar

¼ teaspoon fine sea salt

1 cup packed fresh flat-leaf
parsley (or cilantro)

¾ cup extra-virgin olive oil

½ teaspoon dried oregano

¼ teaspoon smoked paprika

Grated zest of 1 lemon
(optional)

This emerald-green sauce reminds me of Brazil, where it's a *must* with grilled steak. Full of garden-fresh parsley (or cilantro) and lots of garlic, it's as beautiful as it is delicious. If you can make it a few hours ahead, it will taste even better.

In a blender, combine the garlic, vinegar, and salt and blend well. Add the parsley and pulse until evenly chopped. Add the olive oil, oregano, paprika, and lemon zest, if using, and pulse until just combined. (Do not overprocess.)

Allow to rest at room temperature for at least 15 minutes before using. Refrigerate, covered, in an airtight glass container for up to 3 days.

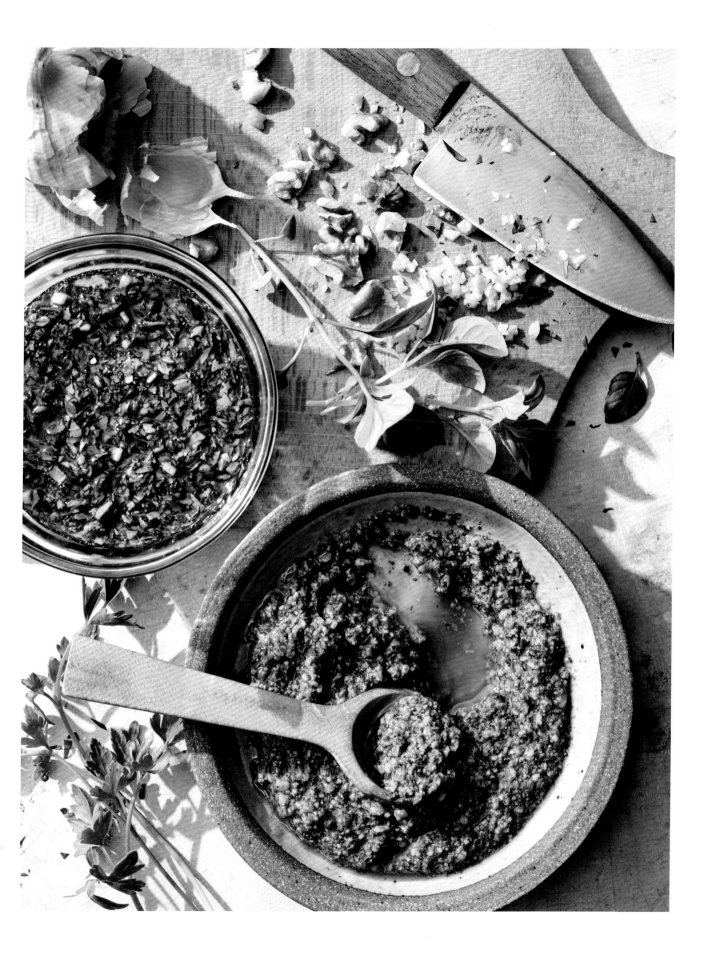

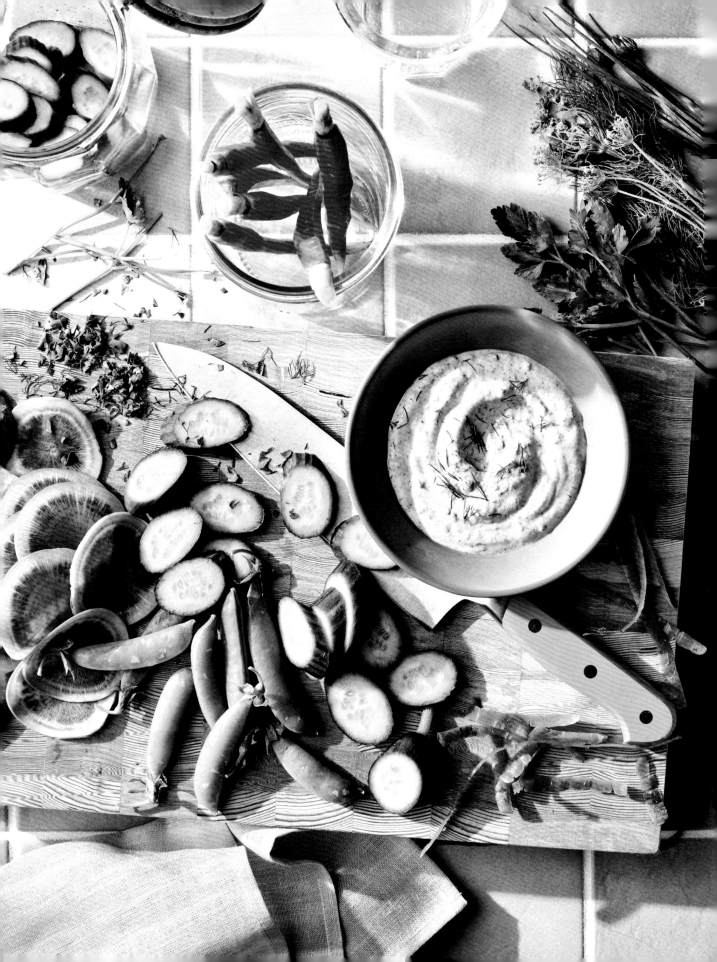

Cashew Ranch Dressing

MAKES 1½ CUPS

1 cup raw cashews

Boiling water

½ cup plain cultured coconut yogurt (or other unsweetened variety)

Juice of 1 lemon

2 tablespoons apple cider vinegar

2 teaspoons granulated onion or 1½ teaspoons onion powder

1½ teaspoons dried dill

1½ teaspoons dried parsley

1¼ teaspoons fine sea salt

1 teaspoon garlic powder

¼ teaspoon freshly ground black pepper

¼ cup filtered water, or more as needed

½ cup chopped fresh parsley or dill, or a combination

2 tablespoons minced fresh chives

My kids and I will happily eat a huge pile of raw or blanched veggies—baby carrots, cucumbers, sugar snap peas, green beans—especially if given a little cup of this dressing to dip them in. It's mostly pantry ingredients (except for the herbs, which I get from the garden) and the cashews need to soak only for a few minutes, so it's easy to whip up whenever there is some produce in my fridge that needs to get eaten. The dried herbs give it a distinct ranch flavor, while the fresh ones brighten it. Make a batch and see how fast your family will consume it.

Place the cashews in a heat-safe bowl or tall measuring glass, and cover with boiling water. Let stand for 15 minutes to soften, then drain and rinse under cold water, and drain again.

In a blender, combine the cashews with the yogurt, lemon juice, vinegar, granulated onion, dried dill, dried parsley, salt, garlic powder, pepper, and ¼ cup water. Blend until very smooth, 30 to 60 seconds. Add up to 4 more tablespoons water, 1 tablespoon at a time, as needed to achieve the consistency you like. Pulse in the fresh herbs and taste for the balance of salt and lemon.

Store, covered, in an airtight glass container for up to 3 days. It will thicken as it sits. Stir before serving, and lighten the consistency as needed by adding additional water by the tablespoon.

USING SAUCES, DRESSINGS, AND DIPS

Sauces and dressings are so versatile. They can be the star of the show, or they can take a plain dish to a new place. Experiment to find which dishes go well with each and the combinations you like best!

Here are some suggestions to get you started with any of the sauces in this chapter:

- Use as a dip for raw, steamed, or blanched vegetables or for Sweet Potato Wedges (page 147).

- Use as a dressing for a salad or over a halved avocado; if needed, thin out with a little extra olive oil.

- Drizzle over Roasted Vegetables (page 144), Miso-Mustard Roasted Whole Cauliflower (page 170), or Sheet-Pan Squash and Chickpeas (page 151).

- Drizzle over a taco (see page 202) or a quesadilla (see page 84), or include in a wrap.

- Serve with Extra-Crunchy Summer Rolls (page 156), Pan-Fried Falafel (page 177), or Vegetable-Quinoa Cakes (page 159).

- Use to dress rice noodles or zucchini noodles, adding a protein or extra vegetables if you like.

- Serve alongside grilled fish or Fish Baked in Parchment (page 188).

Tamari Dressing

MAKES ABOUT 1 CUP

½ cup tamari

⅓ cup unseasoned rice vinegar

2 tablespoons avocado oil

2 teaspoons honey or pure maple syrup

This salty, umami-rich dressing, and all the variations that follow, is a family favorite when we are craving Japanese flavors. The basic version can be used as a dressing or sauce (as in Benny's Shaved Salad, page 102; Veggie Stir-Fry, page 162; or the Ramen-Style Soup, page 136), or even as a marinade for grilled steak, chicken, or salmon. I love this dressing so much that I'm constantly tweaking and changing it. The carrot variation is amazing on crunchy lettuces!

Whisk together the tamari, vinegar, oil, and honey in a small bowl, or shake together in a lidded jar, until emulsified. Refrigerate, covered, in an airtight glass jar or container for up to 2 weeks.

CREAMY TAMARI DRESSING

Whisk or blend the dressing ingredients along with 5 tablespoons cashew or almond butter, or ¼ cup tahini, until smooth.

CARROT-GINGER TAMARI DRESSING

In a blender, combine the dressing ingredients with 2 cups raw, blanched, or steamed carrots (cooked until tender) and 2 teaspoons minced or grated fresh ginger. Blend thoroughly, until completely smooth.

SESAME-SCALLION TAMARI DRESSING

Add 1 tablespoon toasted sesame seeds, 1 teaspoon toasted sesame oil, 1 finely grated garlic clove, and 1 thinly sliced scallion to the dressing and shake until emulsified.

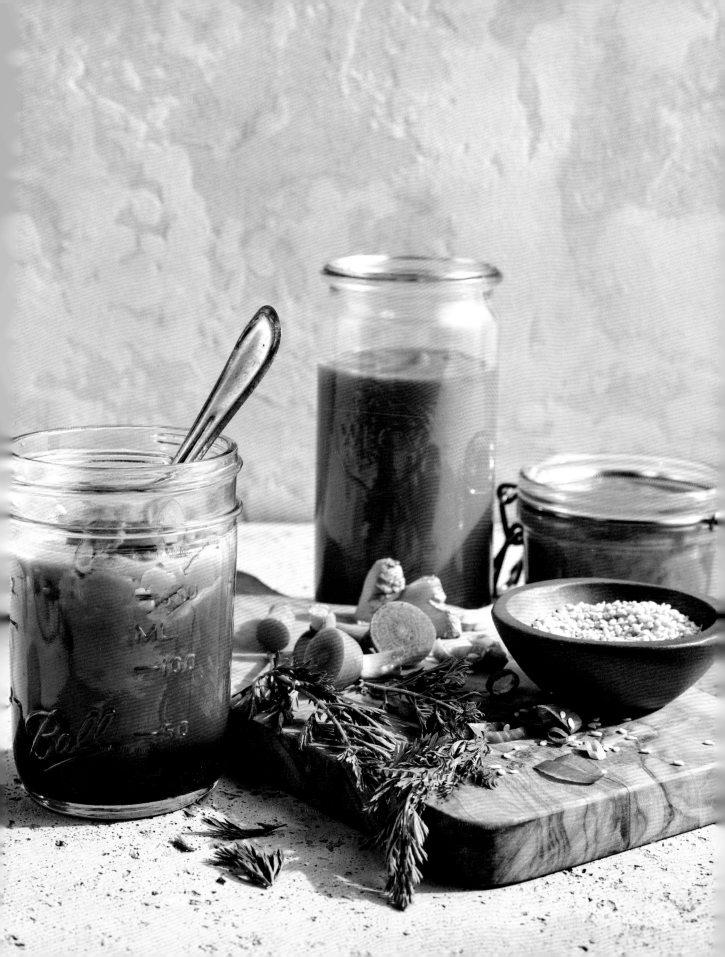

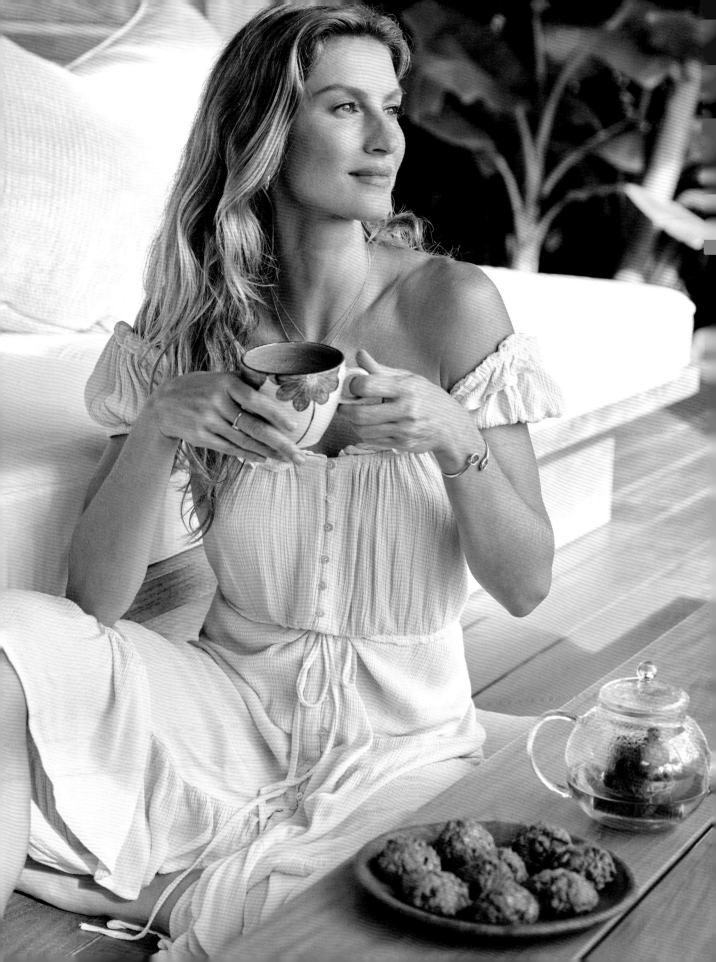

Sweets

What can I say? I love sweets! Here, I've adjusted them to be more nourishing and nutritionally dense so I can love them even more. Made with natural sugars, minimally processed ingredients, and good fats means they are more satisfying and actually give energy. I usually prepare these only on weekends or for special occasions, and when I do, we all really enjoy them!

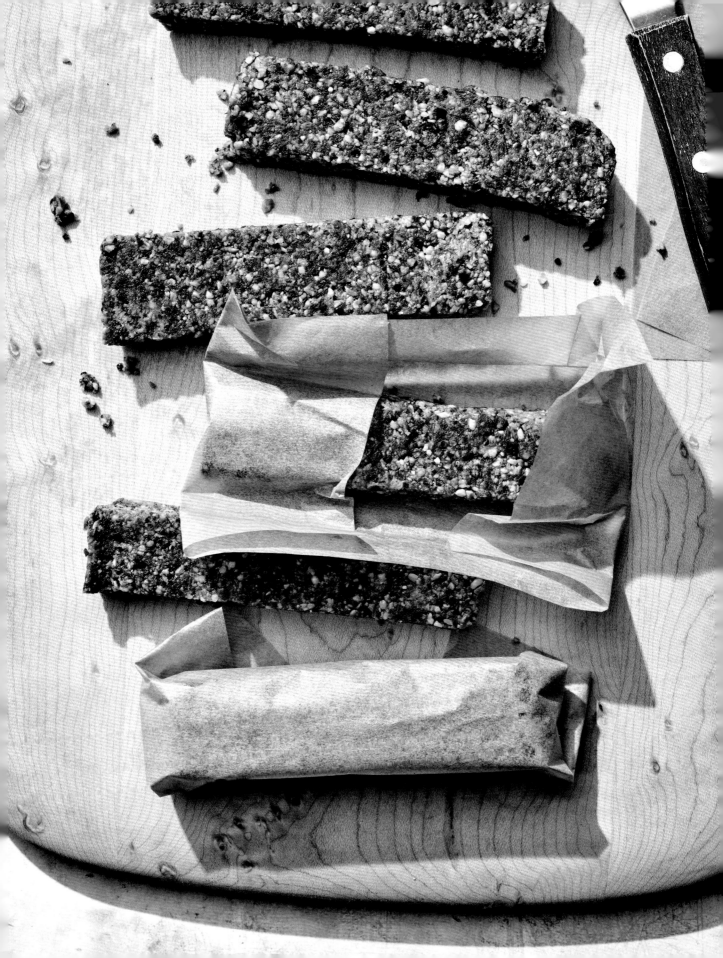

Baru Nut Bars

MAKES 8 BARS

1 cup (about 5 ounces) baru nuts (I like Barùkas brand)

¾ cup pitted Medjool dates (about 5)

¼ cup nut butter (like almond or cashew)

2 tablespoons hemp seeds

1 tablespoon runny mild honey

1 tablespoon unrefined virgin coconut oil, melted

1 teaspoon vanilla extract

¼ teaspoon fine sea salt, or more as needed

Baru nuts are native to Brazil and they grow wild in the Atlantic Forest that extends along the Atlantic coast of South America, but I learned about them only a few years ago, when my friend Mayara brought me some from a Brazilian farmer's market. Because I don't eat peanuts, discovering barus, which taste like something between a peanut and a cashew, was amazing for me. They are now one of my favorite nuts. Lately, it's been easier to find them in the United States, which is good because they are healthy, containing a ton of protein, fiber, iron, zinc, and antioxidants, among other vitamins and minerals. If you can't find them, you can substitute hazelnuts or blanched almonds.

With less fat than other nuts, they are dry and powdery when ground, not pasty. Here, I pulverize them in the food processor with dates and a bit of maple syrup for sweetness and some nut butter to hold everything together. Pressed into a layer in a loaf pan, then cut into bars, these don't require any baking at all—I simply let them set in the fridge. Wrapped in parchment, they provide a ton of awesome plant-based energy: a healthy, sweet treat to throw into your kids' lunchboxes or your bag.

Line an 8½ by 4½-inch loaf pan with a long piece of parchment that hangs over the long sides.

In a food processor, grind the nuts to a coarse powder, 60 to 90 seconds. Add the dates and process until the mixture has an even consistency. Add the nut butter, hemp seeds, honey, coconut oil, vanilla, and ¼ teaspoon salt, and pulse until combined. Taste, adding a few more pinches of salt, if you like. The mixture will appear crumbly.

Add the mixture to the prepared pan and flatten into a compact, even layer. Fold the excess parchment over the top and use a flat-bottomed measuring cup or wide offset spatula to further press down to flatten the mixture. Transfer to the refrigerator for at least 30 minutes or up to 1 hour to firm up.

Lift the bars out of the pan using the parchment overhang and cut into 8 pieces. Stored in an airtight glass container, the bars will keep for 1 week in the refrigerator.

Pecan Bars

MAKES 25 PIECES

For the crust

5 tablespoons unsalted butter or unrefined virgin coconut oil, melted, plus more for the pan

3/4 cup gluten-free flour blend (such as Bob's Red Mill)

1/3 cup coconut sugar

1/4 cup arrowroot powder or tapioca starch

2 tablespoons flax meal

1/4 teaspoon fine sea salt

1 large egg white, beaten (reserve yolk for filling)

For the filling

4 tablespoons unsalted butter or unrefined virgin coconut oil

1/4 cup runny mild honey

1/4 cup coconut sugar

1 tablespoon tapioca starch or arrowroot powder

1 tablespoon vanilla extract

1/4 teaspoon fine sea salt

1 large egg, plus yolk reserved from crust

1 1/2 cups pecan halves or pieces, toasted

4 pitted Medjool dates, slivered or chopped

A regular pecan bar, which is like pecan pie in bar form, usually contains a huge amount of butter, brown and white sugars, corn syrup, and condensed milk, with just a smattering of pecans. Not this version! The dates, honey, and moderate amount of coconut sugar make that quintessential gooey, chewy filling, which is dense with rich toasted pecans (and nutritional value). We make these fresh on Thanksgiving, and everyone raves. Leftovers, eaten straight from the fridge or freezer, are soft, fudgy, and amazing, too.

Preheat the oven to 325°F. Lightly brush an 8-inch square metal baking dish with a little melted butter, and line with a piece of parchment with overhang on the sides.

Make the crust: Whisk together the flour, sugar, arrowroot powder, flax meal, and salt in a medium bowl. Add the melted butter, then stir with a wooden spoon until the mixture becomes moist crumbles.

Spread the dough in the pan and press firmly into an even layer on the bottom and up the sides by at least 1/2 inch (to create a rim that will contain the filling). Bake for 30 minutes. Remove from the oven and liberally brush the crust with the egg white. Return the pan to the oven and bake for 5 minutes more, until dry to the touch and the crust is chestnut brown. Allow the crispiness of the crust to set while you prepare the filling. Keep the oven set at 325°F.

Make the filling: Gently melt the butter in a medium saucepan over low heat, then remove the pan from the heat. Whisk in the honey, sugar, tapioca starch, vanilla, and salt until smooth. Then beat in the egg and reserved egg yolk. Return the saucepan to the stovetop and set over medium heat. Cook, stirring constantly, until the mixture thickens slightly to the consistency of caramel sauce and starts to simmer at the edges of the pan, 4 to 6 minutes; take care to not let it boil. Remove from the heat and stir in the pecans and dates.

Pour the filling into the cooled crust, taking care not to let the filling flow underneath, and gently use a spoon to nudge the nuts and dates into an even layer. Place in the oven and bake until just set in the center, 12 to 15 minutes, rotating the pan halfway through. Set aside to cool completely.

Lift the cooled contents from the pan using the parchment handles. Using a serrated knife, cut into 25 squares (chill first if you want cleaner cuts). In an airtight glass container, the bars will keep for up to 3 days at room temperature or 2 months in the freezer.

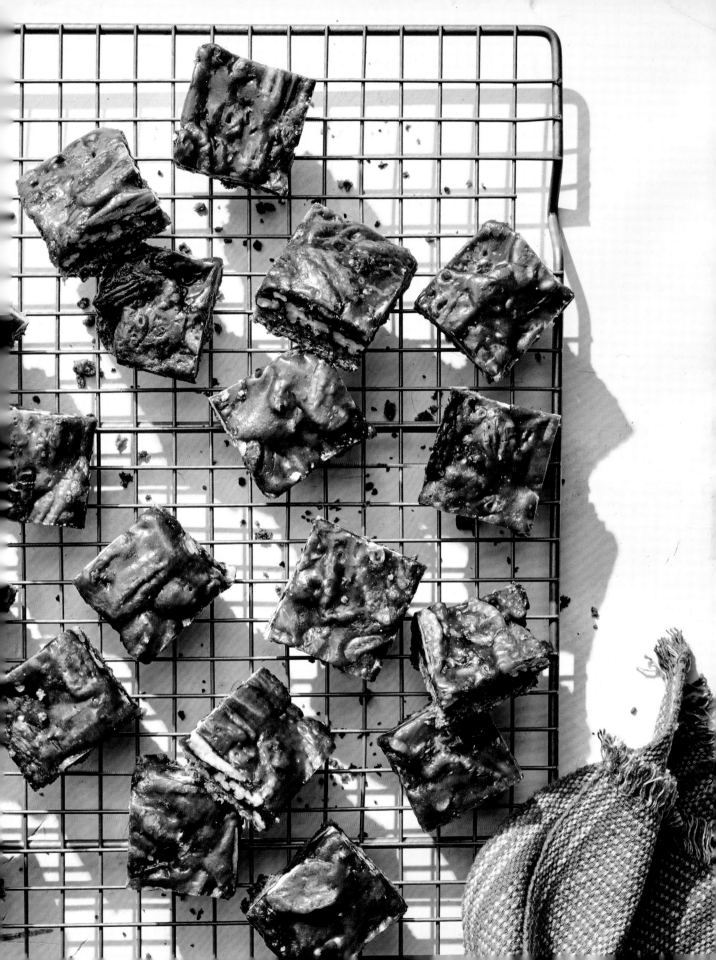

Carrot Muffins

MAKES 12 MUFFINS

½ cup unrefined virgin coconut oil, melted

¼ cup pure maple syrup

¼ cup coconut sugar

1 teaspoon vanilla extract

2 large eggs

1 cup oat flour

¾ cup almond flour

2 tablespoons flax meal

2 teaspoons baking powder

1½ teaspoons ground cinnamon

¼ teaspoon baking soda

¼ teaspoon fine sea salt

3 or 4 medium carrots, coarsely or finely grated

Honey, for topping (optional)

Coconut Whipped Cream (page 237), for topping (optional)

Carrot cake has always been one of my favorite desserts—and this muffin version is a much healthier option that everyone in the family loves. Full of grated carrots and both oat and almond flours, they smell like cinnamon and vanilla and taste just sweet enough to satisfy. The Coconut Dulce de Leche (page 239) is a delicious topping on these instead of the Coconut Whipped Cream.

Preheat the oven to 400°F. Fit a standard muffin tin with 12 paper liners.

In a large bowl, whisk together the oil, maple syrup, coconut sugar, and vanilla, then beat in the eggs one at a time until well combined. In a medium bowl, whisk together the oat and almond flours, flax meal, baking powder, cinnamon, baking soda, and salt. Use a wooden spoon to stir the dry ingredients into the wet, then fold in the grated carrots.

Scoop the batter into the muffin cups, about ¼ cup batter for each one (a spring-loaded cookie scoop works great for this). Place in the oven and bake for 20 to 26 minutes, until the muffins are domed and set in the center and a tester comes out clean. Let cool completely in the tin.

If you like, just before serving, top each cooled muffin with a drizzle of honey or a dollop of whipped cream.

MAKE IT YOURS

For the Kids: Stir together 2 tablespoons of coconut sugar and 1 teaspoon ground cinnamon, then sprinkle that over the muffins before baking.

Coconut Whipped Cream

MAKES ABOUT ½ CUP

1 (13½-ounce) can full-fat coconut milk or coconut cream, chilled at least 8 hours in the refrigerator

2 tablespoons honey or pure maple syrup

1 teaspoon vanilla extract

This whipped cream is also great on top of Sunday Banana Waffles (page 83), pancakes, or Banana Dream Pie (page 245).

Chill the metal mixing bowl of a stand mixer, or a metal bowl if using a hand mixer, for 30 to 60 minutes in the refrigerator.

Carefully open the can of coconut milk or coconut cream, taking care not to shake the contents, and scoop the solidified coconut cream at the top into the chilled bowl. (Pour any liquid at the bottom of the can into a container and refrigerate for another use.) Using the whisk attachment, beat the cold coconut cream for 1 to 2 minutes, until thick and fluffy. Beat in the honey and the vanilla.

Keep the whipped cream cold until you're ready to serve, as any heat will cause it to melt. Can be stored in an airtight glass container for up to 5 days in the refrigerator.

SUGAR FREE—SOMETIMES

When I go home to Brazil for the holidays, sometimes foods that are a treat in normal times—Brazilian Cheese Bread (page 89), Brigadeiros, all kinds of decadent desserts—can temporarily become the norm (on Christmas break 2022, for example!). Even though it all tastes so good when I am eating it, soon after I feel the change in my body. I have less energy, worse sleep patterns, and dysfunctional digestion, all of which are indications that my body needs attention. One simple way to give it that attention is to take a sugar break.

During this reset, I refrain from eating sugar—even naturally derived and minimally processed kinds, including maple syrup, honey, coconut sugar, even fruits. During a typical reset week, I eat lots of veggies and modest amounts of meat and fish, which get my internal systems running back at their best. (If you feel you need some sweets, eating the occasional piece of fruit helps keep those cravings away.) Sometimes I go sugar free for just a few days, while other times it lasts for a few weeks. The key is to listen to your body and look for cues of healing—improved mental clarity, better sleep, digestive regularity. I come out of it refreshed and revitalized, and ready to go!

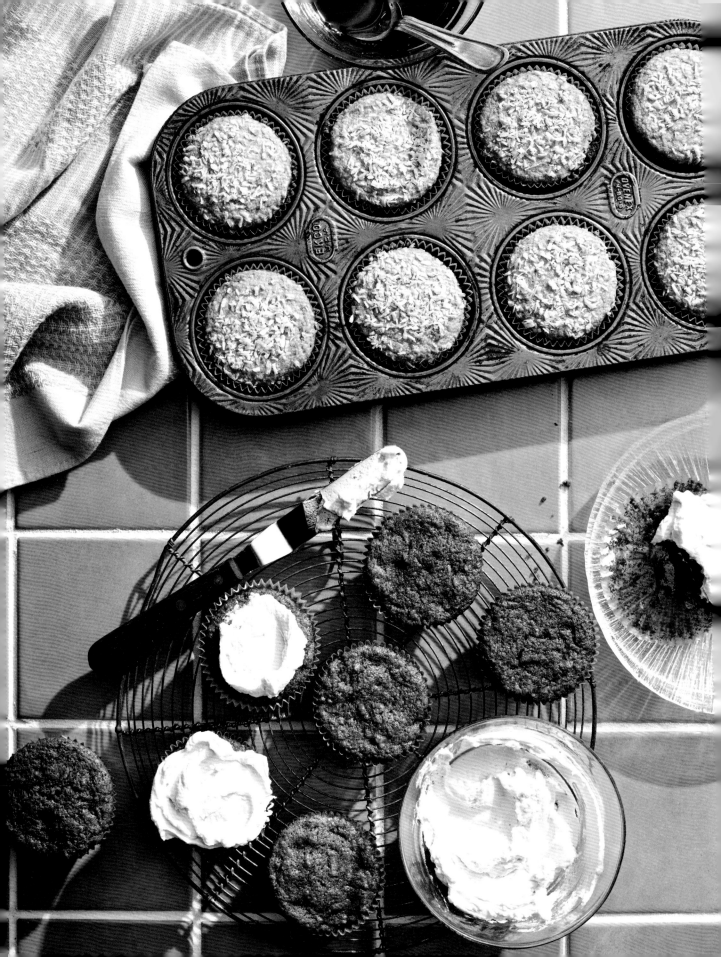

Coconut Muffins
with Coconut Dulce de Leche

MAKES 12 MUFFINS

¾ cup oat flour (see Note)

¾ cup almond flour

2½ teaspoons baking powder

¼ teaspoon fine sea salt

1 (7⅓-ounce) can (⅔ cup) sweetened condensed coconut milk (see Note)

5 tablespoons unrefined virgin coconut oil, melted

¼ cup pure maple syrup

1 teaspoon vanilla extract

⅓ cup milk (any variety), at room temperature (see Note)

3 large eggs, at room temperature (see Note)

⅓ cup shredded unsweetened coconut, plus more for sprinkling

Coconut Dulce de Leche (recipe follows), for topping

These simple muffins are the closest thing to cake that I make in my kitchen. The batter is made with almond and oat flours, and the flavor comes from various coconut products: coconut condensed milk, coconut oil, and shredded coconut. If you like, first make the simple coconut dulce de leche for drizzling on top.

Preheat the oven to 375°F. Fit a standard muffin tin with 12 paper liners.

In a large bowl, whisk together the oat flour, almond flour, baking powder, and salt. In a medium bowl, whisk together the condensed coconut milk, coconut oil, maple syrup, and vanilla extract until smooth. Whisk the room-temperature milk and eggs into the coconut milk mixture, then use a flexible spatula or spoon to fold the wet ingredients into the dry. Fold in the shredded coconut.

Spoon the batter into the muffin cups, each filled about ½ inch from the top rim of the pan (a spring-loaded cookie scoop works great for this). Transfer to the oven to bake for 18 to 22 minutes, until golden brown and a tester comes out clean. Let cool completely in the pan before serving. If you like, drizzle each muffin with coconut dulce de leche and sprinkle with extra unsweetened coconut.

Note: Be sure to buy oat flour labeled "gluten-free" if you are sensitive. And if, after opening the can, the sweetened condensed coconut milk is solid, place the contents in a small saucepan with the coconut oil and warm gently over low heat until just melted; let cool for 5 minutes before adding to the batter. Finally, be sure the milk and eggs are at room temperature so they will not cause the coconut oil to seize up when combined.

Coconut Dulce de Leche

MAKES ABOUT 1 CUP

1 (13.5-ounce) can full-fat coconut milk

6 tablespoons pure maple syrup

Combine the coconut milk and maple syrup in a small saucepan and place over medium-low heat. Bring to a very gentle simmer—just until bubbles appear at the edges—then reduce the heat to low and cook, stirring often with a flexible spatula to prevent scorching on the bottom of the pan, until reduced by half, 70 to 90 minutes. Remove from the heat and cool completely. It will thicken slightly as it cools, and can be kept in an airtight jar in the refrigerator for a week.

Blender Banana Bread

MAKES 2 LOAVES

½ cup unrefined virgin
coconut oil, plus extra
for greasing

4 medium or 3 large bananas,
peeled

3 large eggs

½ cup honey or coconut sugar

1 tablespoon almond butter

1½ teaspoons vanilla extract

1½ cups almond flour

½ cup gluten-free flour

1 tablespoon baking powder

¾ teaspoon baking soda

¼ teaspoon fine sea salt

¼ cup sliced blanched
almonds, toasted (optional)

Emanuel Jimenez, a chef I work with in Costa Rica, taught me this delicious banana bread, and the kids and I go crazy for it. It's so easy to make as it comes together entirely in the blender! It makes two loaves—feel free to freeze one (wrapped in parchment and slipped into a ziptop bag) or give one to a good friend. Sometimes I like to add toasted almonds for a little extra crunch.

Preheat the oven to 350°F.

Brush two 8½ by 4½-inch loaf pans with a little coconut oil, then line with parchment, leaving two ends hanging over the longer sides of the pan like a sling. Brush the parchment with some oil.

Place the bananas, eggs, ½ cup coconut oil, honey, almond butter, and vanilla in the blender and process until just mixed. Add the almond flour and gluten-free flour, baking powder, baking soda, and salt and then pulse, scraping down the sides once or twice, until the batter is fully mixed; do not overprocess (or let the blender run on full speed).

Pour half of the mixture into each prepared pan. If you like, add most of the almonds (reserving a tablespoon or so) to the batter in each pan and use a knife to swirl them in. Smooth the top of the batter and sprinkle with the reserved almonds, if using. Bake until a toothpick or wooden skewer inserted into the center comes out clean (or with just a crumb or two attached), 50 to 60 minutes. Allow to cool before slicing.

Almond Flour–Chocolate Chip Cookies

MAKES ABOUT 20 COOKIES

8 tablespoons (1 stick) unsalted butter or ½ cup unrefined virgin coconut oil

¾ cup coconut sugar

2 teaspoons vanilla extract

1 large egg

2 cups almond flour

1½ teaspoons baking soda

1 teaspoon baking powder

¾ teaspoon fine sea salt

1 cup high-quality, low-additive dark chocolate chips or 4 ounces dark chocolate, coarsely chopped

Flaky salt, such as Maldon, for sprinkling

Plenty of times, a simple date stuffed with an almond will satisfy my sweet tooth. But sometimes a little treat makes life so much sweeter! These are a bit healthier than the average chocolate chip cookie, since they're made with almond flour and use coconut sugar as a sweetener. Coconut oil is delicious and rich, or browned butter gives them a caramelly depth—your choice. I suggest keeping them out of sight, so you don't eat them all in one day. (Trust me, it happens!)

If using butter, in a small saucepan, melt it over medium heat and allow it to bubble away, swirling often, until it darkens a shade, smells nutty, and you can see little flecks of brown milk solids clinging to the bottom of the pan, 4 to 6 minutes. Remove from the heat and let cool for 10 to 15 minutes. If using coconut oil, melt it in a small saucepan.

Add the coconut sugar and vanilla to the cooled browned butter or melted coconut oil and stir until smooth, then vigorously beat in the egg until well incorporated.

In a large bowl, whisk together the almond flour, baking soda, baking powder, and sea salt. Scrape the butter-sugar mixture into the dry ingredients and use a wooden spoon or sturdy spatula to combine until no dry streaks remain. Stir in the chocolate chips. Scrape the batter into an airtight container and chill in the refrigerator for at least 2 hours or up to 3 days; if using coconut oil, chill at least overnight.

Preheat the oven to 325°F. Line two baking sheets with parchment paper.

Spoon heaping tablespoons of dough—a 1½-tablespoon spring-loaded cookie scoop works great for this—onto the prepared baking sheets, spacing them 2 inches apart. (If you like, freeze the unbaked, portioned balls between sheets of parchment in an airtight container to bake off directly from the freezer at your convenience.) Sprinkle each cookie with a little pinch of flaky salt.

Bake for 17 to 20 minutes, until evenly browned and the cookies have puffed all the way to the edges. The cookies are soft right out of the oven, but they will firm up a bit as they cool. Let cool on the sheets for at least 10 minutes before eating. Once cool, they'll keep in an airtight container for up to 3 days.

Avocado-Lime Mousse

SERVES 4

½ cup raw cashews, soaked overnight and drained (see Note)

1 large ripe Hass avocado, halved, pitted, and flesh scooped out

⅓ cup pure maple syrup, plus more as needed

6 tablespoons Coconut Milk (page 72) or store-bought full-fat coconut milk

Grated zest and juice of 3 limes (about ¼ cup juice)

1 tablespoon unrefined virgin coconut oil

½ teaspoon vanilla extract or powder

¼ teaspoon fine sea salt

Pinch of blue spirulina powder (optional)

Coconut Whipped Cream (page 237)

Toasted unsweetened coconut chips, for topping

MAKE IT YOURS

Light Pairing: Try either of these mousses as an ice pop (see page 62).

Hearty Pairing: Gluten-free graham crackers are not especially healthy, but you can use them to bake a simple graham cracker crust and pour the mousse directly into the cooled crust before chilling.

We ate lots of avocados when I was growing up back in Brazil, as we had a huge tree in our backyard. But rather than making them into guacamole or topping toast with them, my mom used to make delicious sweet smoothies with them—they are fruits, after all! Here, the rich velvety avocado flesh is turned into a mousse with a cashew and coconut milk base.

If you've never had avocados like this, you are in for an *amazing* surprise. A pinch of blue spirulina powder doesn't add much flavor, but it does make the color a bit more lime green, which is fun. Served in individual cups or scooped out from one family-style dish, the mousse is creamy, sweet, and just the thing to make ahead if you're having people over (you can even turn it into a pie; see below).

In a food processor, grind the soaked cashews into a smooth paste. Add the avocado, maple syrup, coconut milk, lime zest and juice, coconut oil, vanilla, salt, and spirulina. Process, scraping down the sides of the bowl periodically as needed, until the mixture is smooth, 1 to 2 minutes. (Don't overprocess or the avocado will turn brown.) Taste and add additional maple syrup as needed.

Pour the mousse into a large serving dish or individual dishes. Cover and refrigerate until completely set, at least 1 hour or overnight. Serve cold, with coconut whipped cream and toasted coconut chips, if you like.

Note: If you don't have time to soak the cashews overnight, speed-soak them by bringing to a boil in a saucepan with a few cups of water; allow to cool in the water for about 1 hour, then drain.

AVOCADO-CHOCOLATE MOUSSE

Follow the instructions for making the lime mousse, but instead of lime juice, zest, and spirulina, add ¼ cup organic cacao powder to the food processor along with an extra 2 tablespoons of maple syrup. Process and chill as instructed. If you like, top the mousse with Coconut Whipped Cream (page 237) or with cacao nibs, coconut yogurt, and a drizzle of honey just before serving.

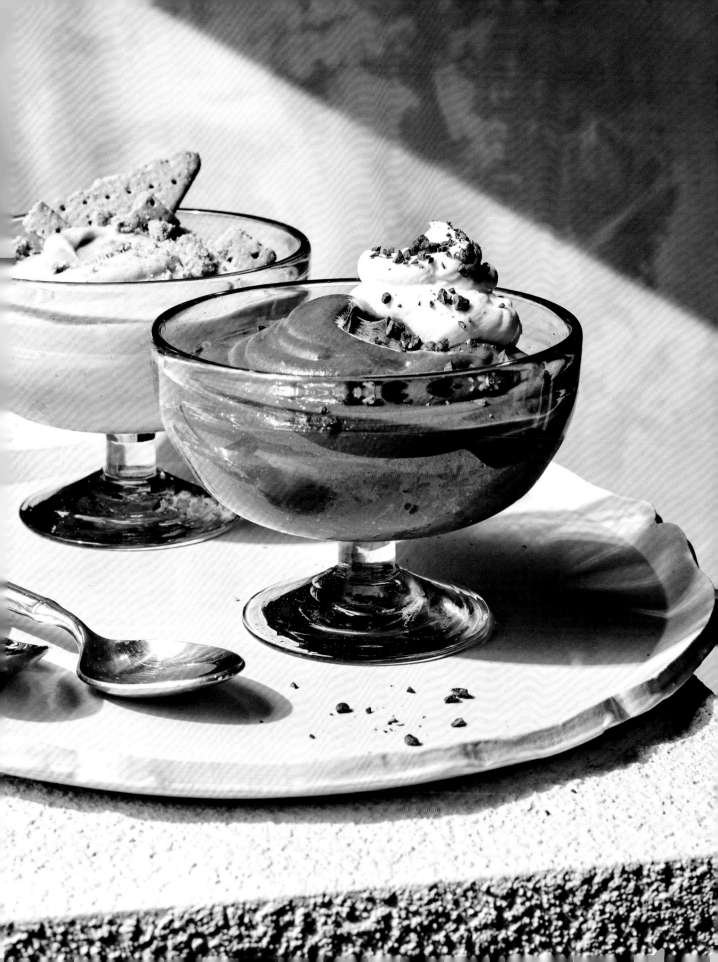

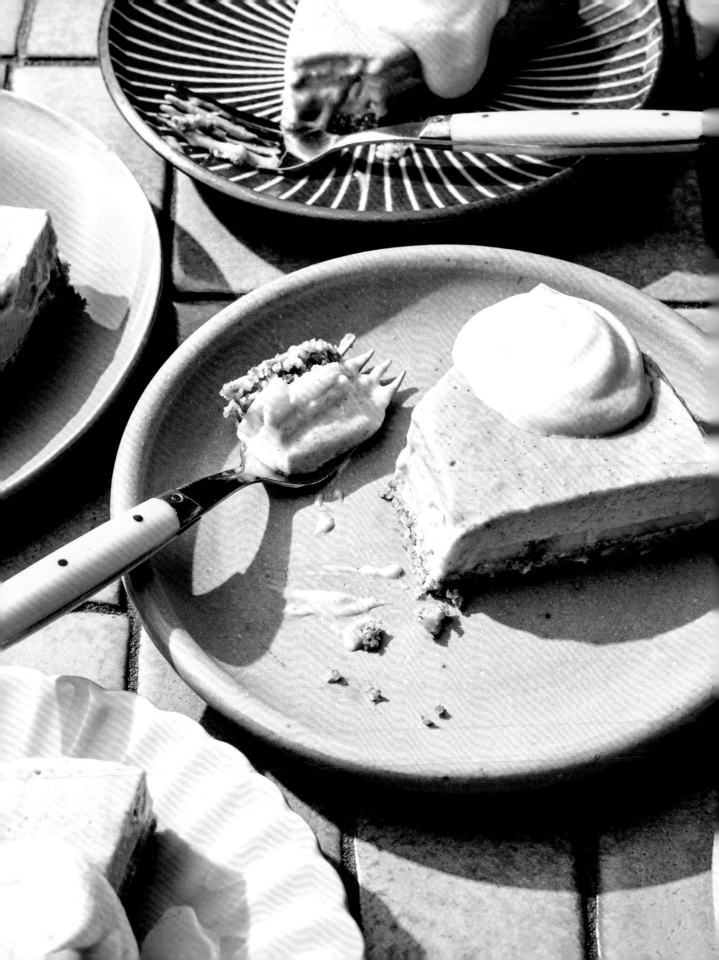

Banana Dream Pie

SERVES 6 TO 8

For the crust

1 cup raw walnuts, almonds, or pecans, soaked overnight and drained; almonds peeled

1 tablespoon unrefined virgin coconut oil, plus more for the pan

½ cup pitted Medjool dates

¼ cup unsweetened dried coconut, toasted

Pinch of flaky sea salt

For the filling

3 ripe bananas

½ cup raw cashews, soaked overnight and drained

⅓ cup pure maple syrup

⅓ cup coconut yogurt

3 tablespoons unrefined virgin coconut oil

Seeds scraped from 1 vanilla bean or 1 teaspoon vanilla extract

½ teaspoon fine sea salt

Coconut Whipped Cream (page 237)

The kids and I are obsessed with this frozen pie, originally found on the Minimalist Baker website. We've altered it quite a bit over the years, but it remains one of our favorites. The filling, made from bananas and soaked cashews sweetened with vanilla and maple, has an amazingly smooth and creamy texture that is perfectly counterbalanced by the crumbly date, nut, and coconut crust—three foods I don't think I could live without. Top this with a dollop of the coconut whipped cream, and you'll see why we call it Dream Pie. Plan ahead, though; the nuts need to be soaked overnight, and if using almonds, their skins should be removed. Also, this pie needs a full overnight chill to set up!

Make the crust: Preheat the oven to 350°F. Add the nuts to a sheet pan and toast in the oven until completely dry, 12 to 15 minutes. Let cool. Brush the bottom and sides of a 8- or 9-inch springform pan with a little coconut oil.

In the bowl of a food processor, pulse the dates until they become a paste; use a spatula to transfer the dates to a medium bowl. Add the nuts, coconut flakes, 1 tablespoon coconut oil, and the salt and pulse until chopped. Return the dates to the processor and pulse until just combined.

Using the bottom of a glass or measuring cup, press the crumb mixture into the pan in an even layer. Place the pan into the fridge to chill thoroughly and set, about 10 to 15 minutes.

Make the filling: Place 2 of the bananas in a blender, then add the cashews, maple syrup, yogurt, oil, vanilla seeds, and salt. Blend until smooth and creamy.

Slice the remaining banana into ¼-inch rounds. Arrange the banana rounds on the crust in a single layer, then pour the filling over the banana slices. Tap the pan lightly on the counter to remove any air bubbles. Cover the pan without touching the top surface and place in the freezer overnight.

Remove the pie from the freezer 10 minutes before serving. Release the pan's clasp and lift off the side of the springform pan. Slice the pie and serve with a dollop of coconut whipped cream, if you like.

Coconut Heaven

SERVES 4

4 cups fresh or frozen coconut meat, defrosted if using frozen

½ cup pure maple syrup

Seeds scraped from ½ vanilla bean or 1 teaspoon vanilla extract

1 cup fresh strawberries, hulled and trimmed, plus more whole berries for topping

¼ cup unsweetened cocoa powder

¼ cup unrefined virgin coconut oil, melted

Joanne Gerrard Young, an amazing raw-food chef, taught me how to make this delicious dessert years ago, and ever since it has remained one of my favorites. Its three beautiful layers—coconut, strawberry, and chocolate—have different textures and tastes. It's creamy and fruity, with a topping that sets hard for that crunch I love.

Instead of making the homemade chocolate layer with cocoa, you could just melt your favorite dark chocolate bar. Make these at least three hours before you plan on serving them.

In a blender, combine the coconut meat, ¼ cup of the maple syrup, and the vanilla seeds until smooth. Put ¼ cup of the mixture into each of the 4 jars or ramekins, smoothing the tops with a spoon.

Add the strawberries to the blender with the remaining coconut mixture and pulse until combined to your liking. Carefully spoon the strawberry-coconut mixture evenly over the coconut layers in each cup and smooth the tops with a spoon.

In a bowl, whisk together the cocoa powder, remaining ¼ cup maple syrup, and the melted coconut oil, stirring until combined. Carefully pour or spoon almost all of it evenly over the strawberry layers in each cup.

Hull the remaining whole strawberries and place on a parchment-lined plate. Spoon the remaining chocolate over each strawberry. Chill the jars and chocolate-covered strawberries in the refrigerator for at least 3 hours, but overnight is best.

When ready to serve, top each dessert with chocolate-covered strawberries and enjoy!

MAKE IT YOURS

Simple Swaps: If you prefer just coconut and chocolate, skip the strawberry and use all of the coconut mixture to make the layer beneath the chocolate. Or, feel free to skip the chocolate topping; then the dessert needs only to chill for 1 hour before serving.

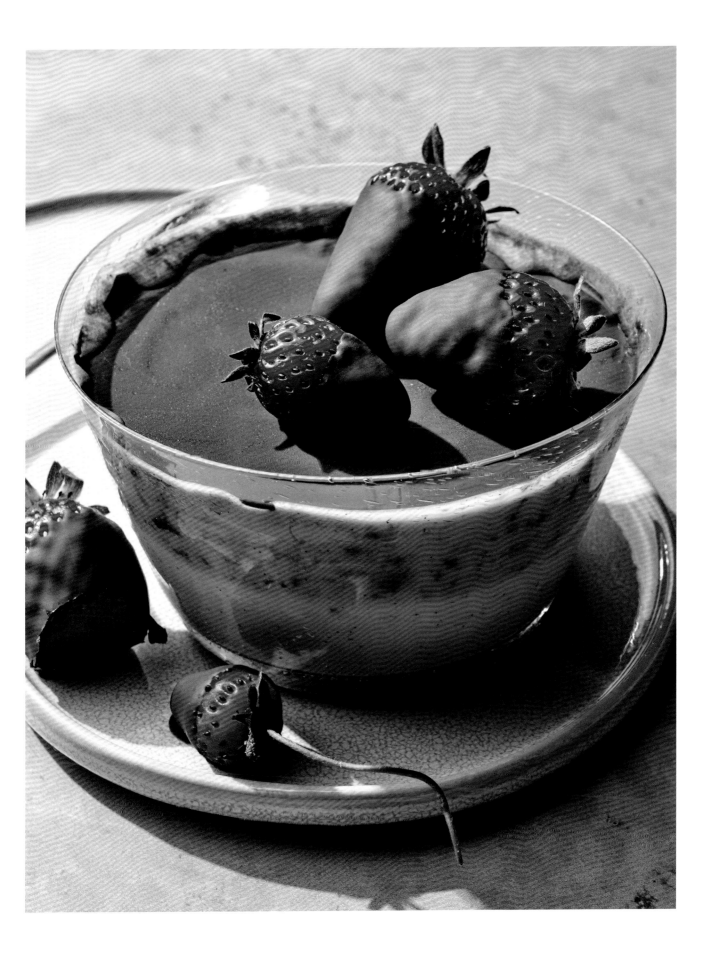

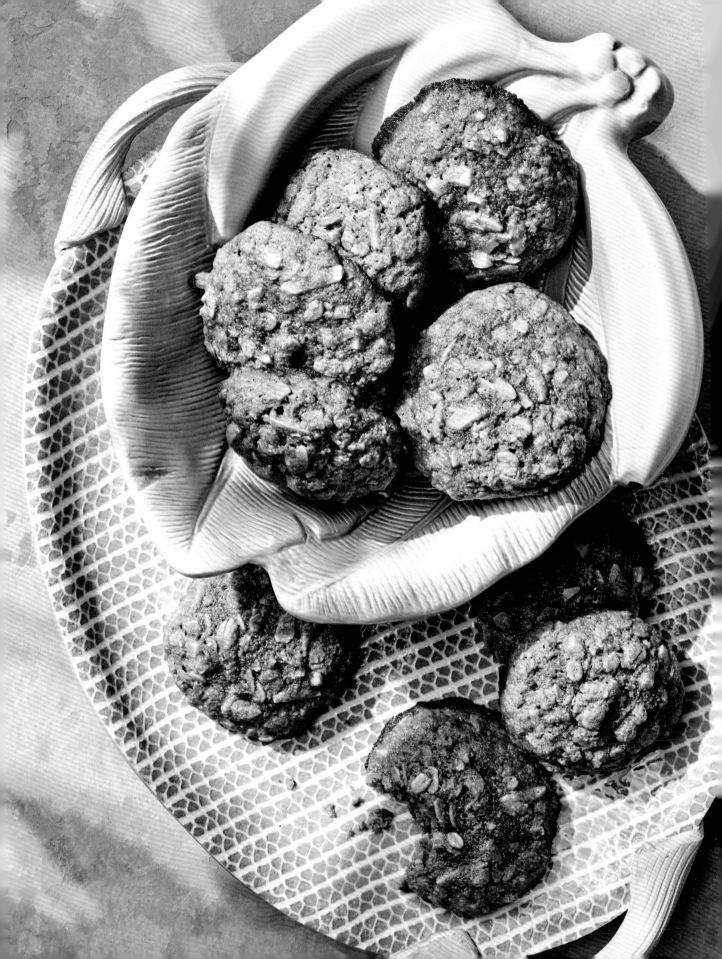

Oatmeal Golden Milk Cookies

**MAKES ABOUT
16 COOKIES**

6 tablespoons unsalted butter, melted and slightly cooled

½ cup coconut sugar

1 large egg

1 teaspoon vanilla extract

2 tablespoons arrowroot powder or tapioca flour

1 to 2 tablespoons golden milk tea powder (I like Gaia brand)

½ teaspoon baking powder

¼ teaspoon fine sea salt

²/₃ cup almond flour

²/₃ cup old-fashioned rolled oats

½ cup toasted slivered almonds or coarsely chopped walnuts or pecans (optional)

Golden milk tea powder (haldi doodh) is a combination of spices, fruit, and roots like turmeric, black pepper, ashwagandha, dates, cardamom, and vanilla that is often used to make an ayurvedic tea. In addition to the health benefits of the turmeric, this particular combination is meant to be stress relieving and calming. I like it as a hot drink, with honey and almond milk, but I really love adding the powder to these oatmeal cookies! Vivi loves them, too. I occasionally add chopped pecans for crunch, but keeping these cookies plain gives the strongest golden milk flavor. (If you love the taste, feel free to use up to 2 tablespoons of the powder.)

In a large bowl, whisk together the melted butter and sugar, then beat in the egg and vanilla. Whisk in the arrowroot powder, golden milk powder, baking powder, and salt until well combined. Then stir in the almond flour, oats, and nuts, if using. Transfer the dough to a bowl and freeze for 30 to 60 minutes to firm up, or place in an airtight glass container and refrigerate overnight.

Preheat the oven to 400°F. Line 2 baking sheets with parchment.

Scoop about 2 tablespoons of the dough into mounds (a spring-loaded cookie scoop works great) and arrange 8 on each of the baking sheets, spacing them about 4 inches apart, since they'll spread quite a bit as they bake.

Place in the oven and bake on the middle racks for 11 to 14 minutes, rotating the sheets halfway through, until browned around the edges and puffed in the centers. They'll be delicate right out of the oven, so make sure you let them cool completely on the baking sheets before removing and eating. Store in an airtight glass container for up to 3 days.

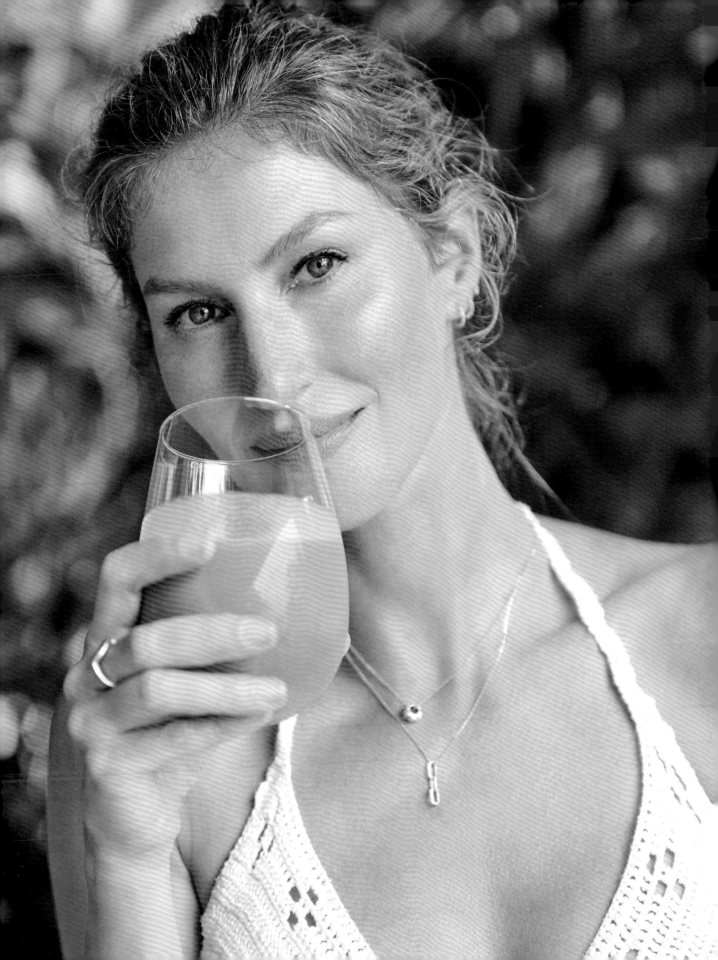

Acknowledgments

My true inspiration for this cookbook is my wonderful mom. She always went the extra mile, even though she was working long hours. As a child, my mom taught me the importance of a well-thought-out plan, conscious shopping, and prepping ahead.

In creating the recipes for this book, I was lucky to work with a few special chefs. I have collaborated with chef James Kelly, who has worked with us in Costa Rica, for over fifteen years. If you know me, you know I have a sweet tooth, and James makes the heathiest and most delicious sweets (like his Avocado-Lime Mousse, page 242). For the last nine years, our family has been fortunate to have chef Susan Ryan with us to create nourishing and flavorful meals. When my kids' friends stay for dinner, the moms always ask how we got them to eat vegetables—it was always Susan's roasted veggies (page 144). Lukas Volger helped me create the delicious Grain-Free Granola (page 76), among other yummy recipes. Years ago, when I was curious about the raw food movement, Joanne Gerrard Young taught me so much. I still incorporate some of her techniques into my recipes. I have learned about the power of optimal digestion from the Valente Brothers (Pedro, Gui, and Joaquim). Their program incorporates special juicing and food-combining techniques that have opened my eyes to new eating habits for myself and my kids.

Thank you, Kevin O'Brien, for making our shoot at home with the kids so easy and fun. Eva Kolenko, thank you for making all of these yummy meals come to life.

And I could not have written this book without Elinor Hutton. She was an incredible partner and confidant and was always so patient. As we worked on this book, she was by my side every step of the way.

This has been a labor of love, and I am so grateful to everyone who helped create this book and make it a reality.

Thank you!

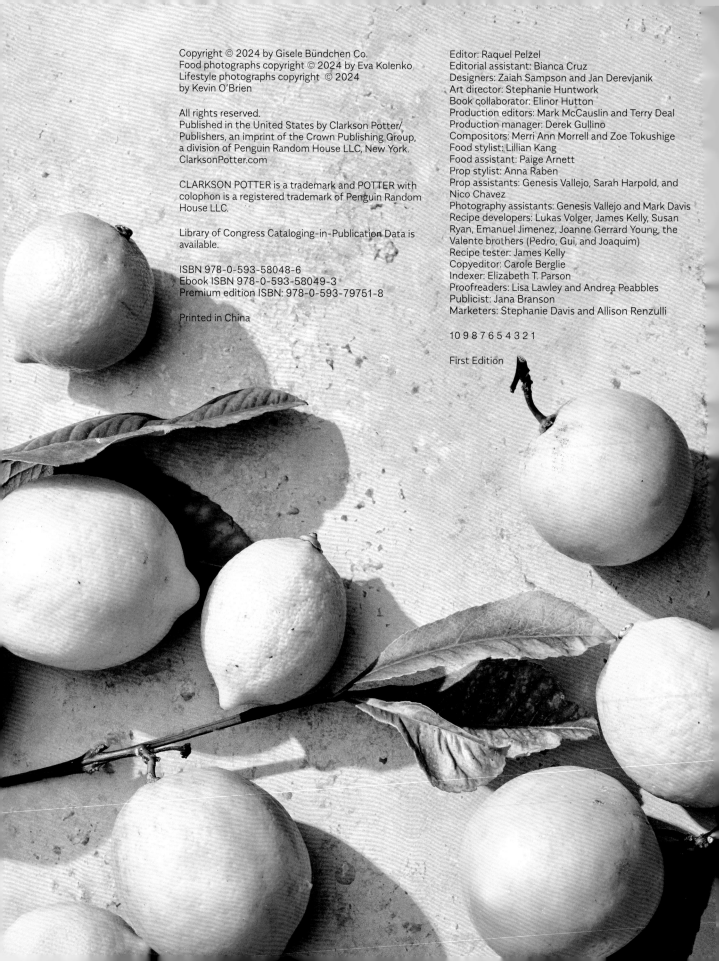

Library of Congress Cataloging-in-Publication Data is
available.

ISBN 978-0-593-58048-6
Ebook ISBN 978-0-593-58049-3
Premium edition ISBN: 978-0-593-79751-8

Printed in China

Editor: Raquel Pelzel
Editorial assistant: Bianca Cruz
Designers: Zaiah Sampson and Jan Derevjanik
Art director: Stephanie Huntwork
Book collaborator: Elinor Hutton
Production editors: Mark McCauslin and Terry Deal
Production manager: Derek Gullino
Compositors: Merri Ann Morrell and Zoe Tokushige
Food stylist: Lillian Kang
Food assistant: Paige Arnett
Prop stylist: Anna Raben
Prop assistants: Genesis Vallejo, Sarah Harpold, and
Nico Chavez
Photography assistants: Genesis Vallejo and Mark Davis
Recipe developers: Lukas Volger, James Kelly, Susan
Ryan, Emanuel Jimenez, Joanne Gerrard Young, the
Valente brothers (Pedro, Gui, and Joaquim)
Recipe tester: James Kelly
Copyeditor: Carole Berglie
Indexer: Elizabeth T. Parson
Proofreaders: Lisa Lawley and Andrea Peabbles
Publicist: Jana Branson
Marketers: Stephanie Davis and Allison Renzulli

10 9 8 7 6 5 4 3 2 1

First Edition

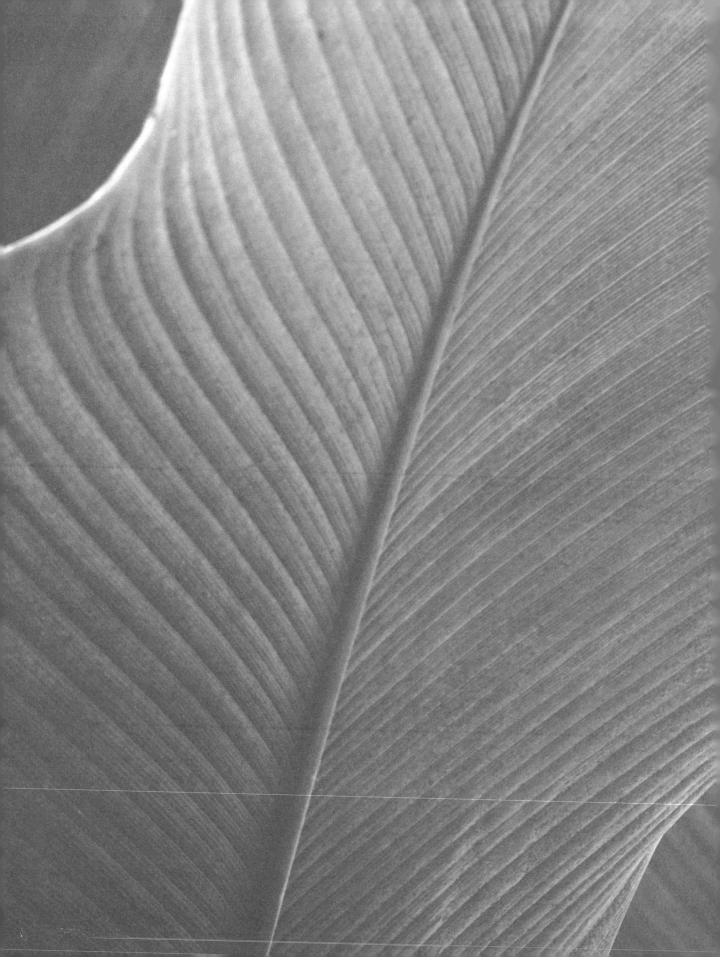